'In this illuminating and comprehensive volume, Dr Joe Tucci and distinguished colleagues present a dazzling compendium of evidence-based knowledge about the multifaceted manifestations of trauma, along with exciting and proven approaches to its treatment.'

– Gabor Maté MD, author, *The Myth of Normal: Trauma: Illness and Healing in a Toxic Culture*

'This rich multidisciplinary book provides us with a deep dive into a trauma transformation paradigm rooted in a thorough understanding of developmental neuroscience and the synthesis of a range of effective interventions of trauma informed practices.'

– Bessel van der Kolk MD, Professor of Psychiatry
BUSM President, Trauma Research Foundation

'Imagine being provided a scientifically solid set of deep dives into the fabric of trauma and being offered actionable steps we can take to help transform human suffering into ways we can connect and flourish. In this magnificent collection of leading world authorities offering concise and insightful overviews of their life's work, our able editors have curated a comprehensive view of how overwhelming adversity impacts development, shapes our neural and relational connections, and leaves us with assaults on trust, hope, and possibility. By summarizing and contrasting each of the chapters' detailed immersions, we, the fortunate recipients of this hard earned wisdom, are provided a practical guide to re-imagining "trauma-informed" approaches and cultivating a focused, in-depth offering of "trauma-transformation" that can alleviate individual distress and offer the potential to put an end to the collective, intergenerational transmission of despair in our lives. A deep bow of gratitude to Joe, Janise, Steve and Ed, for this life affirming work of heart.'

– Dan Siegel, Executive Director, Mindsight Institute;
Clinical Professor, UCLA School of Medicine

'It's a treasure to discover a book that provides a paradigm shift in thinking, informed by knowledge, wisdom, and transgenerational lived experience. In this volume, trauma-informed is transformed into a practice that all services and organisations need to take notice of.'

– Kim S Golding, CBE, Clinical Psychologist,
DDP trainer and author

THE HANDBOOK OF TRAUMA-TRANSFORMATIVE PRACTICE

Emerging Therapeutic Frameworks for
Supporting Individuals, Families or
Communities Impacted by Abuse and Violence

Edited by
Joe Tucci, Janise Mitchell, Stephen
W. Porges and Ed Tronick

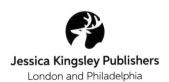

Jessica Kingsley Publishers
London and Philadelphia

First published in Great Britain in 2024 by Jessica Kingsley Publishers
An imprint of John Murray Press

1

Copyright ©:

Chapter 1: Joe Tucci, Janise Mitchell, Stephen W. Porges and Ed Tronick 2024
Chapter 2: Stephen W. Porges 2024
Chapter 3: Louis Cozolino, Chloe Drulis and Carly Samuelson 2024
Chapter 4: C. Sue Carter 2024
Chapter 5: Ed Tronick 2024
Chapter 6: Efrat Ginot 2024
Chapter 7: Paul Gilbert, Deborah Lee and Marcela Matos 2024
Chapter 8: Breanne Kearney and Ruth A. Lanius 2024
Chapter 9: Christine A. Courtois and Julian D. Ford 2024
Chapter 10: Jonathan Baylin and Daniel Hughes 2024
Chapter 11: Judy Atkinson, Margaret Hayes, Carlie Atkinson,
Gerard Webster and Gavin Morris 2024
Chapter 12: Jennifer McIntosh, Jessica Opie and Anna Booth 2024
Chapter 13: Theresa Kestly 2024
Chapter 14: Kevin Creeden 2024
Chapter 15: Maggie Kline 2024
Chapter 16: Janise Mitchell and Noel Macnamara 2024
Chapter 17: Joe Tucci and Janise Mitchell 2024
Chapter 18: Janise Mitchell and Joe Tucci 2024

A CIP catalogue record for this title is available from the
British Library and the Library of Congress

ISBN 978 1 78775 577 2
eISBN 978 1 78775 578 9

Printed and bound in Great Britain by TJ Books Limited

Jessica Kingsley Publishers' policy is to use papers that are natural, renewable
and recyclable products and made from wood grown in sustainable
forests. The logging and manufacturing processes are expected to conform
to the environmental regulations of the country of origin.

Jessica Kingsley Publishers
Carmelite House
50 Victoria Embankment
London EC4Y 0DZ

www.jkp.com

John Murray Press
Part of Hodder & Stoughton Ltd
An Hachette Company

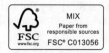

MIX
Paper from
responsible sources
FSC® C013056

Contents

Editor Biographies

Joe Tucci is CEO of the Australian Childhood Foundation, Chair of the National Centre for Action on Child Sexual Abuse, a social worker, a psychologist and a children's rights advocate.

Janise Mitchell is Deputy CEO of the Australian Childhood Foundation, Director of the Centre for Excellence in Therapeutic Care, a social worker and a children's rights advocate.

Stephen W. Porges is Distinguished University Scientist at Indiana University where he is the founding director of the Traumatic Stress Research Consortium. He is Professor of Psychiatry at the University of North Carolina, and Professor Emeritus at both the University of Illinois at Chicago and the University of Maryland. He is the originator of Poly-vagal Theory.

Ed Tronick is a Professor of Psychiatry and Pediatrics at UMass Chan Medical School. He is Founder and Chief Faculty of the Early Relational Fellowship Program at the Chan Medical School. He is a clinical psychologist and human development neuroscientist and developer of the Still-Face Paradigm.

CHAPTER 1

Looking Beyond: Examining the Contribution and Future of the Trauma-Informed Approach

Joe Tucci, Janise Mitchell, Stephen W. Porges and Ed Tronick

Introduction

In *Midnight's Children*, Salman Rushdie's hero Saleem collected 26 pickle jars which he filled metaphorically with the aromas, sensations and experiences of his life's adventures.

> The intricacies of turmeric and cumin, the subtlety of fenugreek, when to use large (and when small) cardamoms; the myriad possible effects of garlic, garam masala, stick cinnamon, coriander, ginger...in the spice bases, I reconcile myself to the inevitable distortions of the pickling process. To pickle is to give immortality, after all: fish, vegetables, fruit hang embalmed in spice-and-vinegar; a certain alteration, a slight intensification of taste, is a small matter, surely? The art is to change flavour in degree, but not in kind; and above all...to give it shape and form – that is to say meaning... (Rushdie, 2008, p.644)

For Saleem, *pickling* is the art of preserving memory, recognizing that the experience itself, what follows, its resonance, its interruptions, its liberations, its inter-relationships, shift and shape how these memories are recalled, relived and sometimes re-imagined. He knew that his memories were not only stored as the fragrance and taste of his chutneys. They came as embodied experiences of the sensory and narrative accumulation of the events he had shared with others. They were stories that he distilled into his jars along with the tasty representations of his experience of events and people.

Saleem's memories included pain, oppression, loss as well as resistance, union and joy. He knew that no single jar held the sum of his life experiences. As he opened and reflected on the collection of his jars, he understood his own magical story that connected the moment of his birth with the stroke of midnight on the day that India achieved its independence.

Looking back, he came to see how his life may have turned out had he been born even an hour later. His life journey became defined by what happened after and as a result of this remarkable historical coincidence.

Trauma, too, forever changes what is experienced after it.

Trauma is a visceral force that resonates through time, often clamping those who have experienced it in moments of their past that are re-enacted and relived in the present, perpetually seeming to reshape their identity, their relationships and their future.

When it occurs in the form of interpersonal violation, it is a betrayal altering the life course of individuals, families and whole communities. It is experienced with an intensity of pain that burns through and overwhelms the adaptations that individuals have to that point used as resources to learn, love and grow.

It distorts trust. In the aftermath of trauma, what can be reliably pre-dicted is put on notice. Many relationships are no longer safe. They have become sources of violation. *Once they have hurt you, they can hurt you again. Your worldview has changed moving forward.* The prediction of safety is absent. Relationships feel strange and frightening. They become the means through which the source of terror may strike again. The way that love is expressed takes on a different possibility. It comes to be associated with distress, control, coercion and powerlessness. Love, care and nurture are used to manipulate what is said, to whom and when. Love becomes a means to justify abuse. It becomes synonymous with dynamics that serve to minimize responsibility by the perpetrator for their actions. Trust becomes a tool for the misuse of power within relationships. It is leaned on to pres-sure victims to submit to their violation, often forcing them to take the blame for the abuse on themselves. It is used to resource contortions of the truth that leave very little space for alternatives. Individuals subject to this falsification do not know who to trust. They are no longer able to rely on what anyone claims to be the truth. They learn to mistrust the motivations of perpetrators. Their belief in the trustworthiness of others is damaged, often irrevocably.

Trauma creates confusion in its wake. Roles and responsibilities change. Children can become protective of their mothers in family violence situa-tions. They step into the middle of a war zone to stop their mothers being abused by a violent partner. They protect their pets, who are sometimes threatened as a way to ensure the silence of family members. Trauma often makes individuals believe that the world no longer has any order left in it. It creates a sense of chaos. Reactions outside consciousness become active in contexts that do not make sense. Powerful emotions cascade without internal or external reference. It feels like mayhem. States of calm and quiet are elusive. Individuals are switched into modes of survival that they do not recognize or are easily understood by others in them. Professionals are drawn in to offer protection and support. But the systems they work in are often fragmented, only allowing them to pursue one part of the problem – the misuse of drugs or alcohol, the mental illness, the suicidality, the homelessness. These services are not integrated and frequently insensitive to the needs of individuals with lived and living experience of trauma. Often, their behaviour is misinterpreted. Victims and survivors withdraw from support they desperately need. Practitioners are left mystified about whether their intervention was experienced as helpfully as they had intended it to be. Those affected by trauma and the service systems designed to assist them are left confounded about what support will work and how it can be offered so that it is helpful.

Trauma hijacks the experience of living and relationships and lets in danger. Children, young people and adults who have suffered trauma have their brain-body systems reorganized around the foreboding presence of threat. The protective mechanisms that the brain-body has at its disposal to prevent the experience of overwhelming pain is switched on and stays on. From that point on in time, these internal systems dominate their feelings, thoughts and behaviour. They close down to change in the event that that such change may in itself lead to the experience of trauma. They become more and more rigid in their application of behavioural routines to ward off the slightest possibility that the violation re-occurs and the pain of the experience floods them all over again. Memory fragments of the experience are stored with intensity markers which link to survival behaviours that can be quickly reactivated in the face of any signs of real or perceived danger. They are no longer who they were before the trauma occurred. They are frightened, enraged, distraught. They clutch on to familiarity, even if that familiarity is harmful and potentially exposes them to more violation.

Trauma isolates people from one another. As part of the aftershock of interpersonal violence, relationships mutate around the dynamics of power and often secrecy. Violation within relationships reinforces and amplifies the power differentials that enabled the abuse to occur in the first place. Individuals do not feel understood or believe that their experiences are valid. They feel different from others. They feel as if they are on their own in a community that does not want to recognize the extent of trauma that is suffered by so many people. They can feel separate to the people they once belonged to because they feel that there is little shared experience to bind them. Even when trauma is collectively shared, there are powerful societal forces which keep it behind walls, away from the gaze of those who cannot bring themselves to bear its presence. Those living with the effects of trauma act as satellites of relationships – never landing, always circling, ready to fall out of orbit and, in the process, break apart. Even when another reaches out with an invitation for connection, the mistrust caused by trauma makes it harder for that connection to be accepted. Individuals affected by trauma can experience being alone even in the context of family, friends and work relationships. The trauma has marked their experience of all current and future relationships with weariness and caution.

Trauma leaves the relational needs of people unmet. In the face of fear, people need reassurance. In the face of distress, they need comfort. In the face of confusion, they need clarity. Trauma blocks these gaping interpersonal holes from being filled. It keeps the individual in a state of waiting perpetually for the need that has never been addressed to be met in the present. It is a timeless experience of anticipation in the hope that those needs will be seen, acknowledged and responded to. For children and young people, their developmental vulnerability only amplifies the impact of unresolved states of need. They are caught in a failed cycle of reliably predicting the extent to which the adults in caring roles know what their needs are, respond to them. They are forced to live with the disorganized internal systems of the adults around them. There cries are left unattended. Their desire to play is rejected. Their invitation to engage is met with indifference or neglected altogether in favour of the adults fulfilling their own needs as a priority. The contingency of the interactions with their carers that children's neurobiological systems crave is absent at best or deliberately and cruelly misattuned. There are only breaches of attention and the flow of love without any opportunity created to restore the intricacies of disappointment and terror that children experience within these daily exchanges. The loop that starts with the experience of a need and the expectancy of a response remains open, unfulfilled. And as they grow, they hold hope for the relief of a soft word or tender embrace that serves them and no other. As adults, childhood abuse is the terror that continues without conclusion.

Trauma evokes shame. It takes the inherent messages from the perpetrator and makes them self-beliefs. *You are worthless. You are vulnerable. You are to blame. You are a nobody. I am in control of you. You have no choice.* They carry with them the power of the violation to reinforce them and ensure that they are experienced as unchallengeable. Individuals living with the effects of trauma carry these truths with them into their interactions with others. They act as if they are what they have been told. Their identity is forever undermined. Shame wipes out other qualities that they experience which are more positive, creative and resourceful. It lets in self-loathing and self-recrimination. Critique and judgement from others are perceived even if they are not present. It is the self that is under attack. It is one of the resonant consequences of trauma. It keeps individuals and communities in states of suspended experiences of failure, often collapsing with the intensity of an internally directed criticism that has no end.

Trauma silences dissent and resistance. Violence acts in ways to impose sanctions on those who speak out or act in opposition to it. It extracts every drop of tenderness, joy and care from relationships. It stifles compassion and ridicules it as overly soft and forgiving. It is how it takes hold in the community and stays. It replicates itself by rendering invisible and inaudible the actions and words of those in the community who challenge its presence, its arguments and its persuasiveness. Trauma follows in its path and serves to weaken even further the individual and collective effort required to make it leave. There is little if any space left for strength and humour to be allowed to oppose its full effects. It undermines all that was resourcing, and amplifies the bedlam of reactions that may have once served as protective but turn into ensconced struggles, breeding additional problems, until violence, as the founding source of social ills, is no longer visible.

Trauma debilitates meaning making. It prevents the formation of narratives that hold the power to make sense of the experiences of the violation. It keeps people from calling out and exposing the motivation of the perpetrators. It stops them from understanding the small steps they took to keep themselves safe, even if those actions were not able to be discerned by anyone else. It breaks down episodic and narrative memories so that timelines are confused and not easy to piece together. It keeps the experiences of violation alive. There is little opportunity to draw out a meaning arch that describes life before the violation, its effects and the changes that result. It withdraws control from the individual and collective to underscore when the experience of living with the trauma may not be as painful, complicated or hard. The meaning of the experiences remains in parts as fragments without integration. In so doing, it obscures the possibility that hope for life with fewer intrusions, more trust and deeper connections is possible.

These descriptions of trauma highlight the emotionality with which the world is altered at its hands. The ways that support is offered to those carrying the ongoing torment of such violation need to incorporate a willingness to touch the intensity of the experience, hold it with respect and engage with the shared humanity of all such pain.

For more than two decades, practitioners, programmes, organizations, systems and, more recently, whole communities have been grappling with the imperative to make sense of and apply an understanding of trauma in their everyday ways of being, doing and organizing themselves to better resource, support, counsel and care for those living with the consequences of trauma. Emanating from the US, this movement has seen efforts to integrate trauma-informed approaches into policy, service, organization and system design across the globe, into differing political and cultural contexts with differing policy and funding drivers and constraints.

Despite the early promise, there are emerging signs that trauma-informed approaches have been limited in their scope of influence (Berliner and Kolko, 2016; Hanson and Lang, 2016; Sweeney and Taggart, 2018).

Practitioners and organizations alike are beginning to face dilemmas about whether the limitations of a trauma-informed approach stem from its very design as it is currently conceptualized or are more reflective of failures in its application and execution.

The next evolution of the trauma-informed paradigm is the focus of this book. The benefit of pausing and reconceptualizing principles and ideas brings with it reflections about clarity, intentionality and impact. For example, drawing on their experience in developing and implementing trauma-informed programmes and services in child welfare and education contexts in Australia, Tucci and Mitchell (Tucci, 2016; Tucci and Mitchell, 2019a) have already offered a glimpse into how the trauma-informed movement could evolve, suggesting the need for an expanded approach that understands the whole person in the sociocultural contexts in which they lived as both an essential part of the meaning making and as offering critical resources in the healing journey. Beyond trauma informed, there may be:

> ...trauma-integrated services which are not only familiar with the knowledge base about trauma...they have fused these principles with their own mission and vision. A trauma-integrated service combines its own value base with its commitment to achieving change. Knowledge of trauma is not separate to the operations of the service – it is at the centre. The evidence from the neuroscience of child development and interpersonal relationships offers resources to practitioners that build on other important principles which include being culturally strong, risk-responsive, rights-oriented and strengths-based. Trauma-integrated services focus away from individual trauma symptoms, and toward the individual, as a whole person, and as part of a network of relationships that are strengthened as the basis for change... (Tucci and Mitchell, 2019b, p.319)

An even further step may involve the development of *trauma-transformative* services and programmes which serve to:

> ...embed two significant additional layers into their orientation. They have thought of, and committed themselves to, a theory of change that realistically supports how children, young people and families affected by violence come to experience their lives differently. The service and its staff believe that the effects of trauma can be changed. They represent hope to service users and the community. They oppose broader community narratives that serve to trap those affected by the effects of trauma in identities that are shaming. Trauma-transformative services connect the community to the pain of violence and resource both understanding and compassion... (Tucci and Mitchell, 2019b, p.320)

Returning to Saleem and his pickle jars provides a playful backdrop for revisiting the origins and story of the trauma-informed paradigm so far. Saleem knew that *pickling functions to preserve and sustain as well as transform*. At its heart, this book serves as an act of pickling. It seeks to recast ideas about trauma-informed practice – maintaining some as they are, adding notes where needed, deepening their value, shifting some meanings, reorganizing their balance. It is also an invitation to reconsider current conceptualizations of trauma-informed approaches and allow deeper consideration of the richness of the core elements of practice that are required to support healing and resource change for individuals, families and communities affected by violence. It privileges a willingness to hold complexity in mind at all times and resist reductionist ideas that too often beset attempts at change, however well meaning and noble their ambition (Piedfort-Marin, 2022).

In this chapter, the evolution of the trauma-informed movement is traced and reconsidered to seek to identify what will come next in the application of trauma-transformative-led design across the multiple dimensions of practice, programme delivery, organizations, systems and communities. In so doing, it sets up what the rest of the book has in store and postulates the contribution it may make.

The origins of trauma-informed practice

In 2001, Maxine Harris and Roger Fallot wrote what is often cited as the original paper arguing the case for human service organizations to consider the implications of the growing acknowledgement that substantial numbers of individuals presenting with support needs had experienced significant levels of trauma at a population level. They differentiated between trauma-specific services (those designed to heal the consequences of abuse and violence) and what would become trauma-informed services (those with broad objectives to offer support and assistance, including mental health, drug and alcohol and housing programmes).

It was the first chapter in a collection of articles that were written to inspire a shift in the planning and delivery paradigm of human service organizations (Harris and Fallot, 2001a, 2001b, 2001c; Fallot and Harris, 2001; Bebout, 2001; Freeman, 2001; Prescott, 2001; Arledge and Wolfson, 2001). It argued, what has been repeated frequently since, that violence and abuse are so commonplace that they should be proactively considered as a significant factor in responding to individuals who present for support at any service. Harris and Fallot chose the phrase 'trauma informed' for two very specific reasons. Being more 'trauma informed' meant that the histories of past abuse and its effects on the lives of victims and survivors should become more central to the ways in which their needs are understood and support is offered to them. More importantly, by appreciating and acknowledging the vulnerabilities and strengths of individuals with trauma in their lives, being 'trauma informed' would promote service users' participation in their treatment. They were particularly interested in the evolution of mental health and substance abuse treatment services, becoming more cognisant of the ways in which traumatic sequelae can be misinterpreted by service systems that are designed traditionally to address a specific problem (e.g. addiction), rather than help to meet the holistic needs of individuals carrying deep pain from past and ongoing experiences of violation.

Harris and Fallot pioneered what has now become the basis on which many subsequent trauma-informed approaches have been developed. They worked in a private not-for-profit adult mental health and substance abuse treatment agency in Washington DC. Their framework was and remains sensitive to collaborative ways to share power, responsibility and authority with service users. It highlighted how a small group of influential and passionate individuals have the power to change one organization, and then help to recalibrate systems towards trauma-informed ways of knowing, being and doing.

Harris and Fallot were the first to identify five clear conditions which need to operate as part of a culture within organizations and/or service systems for them to be considered trauma informed. These were:

- *Administrative commitment to change* – the senior leadership of an organization need to embrace knowledge about trauma and enable it to permeate the policy, resource, and practice settings of the organization. This affirms the direction of an agency to change the ways it interacts with service users so that their needs are visible, acknowledged and collaboratively resourced.
- *Universal screening* – trauma-informed agencies must embed questions about prior experiences of trauma into their screening and assessment processes. Service users will then hear that trauma is recognized as important, creating the space for disclosures, and staff will become more conscious of trauma impacts in their everyday practice. Harris and Fallot acknowledged that service users with lived and living experiences of trauma may still choose not to disclose their histories, possibly having faced unhelpful and further victimizing responses from service providers in the past.
- *Training and education* – a fundamental principle of trauma-informed organizations is to ensure that all staff, regardless of their roles, receive training about the impact of trauma on individuals who are provided with support through their agency. The training is aimed at making staff more sensitive to how trauma manifests in behaviour, how it can compromise the engagement of service users

with the programmes offered by the agency, and how staff can adapt their own language and approach to better suit the needs of individuals with trauma backgrounds. The aim of such training is primarily to mitigate against the risks of the agency further re-traumatizing or making worse the ongoing impacts of trauma for those seeking help.

- *Hiring practices* – the pathway to organizational change should be supported by individuals with a 'trauma-first' orientation. Harris and Fallot were in favour of hiring individuals already with trauma knowledge and those who can act as 'trauma champions' to support the transition to a changed way of practising.

- *Review of policies and procedures* – Harris and Fallot maintained that it would be a natural process for organizations to review their policies and procedures as they become more confident with their knowledge about trauma. This will lead to the replacement of harmful uses of strategies for restraint, seclusion, and involuntary admissions, with fewer intrusive alternatives that respect the needs of services users in crisis. It also will lead to knowledge of the power dynamics of abuse and violation being given more weight in understanding what service users might need and benefit from. In particular, the perspectives of those with lived and living experiences of trauma offer insights about the qualities that service users need in their interactions with workers and agencies. For example, a trauma-informed agency will need to ensure that it challenges the reality that the voices of survivors are often unheard, denied or not validated. Agencies will need to address how secrecy has continued to dictate the way some service users feel about their own experiences of abuse and violence and have policies that ensure confidentiality and the seeking of consent. Procedures may also be necessary for service users to feel safe especially in situations where there is a power differential between them and individual workers.

In the second part of their chapter, Harris and Fallot (2001a) defined a set of principles and a philosophy that underscored a trauma-informed human service system. Using case examples, they proposed the following core elements of such a system:

- Experiences of trauma prompt individuals to understand their meaning and how their lives have changed as a result of the violation.
- Meaning is expressed in behaviour as well as through language. The behavioural routines that individuals used to protect themselves from the immediate threat posed by the violence provide an expression of the meaning that the individual held to survive.

- Service users themselves are not responsible for their problems. They have experienced abuse and violation. Their lives have been disrupted by these experiences. As a result, the focus of a trauma-informed service system is to move away from individual symptomatology to an understanding of the person in their context.
- Trauma survivors have strengths as well as vulnerabilities. Trauma-informed systems facilitate personal agency to the extent to which it is possible.
- Trauma-informed services are designed to promote growth, recognizing that survivors have capacities that they have used to endure in the face of experiences that have overwhelmed their senses with danger.
- Trauma-informed services aim to prevent individuals engaging in behaviour that is problematic for them, their families and their communities in the future.
- Service providers are active in building relationships with service users that are open, genuine and collaborative. Service users have an active voice in setting the directions of the support offered to them, within the timelines that are relevant to them and in ways that are tailored for them, without the expectation that one approach fits all individuals and all presenting problems.
- Service users are encouraged to shape the nature and qualities of the relationships in which support is provided. They are given the space and time to develop the relationships which make most sense to them, allowing them to bring their own understanding of their needs into focus.

In concluding their reflection, Harris and Fallot (2001a) noted that:

> ...the task of making a system trauma informed may at first appear daunting. The shift in philosophy amounts to nothing less than a paradigm shift within service delivery systems...at first, thinking about trauma and its impact seemed like one more thing to be added to the clinician's assessment of every consumer. Slowly, however, in part because consumers responded so positively to our appreciation of the role that violence and victimisation had played and continued to play in their lives, the focus on trauma seemed more integrative and less additive... (p.21)

The potential of trauma-informed practice was taken up by the US Federal Government Substance Abuse and Mental Health Services Administration (SAMHSA), through its funding of what is still the single most significant study aiming to showcase its positive effects. The Women, Co-occurring Disorders and Violence Study (WCDVS) ran between 1998 and 2003, gathering data from nine different sites across the USA. A total of 2729 women were randomly assigned to usual-care group or the trauma-informed care group. Interviews were conducted with most of the women in both groups, with those in the trauma-informed care group showing modestly better and sustained improvements than women in the usual care group on measures associated with drug use, alcohol use and trauma over a 12-month period following completion of the programmes (Noether *et al.*, 2005).

According to McHugo *et al.* (2005), each of the programmes offered in the trauma-informed care programme were required to implement four common key dimensions:

1. Programmes needed to be comprehensive and include eight core service elements: outreach and engagement, screening and assessment, ongoing treatment activities, parenting skills training, resource coordination and advocacy, trauma-specific services, crisis intervention and peer run services.
2. Programmes were required to be integrated at an organizational and clinical level. At an organizational level, programmes needed to connect with other support programmes within agencies, ensuring that service delivery was experienced as continuous and not fragmented by the women participants. As noted, 'clinical integration was defined as the simultaneous and coordinated provision of substance abuse, mental health, and trauma services' (McHugo *et al.*, 2005, p.94).
3. Programmes needed to provide their services in a trauma-informed way which was defined as 'having providers who understand the role of violence and abuse in women's lives, respect women's agency in their own recovery, work collaboratively with women in their services and emphasize women's strengths (McHugo *et al.*, 2005, p.94). These services were required to be designed in such a way as to minimize the possibility of re-traumatization and engage women in their own recovery.
4. All the programmes were required to have the involvement of consumer/survivor/recovering women (CSR) embedded as trauma group facilitators, consultants and other peer-led support activities.

During this period, Jennings (2004) described seven principles encouraging organizations seeking to be trauma informed to follow. They needed to offer safety from harm and re-traumatization; develop and promote an understanding of service users symptoms in the context of their life experiences, history, cultures and society more broadly; facilitate open and genuine collaboration between the agency and service users; emphasize skill building rather than symptom management; appreciate symptoms as ways that service users were coping with the impact of their trauma; adopt the view that trauma is a defining and organizing experience that forms the core of an individual's identity; and focus on the experiences that have service users have had rather than on them as problems.

A year later, Elliott *et al.* (2005) expanded on previous work and identified ten key principles of the trauma-informed approach, noting in particular that its genesis addressed the needs of women survivors of trauma:

1. Recognize the sustained and pervasive effects of violence as a means of validating the restraints survivors face in seeking support.
2. Identify recovery from trauma as a primary goal that is simultaneously integrated with service approaches to other problems facing survivors, rather than providing forms of treatment in a sequential way, dealing with specific problems one at a time.
3. Use an empowerment model that ensures that the objectives and ways of support offered to survivors are established and reviewed collaboratively.
4. Maximize a woman's choices and control over her own recovery.
5. Locate the need for survivors to have relationships with staff that are the opposite to the lived experience of power dynamics in which the abuse and violation took place.
6. Build an atmosphere that is welcoming, respectful and safe for survivors.
7. Emphasize the strengths that survivors hold and understand that trauma-based behaviours are adaptations for survival and not symptoms in need of management.
8. Ensure that the services offered to survivors are not re-traumatizing.
9. Acknowledge the need to understand and consider the cultural background of women as a resource for their recovery.
10. Actively involve service users in the design and evaluation of the supports that they are engaged with.

In 2014, SAMHSA published what is possibly the most cited guide to understanding trauma-informed practice. First, it set out its definition of trauma as resulting from:

> ...an event, series of events, or set of circumstances that is experienced by an individual as physically or emotionally harmful or life threatening and that has lasting adverse effects on the individual's functioning and mental, physical, social, emotional or spiritual well-being... (p.7)

It then describes the four assumptions and six key principles that constitute its approach to trauma-informed practice. The driver for this work stems from its view that:

...trauma researchers, practitioners and survivors have recognized that the understanding of trauma and trauma specific interventions is not sufficient to optimise outcomes for trauma survivors nor to influence how service systems conduct their business... (p.9)

For SAMHSA, the basis of a trauma-informed approach is one in which all staff at all levels of an organization *realize* that trauma is significant and understand how trauma affects individuals, families and communities; *recognize* the signs of trauma and routinely screen for trauma experiences in the background of people who seek support; *respond* in ways that are supportive of individuals who have experienced trauma; and, *resist acts which re-traumatize* both the service users and the staff, and prioritize the well-being of all people with whom the organization engages.

SAMHSA's six key principles which enact trauma-informed practice are given as:

- Ensure physical, emotional and psychological safety.
- Build and maintain trustworthiness and transparency at all levels.
- Provide opportunities for service users to receive and participate in peer support activities.
- Actively facilitate collaboration and act to address power dynamics that result from institutional hierarchy and control of information, funding and other resources; foster a sense of empowerment, voice and choice of staff so that service users are active decision makers in the nature of the support and the way that it is provided to them.
- Integrate wisdom and knowledge that address racist, gender and socio-economic biases in the ways that services are delivered.
- Acknowledge and attend to the lived experience of service users.

There has been a burgeoning list of applications of trauma-informed care and trauma-informed practice since then in many areas:

- Child protection and child welfare (Missouri Department of Mental Health and Partners, 2014; Hanson and Lang, 2016; Lang *et al.*, 2016; Sullivan, Murray and Ake, 2016; Evans and Graves, 2018; Department of Families, Fairness and Housing, 2022).
- Out-of-home care services (Bailey *et al.*, 2019; Mitchell, Tucci and Macnamara, 2020; Mitchell, McPherson and Gatwiri, 2020; Brend and Sprang, 2020; Bargeman, Smith and Wekerle, 2021; Collings *et al.*, 2022).
- Educational settings (Bartlett *et al.*, 2016; McConnico *et al.*, 2016; Chafolueas *et al.*, 2016; Perry and Daniels, 2016; Crosby, Howell and Thomas, 2018; Maynard *et al.*, 2018; Gubi *et al.*, 2019; Thomas,

Crosby and Vanderhaar, 2019; Tucci and Mitchell, 2019b; Miller and Berger, 2020; Fondren *et al.*, 2020; Avery *et al.*, 2021; Brummer, 2022; Howard, 2022).

- Homelessness services (Hopper, Bassuk and Olivet, 2007; Burge, Tickle and Moghaddam, 2021).
- Mental health services (Jennings, 2004; Muskett, 2014; Clark, 2015; Donisch, Bray and Gewirtz, 2016; Sweeney *et al.*, 2016; Kim and Ashmore, 2019; Flavin *et al.*, 2022).
- Adult and youth justice systems (Whittemore and Knafl, 2005; Covington, 2008; McLindon and Harms, 2011; Rozzell, 2013; Crosby, 2016; Levenson, Willis and Prescott, 2016; Skinner-Osei and Levenson, 2018; Levenson and Willis, 2019; Moore, 2022; Silvester, 2022).
- Policing (Evans and Graves, 2018; Lathan *et al.*, 2019; Jones 2022).
- Forensic services (Hocken, Taylor and Watson, 2022; Jones and Willmot, 2022)
- Disability services (Keesler, 2014; Longfellow and Hicks, 2022; Houck and Dracobly, 2022).
- Drug and alcohol rehabilitation services (Pride *et al.*, 2021).

Many of these cite and/or are heavily influenced by the work of SAMHSA. More recently, others have expanded the notion of trauma-informed care/practice to capture local or contextual adaptations.

For example, the US based National Child Traumatic Stress Network (Pynoos *et al.*, 2008), administered by SAMHSA, described seven principles of trauma-informed care:

- Inclusive of routine screening for trauma exposure and effects.
- Promoting the use of culturally appropriate and evidence-based assessment and treatment approaches for trauma and its sequelae.
- Ensuring that information relating to trauma can be accessed by children, families and agency personnel.
- Strengthening the resilience and protective factors for children through interventions aimed specifically at improving developmental vulnerability.
- Addressing parental and caregiver's own histories of trauma.
- Facilitating continuity of care for children with a commitment to collaboration across children's services.
- Actively responding to the impacts of secondary trauma.

These principles expand on the ideas expressed by SAMHSA but with a specific focus on children.

The Office for Health Improvement and Disparities in the UK (2022) issued guidance about trauma-informed principles in response to a perceived need to provide clarity for the health and social care sector. It depicts a working definition of trauma-informed practice that extends beyond the individual, realizing the impact of trauma on individuals, groups and communities, recognizing the scale and nature of trauma and its effects, and preventing re-traumatization. It identified six principles as safety, trust, choice, collaboration, empowerment and cultural considerations.

The Welsh Government (2022) has also identified the need to introduce greater consistency in definitional typology to trauma-informed approaches. It has defined five critical practice principles: relationship focused; resilience and strengths based; inclusive, which recognizes the impact of diversity, discrimination and racism currently and historically; person centred; and adopting a universal approach that does no harm and encompasses therapeutic intervention as well as community-led and preventative initiatives.

For the first time, it also introduced the concept of levels to trauma-informed practice, identifying four levels that refer to the range of roles that professionals and agencies can play in supporting individuals, families and communities affected by trauma and adversity:

> These practice levels are not defined by the profession or setting of the individuals, instead they describe different helping roles to support people of all ages who have experienced trauma. They promote compassionate, empathic and supportive relationships, services and specific personalized and co-produced interventions...They recognize that effective trauma-informed intervention often does not require formal treatment and access to the natural world in Wales has a great capacity to support people... (Welsh Government, 2022, p.11)

The four practice levels are not hierarchical but represent a spectrum of ways in which individuals can and do play a part in providing support.

> ...many people affected by traumatic events will need support from different levels at the same time and a person centred, integrated, interacting system is vital to maximise its effectiveness... (p.11)

The four levels are described as follows:

- *Trauma aware* occurs when individuals understand the role that all members of a community play in appreciating the impact of trauma and adversity and as a result take action to challenge the discourses that maintain oppression and inequality. Within this framework, these individuals respond kindly and empathically to people in distress at the local level within their everyday lives. They help to foster supportive relationships for individuals across families and community networks. They promote the principle that impacts of trauma can be overcome. They take opportunities to reduce stigma, adverse labelling and victim blaming. They act collaboratively to engage community in joint activities that promote healthy and respectful interactions.

- *A trauma-skilled approach* is embedded in the practices of all individuals who provide care or support to people who may have experienced trauma, whether this is known or not. These individuals understand the importance of safe relationships for promoting trust, mitigating the effects of trauma and adversity and preventing the re-traumatization of people. They aim to offer relationships which are 'restorative'. They support individuals and families to determine how support is best offered to them. They help to guide people who have experienced trauma to the best resources for them. They are part of organizational cultures that recognize the effects of trauma on staff and provide them with regular opportunities for reflection, supervision and support.

- *Trauma enhanced* occurs when knowledge and skills are used by staff and carers employed in organizations that provide direct or intensive support to individuals who are known to have experienced traumatic events, with the goal to resource them to better cope with the impact. These staff and carers appreciate when people are overwhelmed with their experience of trauma, and sensitively resource ways to help them with their distress and pain. They are confident about knowing how to inquire about a person's experience of trauma and adversity and offer compassionate responses that make sense and are helpful. They work collaboratively with other services through well-established policies, practise guidance and approaches that enable individuals with trauma experiences to receive individually tailored services that are right for them and their context. There is a shared view among staff and carers about the needs of individuals and families who have been affected by trauma and how to best meet them, including referring them on for more specialist intervention if required.

- *Specialist interventions* are established to meet the needs of people affected by trauma and where possible co-designed with them. There are established ways of assessing the nature and extent of the distress that individuals and families have and continue to experience, taking into account their context. Staff understand the psychosocial determinants of mental health and appreciate the social inequity in the development of difficulties. All these services are genuinely collaborative, empathic and person centred. They support individuals who have experienced trauma to access evidence-based treatment, including pharmacological intervention and other forms of highly specialized resources that are delivered by multidisciplinary teams. These practitioners will lead and support multi-agency care plans as deemed necessary, providing the opportunity to ensure that services are joined up and working with the same intent and purpose.

Interestingly, within this document, acknowledging the investment already made in applying the Adverse Childhood Experiences framework, the Welsh Government proposed an integrated framework – 'TrACE (Trauma and Adverse Childhood Experiences) informed' – believing that the organizational adoption of a 'TrACE informed' approach will result in 'increased ownership for transformational change with their setting' (p.20). This appears to be the first documented attempt to support organizations to integrate a trauma-informed approach in their existing frameworks and models.

Critically, the Welsh Government also introduced the concept of collective action. It makes it clear that 'systems that are trauma informed are the products of collective action' (Welsh Government, 2022, p.22).

While earlier conceptualizations identified the need for systems to be trauma informed, they stopped short of articulating the effort required to achieve this. Trauma-informed systems are not only the focus of public services but should be relevant for individuals, organizations and communities.

Such collective action is effective in challenging and breaking down silo working and restrictive funding and outcome frameworks; reviewing and improving overly bureaucratic processes that serve the functions of the system rather than the person; establishing opportunities for creativity and adaptability for individuals and service systems; promoting equal power sharing through collaboration; avoiding the individualization of personal suffering that results in stigmatization and restricted access to services; understanding that trauma does not affect everyone who experiences it in the same way; ensuring that individuals who seek help are not penalized for doing so; promoting trust in leadership that is trauma informed; and valuing the importance of actions that positively nurture well-being.

Despite the promise of Harris and Fallot's original optimism, the transformation of programmes, organizations and systems and embedding the principles they have articulated is still very much a work in progress. Notwithstanding, their pioneering work has taken trauma from the periphery of practice consciousness and made it a central feature. It has introduced the simple notion that an awareness about the pain that individuals, families and communities have experienced over time arising from violence and forms of oppression can lead to a more sensitive, flexible and compassionate response from service systems which were not originally designed with this knowledge in mind. It has made it more realistic for service users and service providers to share power in creating the way that services are offered. It has demanded greater collaboration between services so that individuals are not lost in between systems with seemingly different aims and approaches. Most significantly, it has moved the locus of individual problems away from a construction of personal failure or inherent limitation to encompass the importance of considering past and ongoing experiences of violation as they affect the life trajectories and outcomes of victims and survivors.

While this effort to trace the history of the trauma-informed movement is not exhaustive, it has highlighted its conceptual elasticity over time. In recent years, there has been a mounting critique of the trauma-informed approach regarding what it is and what it is not, what is important and what is missing (Piedfort-Marin, 2022). The next section of this chapter summarizes this critique and offers further analysis and exploration of the important lessons learned over the last two decades of the trauma-informed paradigm shift, in the hope that it provides some pointers to where its future lies.

Trauma-informed movement – critical reflections on its evolution

It is only recently that critiques have begun to emerge about the extent to which the adoption of trauma-informed practice principles and knowledge is achieving the change it set out to achieve.

In 2013, the Australian Centre for Posttraumatic Mental Health and Parenting Research Centre undertook a study of more than 300 practitioners and organizational leaders in the child and family services sector, revealing that:

> ...although concepts such as complex trauma, trauma-informed care and evidence base were not new to those interviewed, organizational leaders and senior managers identified that the field still lacked clear definitions or understanding of each of these. There was agreement on the need for refinement of how trauma is understood in the field and that greater support could be provided to increase practitioners' knowledge... (p.5)

In 2016, Lucy Berliner and David Kolko commented that:

> ...it is heartening that there has been so much enthusiasm for efforts to be more trauma informed. Increased awareness that so many children suffer victimisation and adversities is good. Society at large, as well as its institutions and professionals working with children, should be knowledgeable about the prevalence of hardship...the challenge for the movement to

instill TIC (Trauma Informed Care) across institutions is to demonstrate that awareness or implementation of other activities associated with TIC initiatives actually makes a difference... (p.168)

They were specifically interested in whether or not the paradigm shift has improved the lives of children, given their areas of expertise. After considering a range of evidence, they concluded that the trauma-informed care movement has had modest benefits with a potential 'positive byproduct' being an increase in the quality of care offered by service systems when practitioners are more empathic and understanding of the needs of children in particular.

However, they point out that so far what have been defined as trauma-informed principles are 'essentially principles of good care and are not specific to trauma per se. For example, safety, trustworthiness, collaboration and mutuality, empowerment, voice and choice should characterise all systems-level responses' (p.169).

Bloom (2019) also noted that 'as I go around the country I find that... there remain large gaps between what is meant by trauma informed care and what actually happens' (p.388).

Sweeney and Taggart (2018) similarly argued that 'despite growing international interest, trauma-informed approaches can seem fuzzy, complex, something that service providers already do, or a theorised call for practitioners to "be nicer"' (p.383).

Quadara and Hunter (2016) expressed the view that the application of trauma-informed care in Australia was best described as:

> ...emergent – practice wisdom and evaluation knowledge have not yet coalesced sufficiently to guide how the principles are put into practice in different settings; enthusiastic – there is significant interest across a range of sectors in becoming trauma informed; opaque – there is a lack of publicly available, coordinated material on the trauma-informed care programs and models being developed and the format they take; and, piecemeal – without strong, collaborative national leadership, the development of trauma informed care models is driven by individual services... (p.8)

In the following section, a number of themes are explored that arise from the evolution of the trauma-informed movement, and questions are raised as to its future effectiveness in resourcing change in the ways that systems serve the needs of individuals, families and communities with lived and living experience of trauma. This thematic analysis begins with an understanding that the social world is inherently complex, dynamic and prone to change. Thus, complexity is an overarching frame within which a nuanced and deeper consideration of these critical issues is explored.

Trauma-informed approaches are most commonly aimed at reducing the impact of complex trauma – trauma that occurs in the context of relational systems that are dangerous, cruel and insensitive, impacting the complex systems of the brain, body and mind of the individual or groups of individuals over time. By implication then, complexity thinking must pervade trauma-informed practice. Trauma-informed approaches are always implemented in complex systems that are emergent, unpredictable, self-organizing, adapting, contextual and multi-dimensional. As argued by Webb (2006) 'wicked problems' such as the amelioration of complex trauma 'are necessarily coupled to the twin processes of uncertainty and complexity as features of changing organizational [and systemic] environments ... uncertainty in the formation of social policy and organizational planning makes error inevitable' (p.191).

Webb's analysis is also helpful in explaining a key cause of what can best be described as a conceptual slippage in the term 'trauma informed'. Hanson and Lang (2016) are among many who have argued that the term lacks consensus of definition making it difficult to evaluate its impact.

Drawing from Rittel and Webber's (1973) earlier work, Webb elaborated on the characteristics of 'wicked problems' in the context of human services:

- They cannot be easily defined so that stakeholders agree on the problem to be solved and the most effective way of approaching this collaboratively.
- They require complex judgements about the level of abstraction at which to define the problem (individual, familial, community, organization, system, sociocultural, political).
- They have no clear stopping rules (e.g. abuse and violence, drug misuse).
- They have better or worse solutions, not right and wrong ones (the constraints on the solution, such as limited resources and political ramifications change over time).
- They have no objective measure of success.
- They require iteration – every trial counts.
- They have no given alternative solutions – these must be discovered.
- They often have a strong moral, political and professional dimension, particularly for failure (violence and abuse, racism, oppressive systems of control based on gender).

Applying the concept and characteristics of 'wicked problems' to the amelioration of trauma renders apparent the complexity of the task of a trauma-informed approach both with respect to its causes and potential solutions. It requires attention to the interactions between micro, meso and macro systems (Mitleton-Kelly, 2002) within which the needs of victims and survivors are viewed as not existing in isolation but as part of complex relational (Ewijk, 2018) and sociocultural contexts. The response to which requires practitioners, programmes, organizations and systems to engage in analysis and explanation, creativity, judgement and the ability to accommodate uncertainty and intricacy. Khoo *et al.* (2020) recently proposed the concept of 'transactional complexity' to explain the interaction between these different complex adaptive systems.

The ambitions of the trauma-informed movement remain relevant – the development of a unifying and working concept in the delivery of human services (SAMHSA, 2014). The future relevance of this movement lies in its capacity to make trauma-informed concepts, frameworks or approaches accessible and 'doable' without becoming too simplistic in their articulation such that their very essence and contribution to 'business as usual practice' is lost.

The evolution of trauma-informed practice is a reaction to the way that violence continues to be minimized in our community consciousness

As noted by a number of authors, trauma-informed practice approaches were developed in response to an increasing awareness among the helping professions of the pervasiveness of violence in the community, in particular interpersonal violence, and the amplifying effects over the lifespan of abuse and violation that occurred during childhood (Fallot and Harris, 2001; Joseph and Murphy, 2014; Knight, 2015; Bloom, 2019; Addis *et al.*, 2022; Champine *et al.*, 2022).

This awareness is not, however, widely shared in the community. This is particularly the case when it comes to child abuse and the complex trauma that results. Many children who have experienced or continue to experience abuse and violation present with a range of social, emotional, behavioural and learning difficulties that are misunderstood or misdiagnosed by the adults responsible for their care, support or education. These children are often viewed as disruptive, disobedient, aggressive, withdrawn, disengaged or risky to themselves or others. Their vulnerabilities and victimhood are often denied such that they become excluded from school, sporting and community activities. Our collective failure to recognize that many of these children are being or have been repeatedly abused and traumatized is in part driven by the pervasive, ongoing ignorance of adults, organizations and systems to the issue of child abuse in the community. Trauma-informed practice has gone some way to recognize the impacts of child abuse cross the lifespan but it masks the critical need for policy and initiatives to empower the community to take action on the issue of child abuse as well as generate compassion for the trauma it causes children, families and communities.

Over the past 18 years, Tucci and Mitchell have examined community awareness and understanding of child abuse and child protection in Australia (Tucci, Goddard and Mitchell, 2001; Tucci and Mitchell, 2021, 2022; Tucci, Mitchell and Goddard, 2003, 2006, 2010). After another round of surveys in 2021 (Tucci and Mitchell, 2021, 2022), they recently drew the conclusion that child abuse remains largely unseen and ignored as a community concern. The results are virtually identical to those found over the past three earlier studies. In 2021, child abuse rated lower than problems with public transport and roads on a list of community concerns.

In 2006, 43 per cent respondents felt so poorly informed on the issue as to be unable to guess the number of reported cases of child abuse, while those prepared to estimate significantly underestimated the problem. In 2021, 56 per cent were so poorly informed that they could not even hazard a guess at the number of reports of child abuse that were received in the preceding year in Australia.

Child abuse appears to remain, at its most basic level, a topic that sits on the periphery of community consciousness. Many people feel sorrow, anger and powerlessness when they come face to face with child abuse in their own families and communities.

A trauma-informed community must embrace the following characteristics: collective acceptance of the need to act to stop violence from occurring; feeling equipped with the knowledge and tools to take confident and capable steps to protect the vulnerable from the trauma caused by abuse and violation; feeling compassion for those experiencing such trauma, and commitment to the provision of effective services and supports to ensure that their needs are met.

A focus by the general and helping community only on compassion and commitment to trauma-informed services for those who have experienced trauma denies the full breadth of collective responsibilities of a trauma-informed community. It is not enough to focus on the end result of violence without engaging with the reality of the violence itself and what is needed to address these acts.

'Trauma-informed practice' is more than a set of principles that are common to 'good practice'

The articulation of the practice principles such as trustworthiness, transparency, power sharing, inclusion of diversity, involvement of service users in service design and person-centred care have not evolved because of trauma knowledge or trauma practitioners. The consumer movement in health and mental health services finds its roots in advocacy to reform institutions and treatment of women in psychiatry. The continuing history of people with lived and living experiences of trauma separately, but similarly, records failures at multiple levels to take into account and respond effectively to their needs within a diverse group of service settings. Of course, there are clear and significant crossovers between movements.

Arguably, trauma-informed practice *should* share principles in common with accepted conventions about what constitutes 'good practice', 'rights-based practice' or plain 'common sense'. However, it is also the case that practice, or an approach of any kind is more than a set of principles. A critical limitation of many attempts to define trauma-informed approaches is their failure to articulate an approach beyond a set of principles. Trauma principles should shape an orientation to what knowledges will be privileged in the process of meaning making with and on behalf of the people served – theoretical trauma knowledge, research, practice wisdom, lived experience, cultural knowledge, procedural knowledge (Thompson and West, 2013). It is the confluence of principles and these knowledges that informs 'why' a practice approach is implemented in a particular way, 'how' it is actually executed in practice, describes 'what' change is being sought, 'who' are the targets of the desired change and 'how' success is understood.

As previously asserted, to engage in trauma-informed practice is to hold complexity. Complex trauma lives in the interpersonal, the spaces in between, and is multi-dimensional. It demands that reductionist thinking is resisted and that practice occurs within a clearly articulated theory of change that embraces both a deep understanding of relevant knowledges and 'transactional complexity'. It also requires that the whole person is understood within their critical relationships and sociocultural context, with an investment of effort to deconstruct professional expertise and work within and across formal and informal systems of influence and control. It involves an understanding of the impact of working with people with trauma and the consequences of secondary trauma or compassion fatigue for the 'helpers', and having systems and processes in place to ensure the well-being and health of the 'helpers'. It encourages organizations to understand that implementing trauma-informed practice is more than a training exercise for its workforce, and that training, in and of itself, does not lead to substantial practice change. It also necessitates critical appraisal and support of its leadership capability to lead and sustain knowledge translation and practice change, and examination of organizational culture and strategic direction. Embedded and sustained practice change takes ongoing investment and effort by organizations and funders that is often poorly appreciated. The emergence of implementation science gives useful pointers to the sustained and comprehensive effort that is required to change 'business as usual' practice.

Indeed, much is left both to the capability of practitioners, programme and service designers, organizations and systems to undertake the complex knowledge translation required to operationalize a trauma-informed approach and the rigor and sustainability of the implementation approach to introduce and embed the new practice paradigm (Becker-Blease, 2017). As Bloom (2016) reflected:

> Just as taking on board the concept of trauma-informed systems necessitates a change in mental models, so too does understanding exactly what it is we are to treat, who to treat when, and what recovery from trauma and adversity actually looks like. As a result of these and other factors, there remain large gaps between what is meant by trauma-informed care and what actually happens, and this means that there is a need for more clarification... (p.388)

The lack of a more fulsome articulation of the complexity that is inherent in a trauma-informed approach leaves it open to criticism. First, there is an emerging perception that it should not be taken seriously, or its validity is questioned, because it is viewed as doing what other paradigms have already marked out or are doing, therefore there is no need to make any changes to service systems. Sweeney and Taggart (2018) noted that:

> ...there is an inevitable risk of co-option: that trauma informed approaches will come to mean little more than treatment as usual repackaged as trauma informed...given the centrality of trust in working with trauma, transparency is crucial and the rebranding of services need to be accompanied by real systemic change... (p.385)

Second, it may be caught up in discourses which criticize identities that are important to victims, such as being innocent children, victims of coercion and manipulation, survivors who have found their own voice in the face of violence. There are disturbing perspectives serving to pathologize trauma through directing all attention to victims who are 'given' the responsibility by the violence to carry the deficits of trauma within them (Gómez *et al.*, 2016; Rosenthal, Reinhardt and Birrell, 2016). This community narrative is already present as a means to cast shame on individuals who have suffered childhood trauma and continue to show distress and other expressions of pain through difficulties identified as mental health, addiction and personality problems. These are the very frames that intensify stigma and shame and form the means through which victims are silenced and abuse of children and other vulnerable groups is kept hidden.

There is the potential for the trauma-informed practice movement to lose legitimacy and eventually fizzle out as it is seen as something that everyone is 'doing' with no scrutiny as to the validity of these claims.

Conceptualizations of trauma-informed practice risk stagnation

In over two decades since the introduction of terms such as trauma-informed practice and trauma-informed care, very little has changed in its conceptualization. There is a growing coalescence about its meaning as noted in the analysis of its history earlier in the chapter. This has not been reviewed, in part because it is difficult to argue with the inherent authority of SAMSHA. It is also not easy to challenge beliefs that have become a form of orthodoxy and for many parts of the world are now driving how decisions about funding are made. Additional terms have been proposed such as trauma specific, trauma skilled, trauma sensitive, trauma aware, and trauma responsive, which has served to evolve a language ecosystem, but to what end? Do they challenge and grow the fundamental tenets of trauma-informed practice or create more delineation and confusion?

Harris and Fallot (2001a) were the first to suggest such a delineation:

> ...systems serve survivors of childhood trauma without treating them for the consequences of trauma: more significant, systems serve individuals without even being aware of the trauma that occurred. This lack of awareness can result in failures to make appropriate referrals for trauma services... (p.3)

They went on to suggest that:

> ...a trauma-specific service is designed to treat the actual sequelae of sexual or physical abuse ... trauma-informed services are not designed to treat symptoms or syndromes related to sexual or physical abuse. Rather, regardless of their primary mission ... their commitment is to provide services in a manner that is welcoming and appropriate to the special needs of trauma survivors... (pp.4–5)

SAMHSA adopted this differentiation, noting that trauma-informed approaches were inclusive of trauma-specific services. This differentiation continues to permeate contemporary conceptualizations of trauma-informed practice. There is a range of assumptions inherent in this differentiation that has received little attention and review. First, there is an inherent focus on the individual to the exclusion of other frames of reference, with the focus on referral of individuals for trauma-specific treatment as the means through which healing symptomatology occurs. This frame excludes more contemporary ways of understanding complex trauma that are inclusive of groups of people who have been traumatized on the basis of 'othering' characteristics such as race, religion or gender. This will be explored in more detail later in the chapter.

Second, it infers that there is a range of trauma treatment modalities in which clinical staff are best equipped to provide to victims and survivors to support their healing and recovery from complex trauma. These approaches are most often rooted in a medical model that pathologizes and decontextualizes the individual, risks re-traumatization through adherence to strict protocols that can remove power and control from people or replicate oppression, and privileges symptom reduction as the primary goal of treatment (Gómez *et al.,* 2016). It is common for people who have experienced complex trauma to also present with a range of other complex needs, including substance abuse, other mental health diagnoses and relationship challenges. Whereas the intent of a trauma-informed approach is to consider the whole person, the implication of trauma-specific treatment is that trauma is treated separately and distinctly from the range of other complex presenting issues, further perpetuating a siloed and fragmented approach to treatment in which people may experience several different treatment modalities targeting their various complex needs that are poorly conceptualized, sequenced or at worst in conflict with each other.

Finally, this differentiation privileges specific trauma treatment as the therapeutic agent of change. In doing so, it denies the potential for 'therapeutic intent' that can arise in environments, networks of relationships and communities. Resourced with knowledge about complex trauma and support to operationalize this knowledge, these relationships and supportive contexts are able to do significant 'heavy lifting' in the process of change and healing. Therapeutic models of out-of-home care for children and young people are offered by way of example of this point (Mitchell, Tucci and Macnamara, 2020; Mitchell, McPherson and Gatwiri, 2020). Early pioneers in what is now more commonly referred to as therapeutic care, Trieschman and colleagues (2002) coined the term 'the other 23 hours' as a counterpoint to the notion of an hour of therapy. Their approach was situated in the key concepts of 'therapeutic milieu', 'life space' and 'therapeutic relationships'. Therapeutic care holds as its central tenet that children come to heal from trauma when the relationship networks around them are resourced with therapeutic intent and hold therapeutic capacity (Mitchell, Tucci and Macnamara, 2020).

> It means that for healing to occur, some of these relationships need to be purposeful and oriented to being used as resources in transformation. Of course, therapists play an important role, too. In this process, the therapist adds the therapeutic effort...locating themselves 'in between' children, their relationship community, their past, their present, their restraints, their strengths... (Tucci, Mitchell and Tronick, 2020, pp.28–29)

While acknowledging the importance of context and relationships, the perpetuation of the distinction between trauma informed and trauma specific serves to limit the power of what a trauma-informed approach can deliver. The integration of the concepts of 'therapeutic intent' and the 'therapeutic effort' that can be found in relationships signals a significant shift away from the current conceptualizations of what a trauma-informed approach is towards one that holds greater coherence and clarity as to a theory of change that is trauma integrative or transformational (Tucci and Mitchell, 2019b).

While the goal of 'do no more harm' is commonplace, the prevention of re-traumatization is more challenging

The trauma-informed practice approach has, as a principle and goal, the prevention of re-traumatization (Harris and Fallot, 2001a; SAMHSA, 2014; Carter and Blanch, 2019). There are built-in assumptions that adherence to a trauma-informed approach will achieve this goal. But do these assumption hold?

For example, Benjamin (2019) noted that the paradigm of trauma-informed care aims to:

> ...provide education about what is reported to be a very common finding in health systems, namely an insensitivity by staff to patients who have been traumatised; most especially in inpatient units and in larger, institutional settings with patriarchal hierarchies... (p.xxxiv)

At its core, the notion of re-traumatization is problematic. The experience of trauma resulting from interpersonal violence is intentional. Perpetrators of violation use power to hurt, cause pain, control and ultimately gain some benefit from their actions. Service systems, in general, can have a deleterious impact on the individuals they try to support. They can send people away because they do not fit rigid criteria for inclusion. They can disempower people in the way they do not share information with service users. They can take over definitions of people's identity and label them with problems they do believe they have. They can misinterpret the meaning of behaviour and attribute intentionality that is not accurate. They can blame people for the problems they are causing to themselves or others. These sorts of experiences for any individual, family or community can cause reverberating impacts that are unhelpful and toxic. For those who have experienced trauma, the impact is likely to be amplified and reactivate biopsychosocial states of defence that they used to protect themselves from the violence in the first place. However, while it is significantly harmful for trauma victims and survivors, it is arguable that it connotes the inherent and purposeful qualities that perpetrators of violence signal to their victims through their behaviour.

This is only important because the primary goal of trauma-informed approaches is explicitly to prevent re-traumatization through the services and systems in which individuals engage for support and assistance. It affords an opportunity to reconceptualize the goals of trauma-informed practice so that they are more oriented to end-state goals that organizations should be aiming for. For example, a more effective objective would be for organizations to understand and meet the needs of service users which arise from the trauma they have experienced. This would still require safety to be a key element of organizational culture, but it would also speak to different areas of interest. For example, it would reorient organizations to understanding how trauma:

- disrupts relational experiences from meeting the needs of the individuals seeking support
- undermines confidence that others will act in ways that are in the interests of the individuals seeking support
- confuses the ways that life narratives are composed and not always consistently told
- introduces fear and threat into every exchange
- requires safety to be absolute in the environments that provide support to individuals who engage with human service organizations.

It is the very nuances of living with the consequences of trauma which need to be imbued into the fabric of human service organizations. It is the way that trauma knowledge is applied in the real world which will lead to organizational cultures that integrate attitudinal and practice shifts, policy changes, re-orientation of funding opportunities and service system design.

In so doing, it would create greater impetus for real change to occur in service systems that continue to challenge basic human rights and dignity; for example, the use of physical restraint to control behaviour (Bonner *et al.*, 2002; Steckley, 2010; Perkins *et al.*, 2012; McGuire, Carlisle and Clark, 2022); the placement of children as young as nine and ten years of age in detention for crimes they are incapable of taking responsibility for given their immaturity and vulnerability (Haysom, 2022; Holland *et al.*, 2022; Myles, 2022); and the removal of children and young people from families of First Nations people at significantly higher rates than non-indigenous populations in countries such as Australia (Creamer *et al.*, 2022; Douglas, 2022; Quinn *et al.*, 2022; Turnbull-Roberts, Salter and Newton, 2022; de la Sablonnière-Griffin *et al.*, 2023).

It should also make explicit, through organizational policies and systems, that there cannot be a repetition of the failures of systems in the past to protect children, calling on organizations to remain vigilant to the possibility that perpetrators of violation of children and vulnerable adults are in fact able to groom and manipulate entire organizations to cover up their abusive behaviour or misdirect attention away from being caught. The lessons of the Royal Commission into Institutional Responses to Child Sexual Abuse in Australia highlighted how organizations allowed predators within a range of institutions caring for children to continue to abuse them without any form of sanction, and even at times enabling them to move to another area where they were able to start all over again (Royal Commission into Institutional Responses to Child Sexual Abuse, 2017; Tucci and Blom, 2019).

It is not enough that trauma-informed organizations are required to ensure safety. The salient lessons from the past, especially in relation to children, must be carried through and implemented. This requires attention paid to safeguarding the interests of all children, young people and vulnerable adults through effective policy and system regimes which are reviewed regularly and integrated deeply into organizational culture.

Effective implementation has limited the impact of trauma-informed practice

Reviews of the evidence to date suggests that the implementation of trauma-informed practice approaches is delivering modest results. For example, Quadara and Hunter (2016) analysed three projects associated with the application of trauma-informed practice with children (the Arkansas Building Effective Services for Trauma training, the Chadwick Trauma-Informed Systems Dissemination and Implementation Project and the Massachusetts Child Trauma Project), finding that the impact was small to moderate. They noted that there are multiple challenges that may be acting as barriers to successful implementation including the need for greater collaboration between services, large caseloads for staff, and stressful, hostile and crisis-driven contexts of service provision (Yatchmenoff, Sundborg and Davis, 2017).

Similarly, Berliner and Kolko (2016) noted that if trauma-informed approaches are intended to produce changes in practice, then there needs to be a shift towards understanding and addressing the need to actually operationalize the ideas into the everyday practices of staff who work in human service organizations. The starting point is the development of a unified definition that can be relevant to all practitioners who interact with and support individuals and families who have experienced trauma, including child protection staff, teachers, mental health practitioners, youth workers, homelessness staff, foster carers and disability workers. The importance of being able to delineate the markers of child, family, community and system level outcomes of the implementation of trauma-informed practice is also tied up with the argument in favour of clearer working definitional frameworks.

The lack of such evidence speaks to the widespread support for the rich interpretive resources that are offered by trauma knowledge about behaviour and experience. But it does not offer insights into how and if such knowledge, training and tied funding actually make a difference to the impact that such services have in the lives of individuals seeking support.

Trauma-informed practice approaches continue to locate problems in the individual and not in the context of relationships and broader sociocultural dimensions of life

The popular maxim that best underscores the paradigm shift of trauma-informed approaches is the reframing of the question 'What is wrong with you?' to 'What happened to you?' It is simple but encourages a seismic change to the way that services built around a biopsychosocial model of health and welfare are delivered. It stops treating the impact of the violence caused by another as the problem owned by the individual victim/survivor and locates the cause of the individual's difficulties with the lasting effects of violation in their lives. Problematic behaviour is understood as being more consistent with adaptations that have enabled the individual to survive the oppressive nature of ongoing threat and danger and continue to function in the best way they can in the face of such overwhelming consequences. Trauma-based behaviours are often acknowledged as functional and adaptive in the context in which the violence was occurring but maladaptive if they continue when the violence is no longer present. Too often, these behaviours become the focus of intervention rather than the relational environments within which change can occur or be supported.

While purporting to acknowledge the relational dimensions of interpersonal trauma arising from violence and abuse, trauma-informed practice elements are more consistent with the societal discourse that serves to reduce accountability for the perpetrators of violence and shifts responsibility for the effects of violence to the victim. The neutral tone of the second question reflects an undervaluing of the inherent dynamics of power on which abuse and violence are facilitated, including the gendered structure of society which privileges male worldviews, racism that discriminates in favour of social groups with histories of colonizing and enslavement, the ways in which children and young people are rendered powerless through adult-centric perspectives and belief systems, and the wrongful perception that abled body frames of reference are more legitimate than those with disabilities.

'What happened to you?' should really become 'How have you been hurt? Who hurt you? How can I understand what it means for you? What do you need from relationships around you?'

As noted by Sweeney and Taggart (2018), the original reframed question was not meant to be literal. Similarly, this proposed revision is designed as an orientation for practitioners to consider as they approach the people who are seeking out their support. Their purpose is to appreciate that the answers which may follow have organized the service user's life course to date, and to find ways to respect that and sensitively interact in ways that offer compassion-driven messages that seek to communicate: *you are understood, you are safe, your pain is validated, your hurt will be tolerated and validated, you are entitled to be cared for.* Even more importantly, victims and survivors need to hear and come to know that practitioners understand that *you were hurt by others who were supposed to care for you, your pain has occurred in relationships that you trusted, you were betrayed by those who you should have been able to rely on.* The relational frame of reference for inter-personal violence resulting in complex trauma needs to be integrated into the very heart of trauma-informed practice.

Screening for trauma is inherently complex

A number of researchers point to evidence that regular trauma screening is not occurring despite it being one of the original practice principles of a trauma-informed approach (Sweeney *et al.*, 2016; Caffrey and Winton, 2022). As argued by Harris and Fallot (2001a), the mere act of asking those seeking support about whether they had experienced any form of trauma during their life had a number of important effects: it kept it on the agenda for staff, reminding them of just how significant a proportion of the population had suffered trauma in their past; it communicated to service users that the organization was willing and able to listen and acknowledge that trauma, even if it had been kept secret, was a topic that could be explored as part of the support offered to them; and it provided vital information to managers about how to adapt their service design to better meet the needs of these service users as they gained important knowledge about their backgrounds and experiences.

However, rates of seeking out this information have remained low. It is not surprising, as pointed out by Sweeney and Taggart (2018), that:

> ...given that health and social care professionals have experienced higher rates of trauma than the general population...and that service providers experience vicarious trauma...there is a challenge to negotiate complex interpersonal dynamics arising from trauma histories... (p.385)

An alternative explanation, of course, is to recognize that adherence to rou-tine screening for trauma imposes a mechanistic procedure to what should be a sensitive and relationally oriented element of practice. Many victims and survivors have never told anyone or have waited years to be ready to disclose. For example, the Royal Commission into Institutional Responses to Child Sexual Abuse in Australia (2017) found that:

> ...many victims do not disclose child sexual abuse until many years after the abuse occurred, often when they are well into adulthood. Survivors who spoke with us during a private session took, on average, 23.9 years to tell someone about the abuse and men often took longer to disclose than women (the average for females was 20.6 years and for males was 25.6 years)... (p.9)

Child USA also reported (2020) that:

> ...while it may seem intuitive that a survivor would disclose abuse when it happened, data reveals a different reality. In a study of over 1,000 survivors, the average age at the time of reporting child sex abuse was about 52 years... (p.4)

Many victims and survivors are not believed the first time they give an indication that they have been violated. Many do not expect to be believed. Some expect to be blamed for the abuse themselves. Talking about their abuse experience is not the same as telling a health professional whether you suffered measles when you were a child. It is not a transactional process aimed at reporting as a matter of fact whether a service user has a trauma history. It is part of a process of expression supported by trust over time and compassion offered as part of a reparative relational experience.

As such, it may be more useful to reconfigure this principle so that it concentrates more on creating the conditions that are conducive to service users deciding for themselves whether to disclose this information about their past. There is restorative power for practitioners and service users alike to co-design service systems with people with lived and living experiences of trauma so that, from the onset, service users know that it is safe to share their experience if they choose to with people with specific roles in the system.

Trauma-informed practice does not adequately differentiate between the diverse experiences of victims and survivors

Sweeney and Taggart (2018) have made a number of very powerful cautionary notes in their analysis of the misconceptions about trauma-informed practice. They acknowledge the need for trauma-informed approaches in mental health services by supporting the assertion that:

> ...although trauma informed approaches are based on the knowledge that trauma is widespread and causal in the development of significant mental

distress, it is not seen as the cause of all mental distress... Instead, it is argued that while everyone is able to use services that are trauma informed and that these services could be considered gold standard, if services are not trauma informed then trauma survivors – who by varying estimates make up the majority of mental health service users – will find it difficult to use them... (p.384)

However, they also warn that strongly prescribed 'trauma-only' explanations of mental health increase the concern that service users will need to be identified primarily as victims, at the very least, in order to access services, negating the possibility that they can engage with less vulnerable identities such as survivors or lived experience experts (Becker-Blease, 2017).

In their anthropological study of the emergence of trauma as a modern post-world-war phenomenon, Fassin and Rechtman (2009) voice an uneasiness that when trauma is expressed in language that is manifestly neutral and universal, it eliminates the diversity and complexity of the violation that is perpetrated in its many forms, its interpretations and its life course consequences. Trauma is assumed to be self-explanatory, as if the damaging experience is the same for everyone. Of course, it is not. Each individual experiences their violation from the perspective of the context of their life to that point. For some, the violation of childhood sexual abuse, as an example, serves to further amplify their vulnerability due to their economic status, gender and cultural background. In carrying the pain from this experience, the layers of historical and ongoing oppression and the relational environment of their lives before and after the violation becomes referenced in the meaning that they come to hold about it.

Trauma-informed practice approaches, despite having the opposite intent, fail to pay adequate attention to the unique circumstances and nature of the violation suffered by people and the way that trauma is shaped by the significance of the dominant social norms and attitudes of the community in which it is experienced (Sweeney *et al.*, 2018). It is understood that trauma-informed approaches are aimed at resourcing the prevailing culture of the human service organization and the way it is operationalized by its staff. It is not able to determine the exact response by specific people in specific roles. But to date, the paradigm leaves knowledge about the distinctiveness of trauma experiences to practitioners who offer specialist trauma-specific intervention. Not one of the principles articulated so far about trauma-informed practice demonstrates the need to listen for the unique narratives of individual victims/survivors, not necessarily about the trauma itself, but about the way in which their lives have unfolded as a result of their experiences. Nor is there a principle that argues the case for staff to not treat individual service users as having an equivalent experience if they identify that they have experienced interpersonal trauma. This can be an orientation that emphasizes greater curiosity and openness to ways in which service users express their need for support.

Trauma-informed practice principles do not have the mechanism to integrate with other frameworks and approaches

Trauma-informed practice approaches do not exist in a paradigm vacuum. It is not as if organizations which attend to disadvantage and poverty should take up trauma-informed approaches to the exclusion of theories about how capitalist structures create social conditions in which the working class are exploited by those with greater financial resources. Or that domestic and family violence services would suddenly jettison their beliefs about the gendered nature of society as it contributes to violence against women and children solely in favour of trauma-informed perspectives. It is not meant to be an 'either/or' but more an 'and'. Indeed, the shared principles that underpin trauma-informed and many other approaches to practice should aid integration.

However, the biggest challenge of the trauma-informed movement is its failure to recognize that there is a need to bring together its trauma knowledge and commitment to improve the experience of trauma victims/survivors with the underlying understandings that organizations are forged with as they start and then continue to adhere to as they transform their philosophical drivers into forms of service delivery.

It is not just a practical application of a way of working that is required but a theoretical exercise that aims to create practice frameworks that are embracing of multiple tenets. It is also a process of capturing the hearts and minds of organizations and their staff who may perceive the introduction of another paradigm as adding yet another layer of complexity or impost on the way they can do their work. It is not surprising that such integration is not adequately explored. It requires that trauma knowledge and other key frames of reference be separated into their core aspects before then being re-assembled in ways that allow for merged forms of conceptualizing to evolve.

The specialist trauma field itself has long been the purview of a pluralist assembly of therapists, theoreticians and researchers who have individually and collectively worked to harness emerging neuroscience, research and evidence about treatment, the cultural wisdom of First Nations peoples around the world, knowledges held by those with lived and living experience and, at times, a reintroduction of older approaches that may have lost their cache. Yet, the emphasis of such work has been the focus on how to support individuals, families and communities to recover and heal. It has been a narrative about how pain and distress can be transformed so that individual suffering can be alleviated. The neuroscience has been a remarkable and powerfully influential story that has enabled trauma to be identified as a real-world problem that creates ongoing difficulties for individuals, groups and communities and ultimately a cost borne by society as a whole. The literature about trauma treatment – what works, how it should be sequenced, what it should involve, how healing occurs – has led to a proliferation of models. The call to prove the effectiveness of any of these interventions is part and parcel of this discourse.

But all of this works against the trauma-informed movement. It makes it harder and harder to keep up with the changing nature of the literature. It privileges treatments that are able to have research funds associated with it. It reasserts the view that experimental design evidence in the form of randomized control studies is preferred. It gives less credence to indigenous ways of understanding and healing trauma than western approaches. It keeps knowledge competing for credibility.

The move beyond trauma-informed practice

Competition about the value of different knowledge frames holds little benefit for victims and survivors. As already noted, the separation of trauma specific and trauma informed is an artificial divide that limits the potential for this knowledge to resource the change that victims and survivors need for their lives. It is only one of the limitations identified in this chapter about trauma-informed practice. After 20 years and a proliferation of applications of the construct, there is an opportunity to reconsider the evolution of the broader trauma knowledge paradigm and how it is interpreted in practice. This book emanates from considering what may not be possible by continuing with trauma-informed practice as it has been conceptualized so far.

The authors of the chapters in this book have a rich history of writing about trauma-related issues in their careers. Some are experts in trauma treatment. Some are researchers who have looked into safety, meaning making and the nature of relational love and attachment. They are part of a group of key influencers in the practice of support and intervention with people who have experienced trauma in their lives. They are bound together in this book because of their shared interest and commitment to alleviating human suffering, in particular when it has been caused by another person through interpersonal violation.

Each chapter offers an exploration about what is important to them. There are theoretical insights. There are research-led perspectives. There are personal amalgamations of work undertaken over decades. At the end of each, there is a reflection provided by the editors about the themes that are relevant to the task of disassembling into their aggregate parts some of the key ideas that are worth considering in resourcing the next evolution of the trauma-informed practice movement.

It as this point that, as editors, we emerge from behind the curtain of our third-person narrative to invite you to join us in our re-examination of trauma knowledge in an endeavour that adopts the metaphor of *pickling* as the simultaneous act of preserving and modifying original flavors into a new taste altogether – a framework that practitioners and organizations can use to transform the lived and living experience of trauma in ways that help victims and survivors to have their pain acknowledged, believed and understood, connecting them to safe and restorative relationships which support their meaning making and, ultimately, their healing.

Our intention is to build out more deeply the construct of *trauma-transformative practice* as a much-needed evolution beyond trauma-informed practice. We believe that the current foundations of trauma-informed practice fail to capture the richness of knowledge that sits in and around the domains that reflect on trauma research and interpersonal neuroscience, the historical and continuing experiences of First Nations peoples, the understandings offered by victims and survivors of violence, the insights from practitioners working with human suffering and pain, and an ongoing analysis of the impact of societal power and oppression. The nature of this effort embraces complexity at its core. It holds multiple perspectives at once, allowing each its own influence while seeking to appreciate different understandings that emerge from their interaction. It is this process that pushes practice forward and allows us to refine and improve.

Through proposing and defining trauma-transformative practice, our hope is to offer a new and reassembled configuration of knowledge that truly realizes the transformational potential of the trauma-informed movement that started over two decades ago with the humble inspiration of Harris and Fallot (2001a).

References

Addis, S., Brierley-Sollis, T., Jones, V. and Hughes, C. (2022). *'Trauma-informed': Identifying key language and terminology through a review of the literature.* Cardiff, ACE Support Hub, Public Health Wales, Wrexham Glyndwr University.

Arledge, E. and Wolfson, R. (2001). Care of the Clinician. In M. Harris and R.D. Fallot (eds), *Using Trauma Theory to Design Service Systems* (pp.91–98). San Francisco, CA: Jossey-Bass/Wiley.

Australian Centre for Posttraumatic Mental Health and Parenting Research Centre (2013). *Approaches targeting outcomes for children exposed to trauma arising from abuse and neglect – Evidence, practice and implications.* Report prepared for the Australian Government Department of Families, Housing, Community Services and Indigenous Affairs. Canberra, Australian Centre for Posttraumatic Mental Health and Parenting Research Centre.

Avery, J.C., Morris, H., Galvin, E., Misso, M., Savaglio, M. and Skouteris, H. (2021). Systematic review of school-wide trauma-informed approaches. *Journal of Child & Adolescent Trauma,* 14(3), 381–397.

Bailey, C., Klas, A., Cox, R., Bergmeier, H., Avery, J. and Skouteris, H. (2019). Systematic review of organization-wide, trauma-informed care models in out-of-home care settings. *Health and Social Care in the Community,* 27(3), e10–e22.

Bargeman, M., Smith, S. and Wekerle, C. (2021). Trauma-informed care as a rights-based 'standard of care': A critical review. *Child Abuse and Neglect*, 119, 104762.

Bartlett, J.D., Barto, B., Griffin, J.L., Fraser, J.G., Hodgdon, H. and Bodian, R. (2016). Trauma-informed care in the Massachusetts Child Trauma Project. *Child Maltreatment*, 21(2), 101–112.

Bebout, R.R. (2001). Trauma Informed Approaches to Housing. In M. Harris and R.D. Fallot (eds), *Using Trauma Theory to Design Service Systems* (pp.47–56). San Francisco, CA: Jossey-Bass/Wiley.

Becker-Blease, K.A. (2017). As the world becomes trauma-informed, work to do. *Journal of Trauma and Dissociation*, 18(2), 131–138.

Benjamin, R. (2019). Introduction. In R. Benjamin, J. Haliburn and S. King (eds), *Humanising Mental Health Care in Australia: A Guide to Trauma-informed Approaches* (pp.xxvi–xlii). London: Routledge.

Berliner, L. and Kolko, D.J. (2016). Trauma informed care: A commentary and critique. *Child Maltreatment*, 21(2), 168–172.

Bloom, S. (2016). Advancing a national cradle-to-grave-to cradle public health agenda. *Journal of Trauma and Dissociation*, 17(4), 383–396.

Bloom, S. (2019). Trauma Theory. In R. Benjamin and J. Haliburn (eds), *Humanising Mental Health Care in Australia* (pp.3–31). New York, NY: Routledge.

Bonner, G., Lowe, T., Rawcliffe, D. and Wellman, N. (2002). Trauma for all: A pilot study of the subjective experience of physical restraint for mental health inpatients and staff in the UK. *Journal of Psychiatric and Mental Health Nursing*, 9(4), 465–473.

Brend, D.M. and Sprang, G. (2020). Trauma-informed care in child welfare: An imperative for residential childcare workers. *International Journal of Child and Adolescent Resilience*, 7(1), 154–165.

Brummer, J. (2022). *Building a Trauma-informed Restorative School*. London: Jessica Kingsley Publishers.

Burge, R., Tickle, A. and Moghaddam, N. (2021). Evaluating trauma informed care training for services supporting individuals experiencing homelessness and multiple disadvantage. *Housing, Care and Support*, 24(1), 14–25.

Caffrey, K.N. and Winton, T. (2022). *Trauma informed care: A multi-modal intervention strategy and effects on staff attitudes toward trauma sensitivity* (NGR6912C project IV report). Miami, Florida State University.

Carter, P. and Blanch, A. (2019). A trauma lens for systems change. *Stanford Social Innovation Review*, 17(3), 48–54.

Chafouleas, S.M., Johnson, A.H., Overstreet, S. and Santos, N.M. (2016). Toward a blueprint for trauma-informed service delivery in schools. *School Mental Health*, 8(1), 144–162.

Champine, R.B., Hoffman, E.E., Matlin, S.L., Strambler, M.J. and Tebes, J.K. (2022). 'What does it mean to be trauma-informed?': A mixed-methods study of a trauma-informed community initiative. *Journal of Child and Family Studies*, 31(2), 459–472.

Child USA (2020). *Delayed Disclosure: A factsheet based on Cutting Edge Research on Child Sexual Abuse*. Philadelphia, PA: Child USA.

Clark, M. (2015). Co-production in mental health care. *Mental Health Review Journal*, 20(4), 213–219.

Collings, S., Wright, A.C., McLean, L. and Buratti, S. (2022). Trauma-informed family contact practice for children in out-of-home care. *The British Journal of Social Work*, 52(4), 1837–1858.

Covington, S.S. (2008). Women and addiction: A trauma-informed approach. *Journal of Psychoactive Drugs*, 40, 377–385.

Creamer, S., Blair, S., Toombs, M. and Brolan, C.E. (2022). Indigenous services leading the way for Aboriginal and Torres Strait Islander children in out-of-home care. *Social Work Education*, 1–25.

Crosby, S.D. (2016). Trauma-informed approaches to juvenile justice: A critical race perspective. *Juvenile and Family Court Journal*, 67(1), 5–18.

Crosby, S.D., Howell, P. and Thomas, S. (2018). Social justice education through trauma-informed teaching. *Middle School Journal*, 49(4), 15–23 de la Sablonnière-Griffin, M., Collin-Vézina, D., Esposito, T. and Dion, J. (2023). A longitudinal study to better understand child protection intervention for First Nations children. *First Peoples Child and Family Review*, 18(1), 97–120.

Department of Families, Fairness and Housing (2022). *Framework for Trauma-informed Practice. Supporting Children, Young People and Families*. Melbourne: Victorian Government.

Donisch, K., Bray, C. and Gewirtz, A. (2016). Child welfare, juvenile justice, mental health, and education providers' conceptualisations of trauma-informed practice. *Child Maltreatment*, 21(2), 125–134.

Douglas, K. (2022). Assimilation through Canadian Child Welfare Policy. *Social Work and Policy Studies: Social Justice, Practice and Theory*, 5(2), 52–64.

Elliott, D.E., Bjelajac, P., Fallot, R.D., Markoff, L.S. and Reed, B.G. (2005). Trauma-informed or trauma-denied: Principles and implementation of trauma-informed services for women. *Journal of Community Psychology*, 33(4), 461–477.

Evans, C. and Graves, K. (2018). Trauma among children and legal implications. *Cogent Social Sciences*, 4(1), 1546791.

Ewijk, H.V. (2018). *Complexity and Social Work*. London: Routledge.

Fallot, R.D. and Harris, M. (2001). A Trauma Informed Approach to Screening and Assessment. In M. Harris, and R.D. Fallot (eds), *Using Trauma Theory to Design Service Systems* (pp.23–32). San Francisco, CA: Jossey-Bass/Wiley.

Fassin, D. and Rechtman, R. (2009). *The Empire of Trauma: An Inquiry into the Condition of Victimhood*. Princeton, NJ: Princeton University Press.

Flavin, L., Hammoud-Milad, M., Labinger, K., Wimberger, N., Stork, C. and Hansen, H. (2022). Using principles of trauma-informed care to address structural racism in psychiatric care. *American Journal of Psychiatry*, 179(2), 94–97.

Fondren, K., Lawson, M., Speidel, R., McDonnell, C.G. and Valentino, K. (2020). Buffering the effects of childhood trauma within the school setting: A systematic review of trauma-informed and trauma-responsive interventions among trauma-affected youth. *Children and Youth Services Review*, 109, 104691.

Freeman, D.W. (2001). Trauma Informed Services and Case Management. In M. Harris, and R.D. Fallot (eds), *Using Trauma Theory to Design Service Systems* (pp.75–82). San Francisco, CA: Jossey-Bass/Wiley.

Gómez, J., Lewis, J., Noll, K., Smidt, A. and Birrell, J. (2016). Shifting the focus: Nonpathologising approaches to healing from betrayal trauma through an emphasis on relational care. *Journal of Trauma and Dissociation*, 17(2), 165–185.

Gubi, A.A., Strait, J., Wycoff, K., Vega, V., Brauser, B. and Osman, Y. (2019). Trauma-informed knowledge and practices in school psychology: A pilot study and review. *Journal of Applied School Psychology*, 35(2), 176–199.

Hanson, R.F. and Lang, J. (2016). A critical look at trauma-informed care among agencies and systems serving maltreated youth and their families. *Child Maltreatment*, 21(2), 95–100.

Haysom, L. (2022). Raising the minimum age of criminal responsibility to 14 years. *Journal of Paediatrics and Child Health*, 58(9), 1504–1507.

Harris, M. and Fallot, R.D. (2001a). Envisioning a Trauma Informed Service System: A Vital Paradigm Shift. In M. Harris and R.D. Fallot (eds), *Using Trauma Theory to Design Service Systems* (pp.3–22). San Francisco, CA: Jossey-Bass/Wiley.

Harris, M. and Fallot, R.D. (2001b). Trauma Informed Inpatient Services. In M. Harris and R.D. Fallot (eds), *Using Trauma Theory to Design Service Systems* (pp.33–46). San Francisco, CA: Jossey-Bass/Wiley.

Harris, M. and Fallot, R.D. (2001c). Designing Trauma Informed Addiction Services. In M. Harris, and R.D. Fallot (eds), *Using Trauma Theory to Design Service Systems* (pp.57–74). San Francisco, CA: Jossey-Bass/Wiley.

Hocken, K., Taylor, J. and Watson, J. (2022). Trauma and the Experience of Imprisonment. In P. Willmot and L. Jones (eds), *Trauma-Informed Forensic Practice* (pp. 298–315). London: Routledge.

Holland, L., Smirnov, A., Hickman, A., Toombs, M. and Reid, N. (2022). Examining incarceration rates of Aboriginal and Torres Strait Islander children. *The Lancet Child and Adolescent Health*, 6(9), 599–600.

Hopper, E., Bassuk, E. and Olivet, J. (2007). *Shelter from the Storm: Creating Trauma-informed Homeless Services*. Washington DC: Department of Health and Human Services (US).

Houck, E.J. and Dracobly, J.D. (2022). Trauma-informed care for individuals with intellectual and developmental disabilities: From disparity to policies for effective action. *Perspectives on Behaviour Science*, 1–21.

Howard, J.A. (2022). *Trauma Aware Education – Essential Information and Guidance for Educators, Education Sites and Education Systems*. Samford Valley, Queensland: Australian Academic Press.

Jennings, A. (2004). *Blueprint for Action: Building Trauma-informed Mental Health Service Systems*. Washington, DC: National Association of State Mental Health Program Directors and the National Technical Assistance Center for State Mental Health Planning.

Jones, L. (2022). Trauma Informed Risk Assessment and Intervention: Understanding the Role of Triggering Contexts and Offence-Related Altered States of Consciousness. In P. Willmot and L. Jones (eds), *Trauma-Informed Forensic Practice* (pp.49–73). London: Routledge.

Jones, L. and Willmot, P. (2022). The Future of Trauma-Informed Forensic Practice. In P. Willmot and L. Jones (eds), *Trauma-Informed Forensic Practice* (pp.413–427). London: Routledge.

Joseph, S. and Murphy, D. (2014). Trauma: A unifying concept for social work. *British Journal of Social Work*, 44(5), 1094–1109.

Keesler, J.M. (2014). A call for the integration of trauma-informed care among intellectual and developmental disability organizations. *Journal of Policy and Practice in Intellectual Disabilities*, 11(1), 34–42.

Kim, I. and Ashmore, T. (2019). The Trauma-Informed Inpatient Facility. In R. Benjamin, J. Haliburn and S. King (eds), *Humanising Mental Health Care in Australia: A Guide to Trauma-informed Approaches* (pp.342–354). London: Routledge.

Khoo, E., Nygren, L. and Gümüscü, A. (2020). From needs to relationships to organizations: Transactional complexity in social work in the Swedish Social Services. *British Journal of Social Work*, 50, 2098–2115.

Knight, C. (2015). Trauma-informed social work practice: Practice considerations and challenges. *Clinical Social Work Journal*, 43(1), 25–37.

Lang, J.M., Campbell, K., Shanley, P., Crusto, C.A. and Connell, C.M. (2016). Building capacity for trauma-informed care in the child welfare system: Initial results of a statewide implementation. *Child Maltreatment*, 21(2), 113–124.

Lathan, E., Langhinrichsen-Rohling, J., Duncan, J. and Stefurak, J.T. (2019). The promise initiative: Promoting a trauma-informed police response to sexual assault in a mid-size Southern community. *Journal of Community Psychology*, 47(7), 1733–1749.

Levenson, J.S., Willis, G.M. and Prescott, D.S. (2016). Adverse childhood experiences in the lives of male sex offenders: Implications for trauma-informed care. *Sexual Abuse*, 28(4), 340–359.

Levenson, J.S. and Willis, G.M. (2019). Implementing trauma-informed care in correctional treatment and supervision. *Journal of Aggression, Maltreatment and Trauma*, 28(4), 481–501.

Longfellow, E. and Hicks, R. (2022). Trauma and Intellectual Disability. In P. Willmot and L. Jones (eds), *Trauma-Informed Forensic Practice* (pp.111–129). London: Routledge.

Maynard, B.R., Farina, A., Dell, N.A. and Kelly, M.S. (2019). Effects of trauma-informed approaches in schools: A systematic review. *Campbell Systematic Reviews*, 15, 1–2.

McConnico, N., Boynton-Jarrett, R., Bailey, C. and Nandi, M. (2016). A framework for trauma-sensitive schools. *Zero to Three*, 36(5), 36–44.

McGuire, F., Carlisle, J. and Clark, F. (2022). Trauma Informed Care in Secure Psychiatric Hospitals. In P. Willmot and L. Jones (eds), *Trauma-Informed Forensic Practice* (pp.348–362). London: Routledge.

McHugo, G.J., Caspi, Y., Kammerer, N., Mazelis, R., Jackson, E. *et al.* (2005). The assessment of trauma history in women with co-occurring substance abuse and mental disorders and a history of interpersonal violence. *The Journal of Behavioural Health Services and Research*, 32, 113–127.

McLindon, E. and Harms, L. (2011). Listening to mental health workers' experiences: Factors influencing their work with women who disclose sexual assault. *International Journal of Mental Health Nursing*, 20(1), 2–11.

Miller, J. and Berger, E. (2020). A review of school trauma-informed practice for Aboriginal and Torres Strait Islander children and youth. *The Educational and Developmental Psychologist*, 37(1), 39–46.

Missouri Department of Mental Health and Partners (2014). *Missouri Model: A Developmental Framework for Trauma Informed Approaches*. Jefferson City, MO: Missouri Department of Mental Health.

Mitchell, J., McPherson, L. and Gatwiri, K. (2020). 'Support and Love and All that Stuff'; Evidence of Impact in the Treatment and Care for Kids Program. In J. Mitchell, J. Tucci and E. Tronick (eds), *The Handbook of Therapeutic Care for Children: Evidence Informed Approaches to Working with Traumatised Children and Adolescents in Foster, Kinship and Adoptive Care* (pp.109–136). London: Jessica Kingsley Publishers.

Mitchell, J., Tucci, J. and Macnamara, N. (2020). What Are the Key Elements of Therapeutic Care? In J. Mitchell, J. Tucci and E. Tronick (eds), *The Handbook of Therapeutic Care for Children: Evidence-Informed Approaches to Working with Traumatised Children and Adolescents in Foster, Kinship and Adoptive Care* (pp.35–58). London, Jessica Kingsley Publishers.

Mitleton-Kelly, E. (2002). Ten Principles of Complexity and Enabling Infrastructures. In E. Mitleton-Kelly (ed.), *Complex Systems and Evolutionary Perspectives of Organizations: The Application of Complexity Theory to Organizations* (pp.25–50). Oxford: Pergamon.

Moore, E. (2022). Trauma and Restorative Justice. In P. Willmot and L. Jones (eds), *Trauma-Informed Forensic Practice* (pp.396–412). London: Routledge.

Muskett, C. (2014). Trauma-informed care in inpatient mental health settings: A review of the literature. *International Journal of Mental Health Nursing*, 23(1), 51–59.

Myles, E. (2022). The over-representation of Aboriginals in Canadian correctional facilities. *Contemporary Issues in Global Criminal Justice*, 219.

Noether, C.D., Finkelstein, N., VanDeMark, N.R., Savage, A., Reed, B.G. and Moses, D.J. (2005). Design strengths and issues of SAMHSA's women, co-occurring disorders, and violence study. *Psychiatric Services*, 56(10), 1233–1236.

Office for Health Improvement and Disparities. (2022). *Working Definition of Trauma Informed Practice*. London: United Kingdom Government.

Perkins, E., Prosser, H., Riley, D. and Whittington, R. (2012). Physical restraint in a therapeutic setting; a necessary evil? *International Journal of Law and Psychiatry*, 35(1), 43–49.

Perry, D.L. and Daniels, M.L. (2016). Implementing trauma-informed practices in the school setting: A pilot study. *School Mental Health*, 8(1), 177–188.

Piedfort-Marin, O. (2022). The need of clear concepts. *European Journal of Trauma and Dissociation*, 6(4), 100302.

Prescott, L. (2001). Defining the Role of Consumer-Survivors in Trauma Informed Systems. In M. Harris, and R.D. Fallot (eds), *Using Trauma Theory to Design Service Systems* (pp.83–90). San Francisco, CA: Jossey-Bass/Wiley.

Pride, T., Lam, A., Swansburg, J., Seno, M. *et al.* (2021). Trauma-informed approaches to substance use interventions with indigenous peoples: A scoping review. *Journal of Psychoactive Drugs*, 53(5), 460–473.

Pynoos, R.S., Fairbank, J.A., Steinberg, A.M., Amaya-Jackson, L. *et al.* (2008). The National Child Traumatic Stress Network: Collaborating to improve the standard of care. *Professional Psychology: Research and Practice*, 39(4), 389.

Quadara, A. and Hunter, C. (2016). *Principles of Trauma-Informed Approaches to Child Sexual Abuse* (discussion paper). Canberra, Royal Commission into Institutional Responses to Child Sexual Abuse and Australian Institute of Family Studies.

Quinn, A., Fallon, B., Joh-Carnella, N. and Saint-Girons, M. (2022). The overrepresentation of First Nations children in the Ontario child welfare system: A call for systemic change. *Children and Youth Services Review*, 139, 106558.

Rittel, H.W.J. and Webber, M.M. (1973). Dilemmas in a general theory of planning. *Policy Sciences*, 4(2), 155–169.

Rosenthal, M.N., Reinhardt, K.M. and Birrell, P.J. (2016). Guest editorial: Deconstructing disorder: An ordered reaction to a disordered environment. *Journal of Trauma and Dissociation*, 17(2), 131–137.

Royal Commission into Institutional Responses to Child Sexual Abuse. (2017). *Final Report – Identifying and Disclosing Child Sexual Abuse, Volume 4*. Canberra: Commonwealth Government of Australia.

Rozzell, L. (2013). *The Role of Family Engagement in Creating Trauma-informed Juvenile Justice Systems*. Los Angeles, CA: National Center for Child Traumatic Stress.

Rushdie, S. (2008). *Midnight's Children: A Novel*. Toronto: Vintage Canada.

Silvester, N. (2022). Developing Trauma-Informed Youth Justice Services. In P. Willmot and L. Jones (eds), *Trauma-Informed Forensic Practice* (pp.333–347). London: Routledge.

Skinner-Osei, P. and Levenson, J.S. (2018). Trauma-informed services for children with incarcerated parents. *Journal of Family Social Work*, 21(4–5), 421–437.

Steckley, L. (2010). Containment and holding environments: Understanding and reducing physical restraint in residential child care. *Children and Youth Services Review*, 32(1), 120–128.

Substance Abuse and Mental Health Services Administration (SAMHSA) (2014). *Trauma-informed Care in Behavioural Health Services – Treatment Improvement Protocol (TIP) Series 57* (HHS Publication no. (SMA 13-4801).

Sullivan, K.M., Murray, K.J. and Ake III, G.S. (2016). Trauma-informed care for children in the child welfare system: An initial evaluation of a trauma-informed parenting workshop. *Child Maltreatment*, 21(2), 147–155.

Sweeney, A., Clement, S., Filson, B. and Kennedy, A. (2016). Trauma-informed mental healthcare in the UK: what is it and how can we further its development? *Mental Health Review Journal*, 21(3), 174–192.

Sweeney, A., Filson, B., Kennedy, A., Collinson, L. and Gillard, S. (2018). A paradigm shift: Relationships in trauma-informed mental health services. *British Journal of Psychiatric Advances*, 24(5), 319–333.

Sweeney, A. and Taggart, D. (2018). (Mis) understanding trauma-informed approaches in mental health. *Journal of Mental Health*, 27(5), 383–387.

Thomas, M.S., Crosby, S. and Vanderhaar, J. (2019). Trauma-informed practices in schools across two decades: An interdisciplinary review of research. *Review of Research in Education*, 43(1), 422–452.

Thompson, L.J. and West, D. (2013). Professional development in the contemporary educational context: Encouraging practice wisdom. *Social Work Education*, 32(1), 118–133.

Trieschman, A., Whittaker, J. and Brendtro, L. (2002). *The Other 23 Hours: Child-care Work with Emotionally Disturbed Children in a Therapeutic Milieu*. New York, NY: Transaction Publishers.

Tucci, J. (2016). What comes after trauma-informed practice? *Prosody*, https://professionals.childhood.org.au/prosody/2016/12/what-next. Accessed 19 July 2023.

Tucci, J. and Blom M. (2019). 'These were terrible years. no love or kindness, no safety or warmth'. Reflections on the outcomes of the Royal Commission into Institutional Responses to Child Sexual Abuse in Australia. *Journal of Trauma and Dissociation*, 20, 373–377.

Tucci, J., Goddard, C. and Mitchell, J. (2001). *More Action – Less Talk: Community Responses to Child Abuse Prevention*. Child Abuse and Family Violence Research Unit, Monash University and Australians Against Child Abuse.

Tucci, J. and Mitchell, J. (2019a). *Making SPACE for Learning*. Melbourne: Australian Childhood Foundation.

Tucci, J. and Mitchell, J. (2019b). Therapeutic Services for Traumatised Children and Young People Healing. In R. Benjamin, J. Haliburn and S. King (eds), *Humanising Mental Health Care in Australia: A Guide to Trauma-informed Approaches* (pp.319–320). London: Routledge.

Tucci, J. and Mitchell, J. (2021). *Still Unseen and Ignored: Tracking Community Knowledge and Attitudes about Child Abuse and Child Protection in Australia*. Melbourne: Australian Childhood Foundation.

Tucci, J. and Mitchell, J. (2022). Still unseen and ignored: Tracking community knowledge and attitudes about child abuse and child protection in Australia. *Frontiers in Psychology*, 4226.

Tucci, J., Mitchell, J. and Goddard, C. (2003). *Tolerating Violence Towards Children – Community Attitudes about Child Abuse and Child Protection*. Child Abuse and Family Violence Research Unit, Monash University and Australian Childhood Foundation.

Tucci, J., Mitchell, J. and Goddard, C. (2006). *Out of Sight, Out of Mind: Tracking Australian Community Attitudes about Child Abuse and Child Protection*. Melbourne: Australian Childhood Foundation and the National Research Centre for the Prevention of Child Abuse.

Tucci, J., Mitchell, J. and Goddard, C. (2010). *Doing Nothing Hurts Children: Community Attitudes about Child Abuse and Child Protection in Australia*. Melbourne: Australian Childhood Foundation and Child Abuse Prevention Research.

Tucci, J., Mitchell, J. and Tronick, E. (2020). The Need for a New Paradigm in the Care and Support of Children in Foster, Kinship and Adoptive Care. In J. Mitchell, J. Tucci and E. Tronick (eds), *The Handbook of Therapeutic Care for Children: Evidence-Informed Approaches to Working with Traumatised Children and Adolescents in Foster, Kinship and Adoptive Care* (pp.21–34). London: Jessica Kingsley Publishers.

Turnbull-Roberts, V., Salter, M. and Newton, B.J. (2022). Trauma then and now: Implications of adoption reform for First Nations children. *Child and Family Social Work*, 27(2), 163–172.

Webb, S.A. (2006) *Social Work in a Risk Society*. Basingstoke: Palgrave Macmillan.

Welsh Government (2022). *Trauma Informed Wales: A Societal Approach to Understanding, Preventing and Supporting the Impacts of Trauma and Adversity*. Cardiff: Traumatic Stress Wales.

Whittemore, R. and Knafl, K. (2005). The integrative review: Updated methodology. *Journal of Advanced Nursing*, 52(5), 546–553.

Yatchmenoff, D.K., Sundborg, S.A. and Davis, M.A. (2017). Implementing trauma-informed care: Recommendations on the process. *Advances in Social Work*, 18(1), 167–185.

CHAPTER 2

Polyvagal Theory: The Neuroscience of Safety in Trauma-Informed Practice

Stephen W. Porges, PhD

Introduction

Contemporary strategies for treating trauma often fail our biological needs by not acknowledging that feelings of threat and safety emerge from inside the body. This chapter focuses on feelings of safety, an elusive construct that has historically been dependent on subjectivity. Although neuroscience has established the impact of threat on the nervous system with consequential degrading impact on mental and physical health, research on the neurobiology of safety has been minimal. This chapter proposes and documents that feelings of safety have a measurable underlying neurophysiological substrate in the state of the autonomic nervous system. Acknowledging that feelings of safety are an emergent property of the autonomic state would shift investigations of feelings of safety from a subjective to an objective science and lead to a focus on feelings of safety in trauma-informed treatment strategies.

Humans, as social mammals, are on an enduring lifelong quest to feel safe and to spontaneously engage and co-regulate their behaviour and physiology with others. This quest appears to be embedded in our DNA and serves as a profound motivator throughout our life. The need to feel safe is functionally our body speaking through our autonomic nervous system – influencing our mental and physical health, social relationships, cognitive processes and behavioural repertoire, and serving as a neurophysiological substrate on which societal institutions dependent on cooperation and trust function are based. Operationally, feeling safe is our subjective interpretation of internal bodily feelings that are being conveyed via bidirectional neural pathways between our bodily organs and our brain. Feelings of safety are not equivalent to an objective measurement of safety, which may pragmatically be defined as the removal of threat. Feeling safe is more akin to a felt sense as described by Eugene Gendlin (2018). Although Gendlin, as a philosopher and psychologist, was not physiologically oriented, he described a 'felt sense' not as a mental experience, but as a physical one.

In understanding the motivation to feel safe, feelings of safety may be conceptualized from Polyvagal Theory. Polyvagal Theory provides an innovative scientific perspective that incorporates an understanding of phylogenetic shifts in vertebrate neuroanatomy and neurophysiology; this perspective identifies neural circuits that downregulate neural regulation of threat reactions and functionally neutralize defensive strategies via neural circuits communicating cues of safety. Feelings of safety are operationally the product of cues of safety, via neuroception (see below), downregulating autonomic states that support threat reactions and upregulating autonomic states that support interpersonal accessibility and homeostatic functions. Basically, when humans feel safe, their nervous systems support the homeostatic functions of health, growth and restoration, while they simultaneously become accessible to others without feeling or expressing threat and vulnerability.

In explaining the profound importance of feeling safe, we are immersed in the ambiguity of our language when it comes to describing feelings and linking feelings to underlying neurophysiological states. This problem dates to the earliest psychologists such as Wundt (Wundt and Judd, 1902), who adopted and standardized introspection techniques to explore sensations, which were essentially limited to external stimuli. Polyvagal Theory leads towards a hierarchical conceptualization of feelings as higher brain interpretations of the neural signals conveying information regarding visceral organs (heart, gut, etc.) to the brainstem. This psychophysiological perspective emphasizes the foundational function of autonomic state in the subjective experiences of global feelings and specific emotions. Within this hierarchical conceptualization, feelings of safety are pre-eminent and form the core of an enduring motivational system that shifts autonomic state, which in turn drives behaviours, emotions and thoughts. The resulting model suggests that feelings of safety reflect the foundational autonomic state, supporting maturation, health and sociality. From a clinical perspective, feelings of safety are the objective of trauma-informed therapy.

In an earlier paper (Porges, 1996), a hierarchical model of self-regulation was proposed to provide insights into optimizing intervention strategies for high-risk infants. The model reflects maturational competencies in neural regulation that provide a substrate for the more complex co-regulatory social behaviours. The main point of the model is that higher behavioural functions, which are frequently intentional, are dependent on the functioning of the more survival-focused foundational systems embedded in the brainstem. The levels are described in Table 2.1 and emphasize the hierarchical nature of specific autonomic states and accessibility of behaviours that we cluster as self-regulation skills. The optimal function of each level is contingent on each of the preceding levels being adequately functioning. Observers of developing children are aware of the strong maturational influence that pushes the child through the sequence. However, few are aware of the parallels between development and evolution and how this information informs us regarding the adaptive functions of specific autonomic states. It is not that a specific autonomic state is good or bad, but rather what adaptive functions ancestral vertebrates accessed while being in a specific autonomic state.

Table 2.1: Hierarchical model of self-regulation (Porges, 1996)

Level I: Neurophysiological processes characterized by bidirectional communication between the brainstem and peripheral organs to maintain physiological homeostasis.
Level II: Physiological processes reflecting the input of higher nervous system influences on the brainstem regulation of homeostasis. These processes are associated with modulating metabolic output and energy resources to support adaptive responses to environmental demands.
Level III: Measurable and often observable motor processes, including body movements and facial expressions. These processes can be evaluated in terms of quantity, quality and appropriateness.
Level IV: Processes that reflect the coordination of motor behaviour, emotional tone and bodily state to successfully negotiate social interactions. Unlike those of Level III, these processes are contingent on prioritized cues and feedback from the external environment.

Dissolution

Consistent with Polyvagal Theory (Porges, 2021a, 2021b), the sequencing of the hierarchy of neural maturation mirrors features of vertebrate evolution. The theory emphasizes the modifications in the neural regulation of the autonomic nervous system that are highlighted through phylogenetic transitions, especially the transition from asocial reptiles to the sociality and co-regulation features of social mammals. Operationally defining feelings of safety as dependent on an autonomic state provides an opportunity to study the potential emergent properties that are dependent on access to this state. Thus, it is proposed that the consequence of feeling safe provides the neural platform for cooperative behaviours, both supporting physiological systems and enabling accessibility to higher brain structures for learning, creativity, appreciation of aesthetics, and even spirituality.

An acknowledgement of this hierarchy results in questions about the sequential unfolding of responses to challenges orienting within the body (e.g. fever and illness) and outside the body (e.g. threat). Disease and injury to the brain have been observed to disinhibit phylogenetically more ancient evolutionary structures, which in the healthy individual are regulated (e.g. inhibited) by newer brain structures. This was described by John Hughlings

Jackson (1884), who stated that 'the higher nervous arrangements inhibit (or control) the lower, and thus, when the higher are suddenly rendered functionless, the lower rise in activity'. Jackson labelled this process 'dissolution' to emphasize that it is evolution in reverse.

While Jackson emphasized a dissolution process that mirrors the reverse of evolution in brain structures (i.e. moving from neocortex to lower brain structures), Polyvagal Theory emphasizes the reverse of evolution in the neural structures and pathways that regulate the mammalian autonomic nervous system. In this hierarchy of adaptive responses, the newest social engagement circuit is used first; if that circuit fails to provide safety, the older circuits are recruited sequentially. The elements of the social engagement system are functional at birth in the full-term infant (see Porges and Furman, 2011) and serve to enable infant and mother to co-regulate autonomic states via reciprocal cues of safety. The product of this co-regulation is the optimization of homeostatic functions, enabling the infant to mature and the mother to recover from the metabolically demanding delivery process. Early in life, this co-regulation provides the neurophysiological platform for mother-infant interactions and attachment (Bowlby, 1988), and the establishment of social bonds, which can be conceptualized as being dependent on associations with feelings of safety.

Autonomic state as an intervening variable

By placing autonomic state at the core of feelings of safety or threat, the pragmatic survival behaviours of fight and flight, as well as complex problem-solving strategies that would lead to escape, are consequential and dependent on the facilitatory function of the autonomic nervous system in optimizing these strategies. Similarly, turning off threat reactions and calming autonomic state, via the ventral cardioinhibitory vagal pathway, will promote interpersonal accessibility, while simultaneously supporting the co-regulation of the autonomic state. This model positions autonomic state as an intervening variable mediating the interpretation of contextual cues and shaping our reactions. Within this conceptualization, depending on the individual's autonomic state, the same contextual cues and challenges may result in different behavioural, cognitive and physiological reactions. For example, recent research documents that indices of autonomic state influenced: the impact the pandemic had on mental health (see Kolacz et al., 2020), perceived stress in college students (Fanning et al., 2020), effectiveness of neurostimulation on abdominal pain (Kovacic et al., 2020), calming behaviour in infants following the still face procedure (Kolacz et al., 2022), and protest behaviours in infants in daycare settings (Ahnert et al., 2021). This would be true both within and between individuals (see Porges et al., 2013). Thus, there may be a range of reactions among individuals who share the same environmental context, but who are in different autonomic states. In addition, the same individual may also have a range of reacting to repeated exposures to the same environmental context that would be mediated by variations in autonomic state. Post-traumatic stress disorder (PTSD) symptoms may be the product of a retuned autonomic nervous system following extreme and/or repeated exposures to threat. Research supports the conceptualization that the mental and physical health consequences of adversity are reflected in a retuned autonomic nervous system locked into states of defence that limit access to the calming pathways through the ventral vagus associated with sociality (Kolacz *et al.*, 2020; Williamson *et al.*, 2013, 2015).

Acknowledging the important role of autonomic state as an intervening variable would have profound consequences on our understanding of behaviour and clinical symptoms of individuals who have survived severe trauma. From a therapist's perspective, the 'intervening' role of autonomic state can be objectified as a determinant of being accessible to therapy and influencing outcome. Often, survivors have been confronted with therapists, colleagues, friends and family who have assumed that intentionality was a major contributor to their asociality and clinical symptoms. In fact, many well-intentioned supporters may have expressed the faulty assumption that a trauma survivor's behaviour was intentional and could be reliably modified by rewards and punishments. During the past decade, trauma-informed therapies have incorporated a somatic orientation that respects the powerful influence that bodily states can have in resisting intentional behaviours and insights. The work of Bessel van der Kolk (2015) highlights the acceptance of this trend.

A polyvagal-informed therapy would emphasize that our cognitive intent and our bodily state can promote competing behavioural outcomes. As an observer of both behaviour and autonomic state, my bet is on the potency of autonomic state. This conclusion is supported by the link between autonomic state and feelings of threat and our embedded biobehavioural programme to survive. Since these states of defence are regulated by primitive neural circuits – circuits which are shared with more ancient vertebrates – intentional self-regulation efforts originating in the cortex are frequently ineffective in downregulating survival-driven reactions to threat, which are dependent on lower brain structures. The survival programme is evolutionarily old, while the programme that turns off threat reactions with cues of safety to promote calmness, sociality and homeostatic functions is a mammalian innovation of a repurposed autonomic nervous system that may be influenced by higher brain structures. Although the calming system is effective in downregulating threat reactions in response to mild threats and effectively enabling feelings of safety, the calming system is difficult to access when the defensive systems are in a highly activated survival mode.

Functionally, we need to conceptualize the model as having both bottom-up and top-down pathways, with the bottom-up pathways being a combination of being both reflexive and derivative of early evolutionary survival processes. The foundational are functionally hardwired via 'neuroception' (see below). Thus, although cues of safety or threat will trigger top-down reflexive changes in autonomic state, the states become associated with thoughts and behaviours. This process is initiated through interoception and then bottom-up feelings of autonomic state are interpreted by higher brain structures, which in turn may initiate intentional behaviours. Interoception is the perception of sensations from inside the body and includes the perception of physical sensations related to internal organ function such as heart beat, respiration, satiety and needs to urinate and defecate. This link between feelings (i.e. autonomic state) and behaviours and thoughts forms the neurophysiological basis for aspects of associative learning.

The premise of many trauma-informed therapeutic strategies is to separate the feelings from the associative thoughts and behaviours. Strategies that are polyvagal-informed focus on enabling the client to experience the feelings without linking the feelings to thoughts or behaviours (see Dana, 2018; Porges and Dana, 2018). Basically, the client learns that the feelings are not intentional or under voluntary control but are part of an adaptive reflexive system that is wired into our nervous system. Thus, although attributes of the sequence are initially reflexive, there are effective portals to modify the association. For example, acknowledging the hierarchy of organization of the autonomic nervous system would suggest that the introduction of cues of safety would be a functional antidote to threat reactions by reducing the associative links between feelings of threat and thoughts and actions.

These speculations are consistent with dissolution, a process in which the cortical influence on regulating (i.e. calming) autonomic state become less effective. Functionally, the repurposed neural system that emerged during the transition from ancient reptiles to early mammals allowed sociality to function as a neuromodulator, calming physiology and optimizing bodily functions. In addition to sociality, positive memories and visualizations associated with positive experiences enable humans to access positive feelings (i.e. autonomic state) to actively inhibit threat reactions.

Access to sociality as a neuromodulator is influenced by both autonomic state and the flexibility or resilience that an individual's autonomic state has in returning from a state of threat to a state that supports homeostasis. We also learn that this accessibility is, in part, dependent on a personal history during which autonomic state may have been retuned to optimize defence. This is frequently observed in individuals with a severe adversity history, whose traumatic experiences have retuned the autonomic nervous system to be locked in states of defence. This is reported by foster parents of children who have been abused and for safety concerns have been removed from their biological parents.

Cultural and philosophical influences divert interest in feelings of safety

Within our educational institutions, we have been culturalized to accept the dictum coined by philosopher Rene Descartes '*I think, therefore I am*' (*cogito, ergo sum*) (Descartes, 1637/1986). This view has led to a cultural expectation that the rational mind defines us, and feelings distort this expectation and need to be constrained.

Polyvagal Theory provides an alternative perspective to this historical proposition. First, the theory leads to a perspective that rather than thinking defining our existence, feeling does. Specifically, a revised polyvagal-informed statement suggests that I feel myself, therefore I am. I frequently use this example in my talks, although I use the French and not the Latin presentation of the dictum. Reflexive verbs are more commonly used in French than in English. Reflexive verbs are actions that the subject is performing on itself. Thus, using the reflexive form of the verb to feel will unambiguously convey internal feelings and not the sensations of feeling (touching) an object. In English, when we use the word feel, it is ambiguous and may reflect either situation. By using *je pense, donc je suis*, it is easily rephrased with the reflexive form of the verb to feel. The modified statement *je me sens, donc je suis* emphasizes that if *I feel myself, I exist* – a statement consistent with the current interest in embodiment and reports from trauma survivors of being disembodied and experiencing a bodily numbness.

Descartes' philosophy led to a partitioning of human experience into separate domains dependent on mind (mental activities) and body (physical structure). Descartes states that mental states or processes cannot exist outside the body and the body cannot think. The separation between mind and body, often labeled as Cartesian dualism, has been consistent with our contemporary cognitive-centric world view that is mirrored in a cortico-centric brain-body separation that dominates much of medical and mental health treatment models. Descartes argued that rational decision making can only be developed when judgements are based not on passion (i.e. bodily feelings). This dualism is still prevalent in current medical practices, especially when illness cannot be linked to a specific organ dysfunction. When objective clinical assessments of bodily fluids and tissues do not provide a positive clinical indicator leading to an understood disorder, physicians often assume that the disorder is psychiatric or psychosomatic and the patient should get psychiatric consultation and care.

According to Damasio (1994), Descartes' perspective had a fatal error in not acknowledging the interaction of feelings (i.e. body) with the mental activities (i.e. brain). Consistent with Polyvagal Theory, Damasio emphasizes that bodily feelings can have a powerful influence on mental processes. Thus, rational thought espoused by Descartes would be a special case of mental processing in which the autonomic nervous system is not disrupting cognitive function. Perhaps, this special case is dependent on an autonomic state associated with feelings of safety.

The phylogenetic journey

Feelings of safety form the foundational neural platform for sociality. Through the lens of evolution, Polyvagal Theory focuses on how mammals adapted many of the phylogenetical ancestral structures that evolved to support survival in a hostile world. Note that the title of the initial publication presenting the theory (Porges, 1995) is a synopsis of the theory: 'Orienting in a defensive world: Mammalian modifications of our evolutionary heritage. A Polyvagal Theory'. The title summarizes a phylogenetic narrative in which the survival of mammals was dependent on an ability to downregulate and modify the innate defensive systems that were inherited from their reptilian ancestors. These embedded vestigial circuits with their emergent adaptive strategies are embedded in the genes of mammals. For mammals, whose survival is dependent on their sociality to cooperate, to connect, and to co-regulate (Dobzhansky, 1962), the ancient defence programmes had to be harnessed and repurposed to enable the expression of several defining features, including signals of safety and calmness in proximity to another trusted mammal.

Polyvagal Theory's interest in investigating mammalian autonomic regulation from a phylogenetic perspective does not focus on the obvious similarities with more ancient vertebrates. Rather, it focuses on the unique modifications that enabled mammals to optimize their survival. Consistent with this theme, Polyvagal Theory focuses on the evolved neural circuits that enabled mammals to downregulate the sympathetic activation that could support mobilization to fight or flee, to reduce psychological and physical distance with conspecifics, and to functionally co-regulate physiological and behavioural state.

The theory focuses on the transition from reptiles to mammals and emphasizes the neural adaptations that enable cues of safety to downregulate states of defence. Within Polyvagal Theory, the evolutionary trend has led to a conceptualization of an emergent and uniquely mammalian social engagement system in which a modified branch of the vagus is integral. Neuroanatomically, this system is dependent on a brainstem area known as the ventral vagal complex. This area regulates not only the mammalian ventral cardioinhibitory vagal pathway, but also the special visceral efferent pathways controlling the striated muscles of the face and head. This does not preclude other structures being involved in mammalian social engagement behaviours or homologous structures in other vertebrates that do not share our phylogenetic history being involved in social engagement behaviours.

The relationship between mothers and their nursing offspring illustrates the social engagement system in action. To survive, mammalian offspring must initially nurse as the primary mode of ingesting food. To nurse, the infant must suck, a process dependent on a brainstem circuit involving the ventral vagal complex. Survival is dependent on the infant's nervous system efficiently and effectively coordinating suck-swallow-breathe-vocalize behaviours with vagal regulation of the heart through the ventral vagal pathways originating in the nucleus ambiguus. Through maturation and socialization, this 'ingestive' circuit provides the structural neural platform for sociality and co-regulation, as major mediators, to optimize homeostatic function leading to health, growth and restoration (see Porges and Furman, 2011). For mammals, there is a dependency between reactions to contextual cues and the function of this circuit. Cues of threat may disrupt, while cues of safety may support or enhance function. The sensory branches of the facial and trigeminal nerves provide major input into the ventral vagal complex. Functionally, changes in the state of this circuit, through the process of dissolution, will either disinhibit phylogenetically older autonomic circuits to support defence (e.g. predator, disease, physical injury) or inform all aspects of the autonomic nervous system, including the enteric system to optimize homeostatic function (Kolacz and Porges, 2018; Kolacz, Kovacic and Porges, 2019).

Mammals uniquely have detached middle ear bones, which distinguish them from reptiles in the fossil record. Detached middle ear bones delineate the frequency band that mammals can hear species-specific vocalizations associated with social communication and provide a 'safe' frequency band in which they can socially communicate without detection by reptiles. Middle ear bones are small bones that separated from the jawbone during gestational development and form an ossicle chain that connects the eardrum to the inner ear. Small muscles regulated by branches of the trigeminal and facial nerves regulate the transfer function of the middle ear and determine the acoustic properties of the sounds transduced through middle ear structures by controlling the stiffness of the ossicle chain. When the chain is stiff, the eardrum is tighter and low frequency sounds are attenuated; when the muscles relax, lower frequency sounds pass into the inner ear. In all mammalian species, based on the physics of their middle ear structures, there is a frequency band of perceptual advantage that is expressed when the middle ear muscles contract (see Kolacz, Lewis and Porges, 2018). It is within this frequency band that social communication occurs, while the low frequencies that through evolution have been associated with predators are attenuated (see Porges and Lewis, 2010).

Interestingly, the coordination of the contraction and relaxation of these small muscles is frequently co-regulated with autonomic state and they contract when there is strong ventral vagal tone to promote social communication and co-regulation. This coordination between listening to specific sounds and autonomic regulation provides the neurophysiological basis for sound to communicate cues of safety and trust. In contrast, when the autonomic nervous system shifts to a state of defence the muscles relax, allowing detection of low-frequency predator sounds, which support defence strategies with auditory cues. In this state, the acoustic perception is biased towards detecting cues of threat.

The link between behavioural and autonomic state and listening is obvious in the study of language delays and auditory processing problems in children. Many children with problems in auditory processing also have behavioural state regulation limitations. This neurophysiological link provides a portal to regulate autonomic state through acoustic stimulation, which is easily observable when a mother calms her infant using prosodic vocalization. In a recent study (Kolacz *et al.*, 2022), we documented that the acoustic parameters of mothers' vocalizations had differential influences on calming their infants, following an experimental manipulation known as the 'still face' procedure (Tronick *et al.*, 1978). Prosodic maternal vocalizations were more effective in calming behaviour and reducing heart rate following the social disruption of the still face procedure. Of course, parents and pet owners are familiar with the impact of their voices on calming their children and mammalian pets.

Based on this link between prosodic vocalizations and calming, a listening intervention, known as the Safe and Sound Protocol™ (SSP), was developed to reduce auditory hypersensitivities, improve auditory processing and calm the autonomic nervous system. The SSP functionally amplifies the embedded prosody in music by applying dynamic filters to pre-recorded music. Preliminary publications document the effectiveness of this strategy (Porges *et al.*, 2013, 2014). The technology embedded in the SSP has received three patents and is marketed by Unyte/Integrated Listening Systems. One of the awarded claims on the patents is for the application of technology as an acoustic vagal nerve stimulator.

Through the evolution of vertebrates there were strong trends in the structures involved in regulating autonomic function. These trends may be summarized as moving from chemical to neural and then evolving greater specificity, efficiency and speed through feedback circuits that relied on myelinated pathways. Evolution is a process of modification in which existing structures and circuits are modified to serve adaptive functions. In mammals, three primary autonomic states with specific neural circuits are observable and emerge at different times within the evolutionary history of vertebrates. In polyvagal terms, the newest is labelled the *ventral vagal complex*, the oldest is the *dorsal vagal complex*, and in between is the spinal *sympathetic nervous system*. Thus, evolution informs us of the sequence through which the three phylogenetic dependent circuits regulate autonomic function in response to survival-driven threat reactions.

Neuroception

Polyvagal Theory proposes that the neural evaluation of risk and safety reflexively triggers shifts in autonomic state without requiring conscious awareness. Thus, the term 'neuroception' was introduced to emphasize a neural process, distinct from perception, capable of distinguishing environmental and visceral features that are safe, dangerous or life-threatening (Porges, 2003, 2004). A form of neuroception can be found in virtually all living organisms, regardless of the development of the nervous system. In fact, it could be argued that single-celled organisms and even plants have a primordial neural or neurochemical system that responds to threat. As mammals, we are familiar with reactions to pain, a type of neuroception. We react to pain prior to our ability to identify the source of the stimulus or even of an awareness of the injury. Similarly, the detection of threat appears to be common across all vertebrate species. However, mammals have an expanded capacity for neuroception in which they not only react instantaneously to threat, but also respond instantaneously to cues of safety. It is this latter feature that enables mammals to downregulate defensive strategies to promote sociality by enabling psychological and physical proximity without an anticipation of potential injury. It is this calming mechanism that adaptively adjusts the central regulation of autonomic function to dampen the metabolically costly fight/flight reactions dependent on sympathetic activation and to protect the oxygen-dependent central nervous system, especially the cortex, from the metabolically conservative defensive reactions of the dorsal vagal complex (e.g. fainting, death feigning).

Polyvagal Theory proposes that neuroception functionally involves both top-down and bottom-up mechanisms. The process of neuroception, consistent with Level II in Table 2.1, is assumed to be initiated via top-down pathways involving cortical areas located in or near the temporal cortex – components of the central nervous system that reflexively interpret cues of threat and safety. These areas of the cortex are sensitive to the intentionality of biological movements, including voices, faces, gestures, and hand movements. Embedded in the construct of neuroception is the capacity of the nervous system to react to the intention of these movements. Neuroception functionally decodes and interprets the assumed goal of movements and sounds of inanimate and living objects. Thus, the neuro-ception of familiar individuals and individuals with appropriately prosodic voices and warm, expressive faces frequently translates into a positive social interaction, promoting a sense of safety. The autonomic state responds to the top-down detection of risk or safety. The autonomic reactions send sensory information regarding bodily feelings to the brain where they are interpreted and consciously felt. The bottom-up limb of the neuroception is functionally equivalent to interoception. Thus, although we are often unaware of the stimuli that trigger different neuroception responses, we are generally aware of our body's reactions (i.e. visceral feelings) embodied in other autonomic signatures that support adaptive behaviours (i.e. social engagement, fight/flight, shutdown).

Social connectedness: A biological imperative

A biological imperative identifies a need that must be fulfilled for a living organism to perpetuate existence and survival. Polyvagal Theory suggests that social connectedness is a core biological imperative for humans, since human survival is dependent on trusted others and is wired into our genetics and expressed throughout the lifespan, starting from the moment of birth.

Polyvagal Theory proposes that social connectedness is tantamount to stating that our body feels safe in proximity with another. The theory elaborates that the neural structures involved in the social engagement system (Porges, 2009) orchestrate the autonomic states of the interacting dyad to both broadcast and receive cues of safety that downregulate threat reactions of defence and promote accessibility and co-regulation.

To be socially connected via a functional social engagement system (Porges, 2009), common brainstem structures must appropriately coordinate the striated muscles of the face and head with the vagal regulation of the viscera, originating in a brainstem region known as nucleus ambiguus. Interestingly, neuroanatomically the special visceral efferent pathways regulating the striated muscles of the face and head originate in and communicate with the brainstem area (i.e. ventral vagal complex) that regulates the ventral vagal cardioinhibitory pathway. The ventral vagal cardioinhibitory pathway provides the neural pathways that are expressed as the vagal brake and can be monitored by quantifying the amplitude of respiratory sinus arrhythmia (RSA). RSA is the rhythmic component in heart rate variability observed at the frequency of breathing.

An optimally resilient individual has opportunities to co-regulate their physiological state with a safe and trusted other. Ideally, the 'other' person projects positive cues regarding their autonomic state through prosodic voice, warm welcoming facial expressions, and gestures of accessibility.

From an evolutionary perspective, the integration of the neural regulation of the viscera with the regulations of the striated muscles of the face and head enable the visceral state to be projected in vocalizations and facial expressions. This also allows vocalizations and facial expressions, modulated by autonomic states, to serve as cues of safety or threat to others. Together, these pathways connect behaviour to the nervous system and form the basis for social communication, cooperation and connectedness.

This system also produces, via a ventral vagal cardioinhibitory pathway, an autonomic state that produces feelings of safety and reflects an adaptive mastery of Level II processes (see Table 2.1).

Polyvagal Theory, by articulating an evolutionary hierarchy (i.e. based on Jacksonian dissolution) in the function of the autonomic nervous system to challenges, provides a guide to dynamically monitor adaptive autonomic responses. The autonomic state of an individual serves as a functional map of the foundation for emergent behavioural, emotional and physiological reactivity that an individual may have in response to threat or alternatively to positive experiences. The state of the autonomic nervous system provides a neural platform for an expanded range of feelings from threat to safety that in turn provides a neurophysiological substrate for higher brain structures to elaborate these feelings. If the feelings are negative and dependent on autonomic states supporting defence, the feelings may evolve into diffuse states of anxiety or specific emotions such as fear or anger. Alternatively, if the feelings are positive and dependent on an autonomic state of calmness, thus enabling interpersonal accessibility and co-regulation, then these feelings may be associated with trust, love and intimacy.

Clinical implications

From a polyvagal perspective, it may be helpful to investigate how challenges move us into physiological states of threat that disrupt our connectedness and place our mental and physical health at risk. But, more relevant to both to clients and personal survival, therapists need to identify and emphasize the innate resources their clients have available to mitigate the potentially devastating reactions to threat, which in turn can destabilize the autonomic nervous system, sometimes resulting in visceral organ dysfunction and compromised mental health.

Awareness of the neural systems underlying Polyvagal Theory informs both therapists and clients regarding the threats to survival that can shift autonomic state, moving it through sequential neural platforms or states that mimic evolution in reverse or dissolution (Jackson, 1884). Functionally, to inhibit the trajectory of dissolution to calm, we must first use the competence of our social engagement system (a uniquely mammalian myelinated vagal pathway involving brainstem structures regulating vocal intonation and facial expressions) to connect with others and calm our physiology. Without these resources, we are vulnerable to move into adaptive defensive states.

Our defence repertoire is first expressed as chronic mobilization requiring activation of the sympathetic nervous system and then expressed as immobilization, which is controlled by an evolutionarily older unmyelinated vagal pathway. In the absence of an active social engagement system, the mobilized state provides an efficient neural platform for fight and flight behaviours. For many individuals, this state will reflect chronic anxiety or irritability. When mobilization does not successfully move the individual into a safe context, then there is the possibility that the nervous system will shift into an immobilized state. Immobilization with fear can be associated with features of death feigning, syncope, dissociation, withdrawal, loss of purpose, social isolation, despair and depression.

Although the two defensive strategies have adaptive values in protecting the individual, they are dependent on different neural pathways (i.e. high sympathetic tone or high dorsal vagal tone). Activation of these systems, independently or simultaneously, will interfere with interpersonal interactions, co-regulation, accessibility, trust and feeling safe with another person. Thus, defensive states emerge from neural platforms that evolved to defend, while simultaneously compromising capacities to downregulate our defences through co-regulation with a safe and trusted individual. Basically, the theory emphasizes that in the presence of cues of safety, which we associate with positive social interactions, the mammalian social engagement system can downregulate our innate reactions to threat, whether the threat is tangible and observable or imagined and invisible.

Resilience: An emergent property of connectedness and feelings of safety

Polyvagal Theory informs us that sociality is a neuromodulator and supports homeostatic functions that serve as a neurophysiological foundation for the positive emergent emotional and social consequences. In this chapter, several related processes have been associated with feelings of safety or threat. In a sense, we could say that Polyvagal Theory emphasizes that resilience reflects a physiological state, which is sufficiently flexible to recover from disruptions, support feelings of safety, and connect with others via an active social engagement system. Moving into this state has positive outcomes that are not solely reflected in sociality and trust, but also in prosocial actions of compassion, benevolence and generosity that enable humans to actualize their biological imperative of connectedness. The narratives highlighted the possibility that resiliency might be a product of a nervous system with sufficient resources to move out of the self-oriented focus of threat and stress to another oriented focus of feelings of safety that naturally emerge into actions of sociality and compassion.

Resilience is a complex construct that appears to embody the successful integration of several skills and underlying neurophysiological mechanisms to recover from severe survival-related challenges. Considering the focus and organization of this chapter, resilience and feelings of safety share a common neurophysiological substrate. On its most foundational level, resilience reflects behavioural, physiological, emotional and social processes that are dependent on the recovery of autonomic function to a state that supports social engagement as an adaptive strategy to co-regulate with others and to mutually support health, growth and restoration. The antithesis of resilience might be thought of as being locked in an autonomic state that would support threat reactions within the body (e.g. injury and infection) and from others. This foundational level would be reflected in the descriptions of Levels 1 and 11 in Table 2.1. When these foundational levels are functional, the nervous system can support coordinated, goal-directed behaviours (Level 111) and social interactions (Level 1V).

An optimally regulated autonomic nervous system would support homeostasis and appropriately respond to challenges with an efficient vagal brake (i.e. enhanced vagal efficiency) by reacting and recovering to transitory challenges. But these narratives of resilience emphasize that there is a more integrative mechanism involved that is linked to fulfilling the biological imperative of social connectedness. This capacity for connectedness requires an active social engagement system, which broadcasts the individual's accessibility through voice and facial expressivity. In a simplistic manner, the face and voice, via brainstem pathways in the ventral vagal complex, provide a mechanism through which the autonomic state of two individuals can be shared and functionally transmit feelings of safety, trust and accessibility that lead to effective co-regulation. The ability to co-regulate is not simply a collection of voluntary operant behaviours involving facial expressions and vocalizations but seems to require the transmission of veridical cues of safety that are sufficient to elicit a neuroception of safety. It is hard to calibrate these cues, although we subjectively know through our personal reactions that with some we feel safe and accessible, while with others we feel uncomfortable. I have come to label people whose presence triggers a smile with feelings of accessibility and connection, as super co-regulators. Perhaps, resilience, as a process, reflects the successful biobehavioural navigation of the four levels described in Table 2.1 and could succinctly be summarized as the capacity to spontaneously foster feelings of safety in both self and other.

Concluding remarks: Claiming our phylogenetic heritage

Feelings of safety play a fundamental role in enabling humans not only to survive, but to thrive. This supposition poses the important scientific question of how a feeling could be so critical to the survival of our species. To answer this question, it is first necessary to understand the relationship between feelings of safety and the specific neurophysiological architecture that underlies this specific category of feelings. Unfortunately, historical attempts to answer these types of questions have been elusive. Attempts to identify neurophysiological signatures of specific feelings, emotions, thoughts, or even global processes such as sociality, have produced, at best, confusing and ambiguous results (e.g. Cacioppo *et al.*, 2000; Levenson, 2003).

Central to the solution of this problem is how terms and constructs are used in different disciplines. In general, attempts to translate from psychological to physiological phenomena have focused on a strategy that could be succinctly labelled as 'psychophysiological parallelism.' Psychophysiological parallelism is an intriguing strategy with a strong assumption that it is possible to identify unique neurophysiological signatures of specific mental processes (e.g. feelings, emotions, thoughts). In the 1960s, psychophysiology emerged as an interdisciplinary science with historic roots embedded in this assumption.

Although Polyvagal Theory (Porges, 1995) emerged from traditional psychophysiology, it provided a theoretical demarcation from parallelism. In a sense, psychophysiological parallelism implicitly assumed that the constructs employed in different domains were valid (e.g. subjective, observable, physiological) and focused on establishing correlations across domains that optimistically would lead to an objectively quantifiable physiological signature of the construct explored in the psychological domain. In contrast, Polyvagal Theory emphasizes the interactive and integrative aspect of different levels of the nervous system. The theory emphasizes a hierarchical organization that mirrors phylogenetic shifts among vertebrates. The evolutionary changes are also reflected in maturational trends. Thus, what appears to be more complex and related to higher brain structures, such as language and sensitivities to another's physiological state via intonation of voice and gesture, is reflecting the functional and structural changes mapped into the evolutionary history of vertebrates. Frequently missed with our cortico-centric and cognitive-centric orientation is the importance of lower brain mechanisms in managing our basic survival-oriented reactions. Although the less complex earlier-evolved systems are often repurposed in mammals, they remain survival oriented and are efficiently available to support states of defence when survival is challenged.

Polyvagal Theory focuses on the functional consequences of how the autonomic nervous system was repurposed during the evolutionary transition from asocial reptiles to social mammals. This focus had a serendipitous benefit, since the brainstem area is relatively small and there was sufficient comparative neuroanatomy conducted to map the changes in the brainstem pathways and their potential adaptive functions. The theory focuses on how phylogenetic changes in the neural regulation of the heart provided the foundational properties for feelings of safety and emergent sociality. This chapter emphasizes that these two 'psychological' constructs have a dependence on an evolved link between social engagement behaviours and vagal regulation. However, there are convergent evolutionary changes in how the neuropeptides of vasopressin and oxytocin function to support the advent of sociality in mammals (Carter, 2021; Porges, 2001). Specifically, oxytocin plays an important convergent role with the autonomic nervous system in enabling mammals to immobilize without fear, give birth and experience intimacy without recruiting physiological defensive reactions through dorsal vagal pathways (e.g. bradycardia, syncope and diarrhea).

Information from three scientific strategies leads to an understanding of the critical role that feelings of safety play in human survival. Complementing the evolutionary and developmental trends introduced above there is a third strategy, an unfolding or de-evolution of the hierarchy in response to threat. This third strategy represents the study of pathology and adaptive reactions to challenges including threat and illness. Jackson (1884) formally introduced de-evolution as dissolution to emphasize the functional impact of disease or damage to the brain. He noted that as evolutionarily newer circuits became dysfunctional, they no longer inhibited the actions of older circuits, and the older circuits became active. Threat is a generalized reaction that can occur in response to a physical challenge, a pathogen or even an inaccurate interpretation of context. The elements resulting in a threat response do not have to be valid from an objective interpretation of threat. Rather, threat responses reflect the nervous system's interpretation of risk. In polyvagal terminology, threat responses are due to a neuroception of danger or life threat in which the nervous system determines risk outside conscious awareness.

From a polyvagal perspective, threat reactions represent a disruption of homeostatic function regardless of the validity of threat. Conversely, a neuroception of safety results in an autonomic state that supports homeostatic function with emergent feelings of safety.

Feelings of safety and threat recruit different autonomic resources to optimize survival. However, survival as a construct is overly broad and confusing. Survival can initially be deconstructed into two domains of competence: one within the body and the other outside the body. Although adequately responding to both challenges is necessary, *internal competence needs to precede external competence*. The internal processes focus on how the nervous system manages the regulation of bodily organs and supports the basic homeostatic processes of health, growth and restoration. This is obvious when observing the challenge to survival of being born premature, basically born too soon for the nervous system to effectively manage homeostatic demands. The external processes focus on how the nervous system supports responses to challenges. For humans, this starts with mastering the coordination of suck-swallow-breathe-vocalize behaviours that enable ingestion and social signalling.

On the most basic level, feelings of safety are a direct reflection of autonomic state when it is efficiently supporting homeostatic functions. But there is a consequential factor. Being in a calm autonomic state provides neural access to the regulation of the muscles of the face and head that form an integrated social engagement system. This system utilizes the same neural network that coordinates sucking, swallowing, vocalizing, and breathing at birth. Interestingly, access to this system is also a portal to calm as evidenced by the overlap between social behaviour and ingestion.

Thus, feelings of safety not only reflect a calm autonomic state supporting homeostatic functions that is effectively regulated via the ventral vagus, but also provide access to the special visceral efferent pathways that also originate in the ventral vagal complex and enable social communication.

Frequently missed is the understanding that the brainstem area regulating the autonomic state supporting feelings of safety also regulates the muscles of the face and head that we use for ingestion, social communication, and signalling that we can be trusted and are safe to approach. For example, the intonation of voice reflects our autonomic state. If we are calm and our heart rate is slow and rhythmically variable, our voice is prosodic. The intonation of voice reflected in prosody is the product of vagal pathways regulating laryngeal and pharyngeal muscles. When we are frightened or angry, our voice loses prosody, and our heart rate is fast and loses rhythmic variability. Feeling safe, by being in an autonomic state, enables us to efficiently use the social engagement system and to convey the feelings of safety to another. This is universally observed as a mother calms her infant with melodic vocalizations, gentle reassuring gestures and warm facial expressions. Underlying the effectiveness of the mother's vocalizations and facial expressions in calming the infant is the fact that these cues of safety are actively both reflecting the mother's autonomic state and directly impacting on the nerves that regulate the infant's autonomic nervous system, and are being regulated by the same brainstem structures located in the ventral vagal complex. However, access to the structures involved in ingestion and social engagement behaviours is limited by autonomic state.

These structures are efficiently accessible when the autonomic nervous system is calm, not in a state of defence, and under the regulation of the ventral vagal pathway.

This chapter has emphasized the common theme that feelings of safety reflect a core fundamental process that has enabled humans to survive through the opportunistic features of trusting social engagements that have co-regulatory capacities to mitigate the metabolically costly defence reactions. The short-term outcome is obvious in terms of the support of homeostatic functions. However, there is also a long-term consequence of feelings of safety that is reflected in the emergence of communities in which feelings of safety expand through spontaneous social engagement. Prosocial behaviours among a collective become the norm. Thus, our sociality enables an expansion of those with whom we feel safe and trust. This, of course, is the underlying premise of communities including legal systems, business transactions, political negotiations and international treaties.

Through the study of neural development and phylogeny, we can extract foundational principles and their underlying mechanisms through which the autonomic nervous system leads to feelings of safety and opportunities to co-regulate. The study of mental and physical illnesses provides a convergent research strategy to confirm these principles, since illness is a trigger of dissolution, which functionally disrupts autonomic regulation and compromises social engagement behaviours.

In Table 2.2 below, the foundational principles are outlined. The principles succinctly form a hierarchy that leads to an optimization of health as well as mental, social and behavioural processes. An acknowledgment of these principles in daily interactions and societal institutions would reinstate processes that would support the qualities of human experience, in which feelings of safety form the foundation of a healthier and more productive society. These principles highlight the validity of a science of safety that when implemented in societal institutions, ranging from healthcare to education, would enhance health and sociality, and lead to greater productivity, creativity and a sense of well-being. In a way, by respecting our need to feel safe, we respect our phylogenetic heritage and elevate sociality as a neuromodulator, and provide the scientific validation for a societal focus on promoting opportunities to experience feelings of safety and co-regulation.

In summary, feelings of safety and threat are subjective interpretations of the autonomic nervous system communicating via interoception with higher brain structures. As humans, we are on a lifelong quest to feel safe. Polyvagal Theory deconstructs this intuitive truth into a plausible neuroscience with testable hypotheses and objective neurophysiological indices. Functionally, this quest to feel safe is the product of respecting the important functions of neuroception and the powerful role of co-regulation and other attributes of sociality as a neuromodulator that can optimize health, growth and restoration.

Table 2.2: Principles of a science of safety

1. Feelings of safety are a subjective interpretation of a calm autonomic state regulated by the ventral vagal pathway that supports homeostatic functions (i.e. health, growth and restoration).
2. Feelings of threat, stress, or anxiety are subjective interpretations of a shared defensive autonomic state that disrupts homeostatic function.
3. Feelings of safety provide access to the social engagement system.
4. When recruited, the social engagement system sends signals of safety (e.g. intonation of voice, facial expressions) to others that functionally downregulate (via neuroception) autonomic states of defence to states of calmness and accessibility, mitigating the metabolically costly threat reactions through co-regulation.
5. Co-regulation provides the neural state that supports the establishment of trusting relationships.
6. Autonomic states of calmness (e.g. feelings of safety) enable efficient access to the higher brain structures involved in cognitive processes and mental health.
7. The reciprocal benefits of co-regulation form the basis of sociality and support the neural systems, optimizing health and performance.

KNOWLEDGE AND PRACTICE REFLECTION

Janise Mitchell, Joe Tucci, Ed Tronick and Stephen W. Porges

In this chapter, Porges offers a deep dive into what interpersonal safety really feels like, is like and how it is created. As Porges has said here and in much of his writing, safety is a biological imperative. It is the substrate of human relationships. It is not merely the absence of threat and danger. It is an evolutionary drive to co-ordinate, collaborate and co-operate with the social engagement systems of others who live and act in close proximity with us.

Safety is more than a feeling or some kind of esoteric quality. It is a real bodily state that is interpersonal by nature. As Porges highlights, the resources of the body's calming system that are conscious and deliberate are effective in downregulating threat reactions when the danger is mild. However, this biologically younger part of the calming system is ineffectual when the defence systems are in highly activated survival mode. When faced with overwhelming danger, evolutionary older pathways set off all sorts of internal physiological changes that mobilize the body to take action to protect itself from threat. As the danger continues, as is the case when the source of that danger is another person or group of people with whom humans co-exist in relationships, the body changes again responding to the ongoing jeopardy by becoming immobilized with fear, conserving its energy in order to keep functioning.

Porges is matter of fact about how the body can instantaneously respond to cues of safety, as it does to signs of danger. These cues are tangible, visible and available through learning from the signals of care and love that parents show to their newborn infants, who cannot access language as a primary form of communication. So instead, carers of babies use the prosody of their voice (cooing, clicking, little giggles, ahhhhs, tickety boos), warm, welcoming facial expressions (smiles, eye opening, slightly exaggerated nodding) and gestures of accessibility (mimicking, open body orientations, tickling) as ways of connecting and shaping the infant's state of arousal. In turn, the infant's responsive interactions shape the state of being of the carer.

The work of Stephen Porges has created the science of safety as an area of deep significance to practitioners and organizations working to support those who have and continue to experience trauma in their lives.

As one of the key principles of trauma-informed practice, safety appears to focus mainly on the tangible dimensions of an organization. There are a number of examples of calls to eliminate involuntary interventions, such as seclusion and physical restraint in mental health services (Kim and Ashmore, 2019; Watson *et al.*, 2014; Kontio *et al.*, 2012). There is an understanding of the need to ensure that the vulnerability of children, young people and adults is not exploited by individuals who move into organizations in ways that manipulate the policies and protocols already in place in order to abuse and victimize (Tucci *et al.*, 2015). Some examples highlight how the physical environments can be adapted to be more welcoming, with touches of homelike furniture, fabrics and styling making places feel more familiar.

But it is the interpersonal nature of safety cues and the inherent centrality of relationships that has yet to be fully explored in the trauma-informed literature. At best, especially in educational settings, teachers are urged to keep themselves calm in order to attend to the arousal needs of their students. Similarly, foster carers and residential care workers in out-of-home care services are encouraged to be present and calm in the face of children and young people's activated states arising from experiences of everyday living.

Porges points to it being more than that. Safety comes from the way that intent (of an individual or a group of individuals) is signalled and perceived and the interaction of this knowing with memory states from the past about the trajectories of such intent. A young person can pick up if their youth worker looks as if they have other things on their mind on a particular day, and may react by storming away. Or the adult living with the effects of trauma senses that they have to face talking to another doctor about the symptoms of their headaches, even though they have described them 50 times before.

He also expresses some caution about the use of the word *survival* in relation to what the mind-body is purporting to struggle for in its reaction to overwhelming threat. It is, as he maintains, a broad and confusing construct. He prefers the orientation that humans are on a lifelong quest for safety. In the face of interpersonal violence, he describes the physiological changes that occur as a result of the nervous system interpreting risk outside conscious awareness in an effort by the body to return to an internal equilibrium that is perceived from *within* as having the qualitative experiences of safety.

As such, beyond ensuring the absence of physical threat or danger, safety is an inherent critical goal for good practice in all human service organizations. It is what should become interwoven into the organizational fabric if personnel learn and appreciate that the experience of safety rests in the way they interact with service users and with the intent behind their behaviour being as significant as what they do. Indeed, without the experience of safety, trust cannot be built. The current literature describing trauma-informed approaches fails to explore the central relationship between safety and trust. There is nothing more important than appreciating how interconnected everyone is to each other and how reliant we are on each other to know and experience safety. It also hinges on an awareness that we communicate signals to victims and survivors through the state of our nervous system and this occurs outside our consciousness. So, it is not hard for them to pick up on cues that reflect the underlying states of our bodies, such as indifference, fear, joy, distress, warmth and anger.

Deb Dana (2021) has been instrumental in helping to make the science of safety more tangible and able to be implemented in the everyday. The three mechanisms that engage safety are:

- the hierarchical and evolutionary nature of the autonomic nervous system (as explained by Porges)
- the capacity of humans to be aware of the state of their body in relation to safety and danger (neuroception). There are three streams of awareness – inside (heartbeat, breath rhythms, muscle action, digestive organs), outside (awareness of your physical environment in your home, neighborhoods and community) and between (perceptions of the way your nervous system communicates and interrelates with the nervous system of others as individuals and in groups)
- the opportunity to co-regulate with others, share feeling states, shape each other's reactions and internal levels of arousal.

More interestingly for the construct of trauma-transformative practice are the three aspects of well-being that Dana argues help to anchor the nervous systems in safety and regulation: 'context, choice and connection...when these three elements are present, we more easily find the way to regulation. When any of these elements is missing, we feel off balance and experience a sense of unease' (Dana, 2021, p.23).

Context involves coherence. It is the perception of the difference between the explicit environmental cues about safety or danger and the implicit cues which are communicating outside our awareness of how safe the environment is perceived: '...without explicitly stated information, we are more likely to sense unsafety and move into patterns of protection' (Dana, 2021, p.23).

Choice is the second element of well-being – a quality that has been identified in trauma-informed literature already (Harris and Fallot, 2001; SAMHSA, 2014). Dana argues that choice is experienced in micro-moments:

> ...with choice, it is possible to be still or move, approach or avoid, connect or protect. When choice is limited or taken away, or when we have a sense of being stuck or trapped without options, we begin to look for a way out... (p.24)

Connection is the experience of relatedness and relationship. According to Dana, it has four dimensions:

- Connection to self
- Connection other people
- Connection to nature
- Connection to spirit.

We would add that connection to culture is an important element of connection. Over and over again, First Nations people, in particular, have maintained that connection to culture is intrinsic to their well-being. As Kickett, Chandran and Mitchell (2020) have pointed out:

> Understanding the dynamics of culture is not just about seeing the 'tip' of the cultural identity 'iceberg' of food, dress, music, language, and art, but is concerned with the more subtle ways in which culture impacts on how individuals and communities see and engage with the world (St. Onge, Cole and Petty 2003, as cited in Bamblett et al., 2010). It defines identify, beliefs and values, forms of communication and the ways in which relation-ships are formed and maintained. It is passed down the generations in the complexity of relationships, protocols, languages, social organization and life experiences that bind diverse individuals, families and communities together... (p.164)

Culture is a dynamic, living process. It changes over time to reflect the changed environments and social interactions of people living together (Atkinson, 2002). First Nations cultures have many elements which connect and interconnect children and young people to their family, extended family and country through language, stories, songs and dance. First Nations children and young people who can grow up strong in a culture develop a sense of strength, confidence, pride, belonging, peace and security that has the potential to guide and protect them through adolescence and adulthood (Bamblett, Harrison and Lewis, 2010; Bamblett, 2013). Connection to culture is a key dimension of what helps First Nations people, but really all of us, feel and be safe.

In summarizing the impact of connection, Dana (2021) comments that:

> ...with connection, we feel safely embodied, accompanied by others, at home in the environment, and in harmony with spirit. When there is rupture in our sense of connection, our ability to anchor in safety and regulation is challenged, and we turn to communication and social engagement to try and find our way back into connection. When there is an ongoing disruption of connection, we often reach out in desperation before retreating into despair... (p.25)

For a practitioner or an organization aiming to support those who have experienced trauma to achieve its vision, safety needs to be translated into practical applications that are built on the science that Porges has been defining over the course of his career. In effect, safety is a quality that must be integrated into the core design of practice and services, answering the following sorts of questions:

- What is the organization's tone of voice? How does it signal safety? How can its communication be interpreted? Are its intentions clear and repeated? Are its intentions and its actions congruent?
- How much time is allowed for safety to emerge and be experienced before a service user is expected to engage and trust?
- What choice is offered to an individual about when, with whom and for what purpose do engagements begin and continue with an individual practitioner or as a whole?
- What connections are offered to the individual service user that keep them attuned to cues of safety rather than signals of possible danger?
- How much respect is there for and commitment to the cultural background of the service user and is this communicated explicitly and implicitly?
- What is the first experience that service users with trauma backgrounds have as they approach the organization? What are the staff

aware of as they interact with service users? How is collaboration with service users viewed?

- As a service or programme, how is an understanding of trauma made explicit in the documentation describing the operational model? How is safety built into this? What are the considerations for how safety is negotiated?

Safety is not an end state. Safety is a process – a quest, as Porges has posited. It is relational quality that facilitates trust in others. The external dynamics of interpersonal interactions which are perceived as safe resonate with internal systems that are the preference of human physiology – calm, resourced, connected. There are no surprises. There is no sudden move to defence. The body's interpretations of risk are more neutral. This experience is in itself reparative for those with lived and living experiences of trauma.

At its heart, the experience of safety is reparative because it reduces the reliance on old patterns of reactivity that have been useful for the individual in the past to protect them in the face of danger and violation (Tucci, Weller and Mitchell, 2018). This is all part of the way that trauma-transformative practice can work. Safety works all the time in the background. It recognizes that trauma-specific interventions, as they have so far been conceptualized, are not the only opportunities for healing.

Transformational experiences occur in the everyday, where relationships communicate safety in a congruent and consistent way over time.

References
References for chapter

Ahnert, L., Eckstein-Madry, T., Piskernik, B., Porges, S.W. and Lamb, M.E. (2021). Infants' stress responses and protest behaviours at childcare entry and the role of care providers. *Developmental Psychobiology*, 63(6), e22156.

Bowlby, J. (1988). *A Secure Base: Parent-Child Attachment and Healthy Human Development*. New York, NY: Basic Books.

Cacioppo, J.T., Berntson, G.G., Sheridan, J.F. and McClintock, M.K. (2000). Multilevel integrative analyses of human behaviour: Social neuroscience and the complementing nature of social and biological approaches. *Psychological Bulletin*, 126, 829–843.

Carter, C.S. (2021). Oxytocin and love: Myths, metaphors and mysteries. *Comprehensive Psychoneuroendocrinology*, 9, 100107.

Damasio, A.R. (1994). *Descartes' Error: Emotion, Reason, and the Human Brain*. New York, NY: G.P. Putnam.

Dana, D. (2018). *The Polyvagal Theory in Therapy: Engaging the Rhythm of Regulation*. New York, NY: W.W. Norton and Company.

Descartes, R. 1596–1650. (1986). *Discourse on Method*. New York, NY: Collier Macmillan.

Dobzhansky, T. (1962). *Mankind Evolving*. New Haven, CT: Yale University Press.

Fanning, J., Silfer, J.L., Liu, H., Gauvin, L. *et al.* (2020). Relationships between respiratory sinus arrhythmia and stress in college students. *Journal of Behavioural Medicine*, 43(2), 308–317.

Gendlin, E. (2017). *A Process Model*. Evanston, IL: Northwestern University Press.

Jackson, J.H. (1884). The Croonian lectures on evolution and dissolution of the nervous system. *British Medical Journal*, 1, 703.

Kolacz, J., daSilva, E.B., Lewis, G.F., Bertenthal, B.I. and Porges, S.W. (2022). Associations between acoustic features of maternal speech and infants' emotion regulation following a social stressor. *Infancy*, 27, 135–158.

Kolacz, J., Hu, Y., Gesselman, A.N., Garcia, J.R., Lewis, G.F. and Porges, S.W. (2020). Sexual function in adults with a history of childhood maltreatment: Mediating effects of self-reported autonomic reactivity. *Psychological Trauma: Theory, Research, Practice and Policy*, 12(3), 281.

Kolacz, J., Kovacic, K., Lewis, G.F., Sood, M.R. *et al.* (2021). Cardiac autonomic regulation and joint hypermobility in adolescents with functional abdominal pain disorders. *Neurogastroenterology and Motility*, 33, e14165.

Kolacz, J., Kovacic, K.K. and Porges, S.W. (2019). Traumatic stress and the autonomic brain-gut connection in development: Polyvagal theory as an integrative framework for psychosocial and gastrointestinal pathology. *Developmental Psychobiology*, 61, 796–809.

Kolacz, J., Lewis, G.F. and Porges, S.W. (2018). The integration of vocal communication and biobehavioural state regulation in mammals: A polyvagal hypothesis. *Handbook of Behavioural Neuroscience*, 25, 23–34.

Kolacz, J. and Porges, S.W. (2018). Chronic diffuse pain and functional gastrointestinal disorders after traumatic stress: Pathophysiology through a polyvagal perspective. *Frontiers in Medicine*, 5, 145.

Kovacic, K., Kolacz, J., Lewis, G.F. and Porges, S.W. (2020). Impaired vagal efficiency predicts auricular neurostimulation response in adolescent functional abdominal pain disorders. *Official Journal of the American College of Gastroenterology*, 115(9), 1534–1538.

Levenson, R.W. (2003). Autonomic specificity and emotion. *Handbook of Affective Sciences*, 2, 212–224.

Porges, S.W. (1995). Orienting in a defensive world: Mammalian modifications of our evolutionary heritage. A polyvagal theory. *Psychophysiology*, 32, 301–318.

Porges, S.W. (1996). Physiological regulation in high-risk infants: A model for assessment and potential intervention. *Development and Psychopathology*, 8, 43–58.

Porges, S.W. (2001). The Polyvagal theory: Phylogenetic substrates of a social nervous system. *International Journal of Psychophysiology*, 42, 123–146.

Porges, S.W. (2003). Social engagement and attachment: A phylogenetic perspective. *Annals of the New York Academy of Sciences*, 1008, 31–47.

Porges, S.W. (2004). Neuroception: A subconscious system for detecting threats and safety. *Zero to Three*, 24, 19–24.

Porges, S.W. (2009). The polyvagal theory: New insights into adaptive reactions of the autonomic nervous system. *Cleveland Clinical Journal of Medicine*, 76, S86.

Porges, S.W. (2021a). *Polyvagal Safety: Attachment, Communication, Self-regulation*. New York, NY: W.W. Norton and Company.

Porges, S.W. (2021b). Polyvagal Theory: A biobehavioural journey to sociality. *Comprehensive Psychoneuroendocrinology*, 100069.

Porges, S.W., Bazhenova, O.V., Bal, E., Carlson, N. *et al.* (2014). Reducing auditory hypersensitivities in autistic spectrum disorder: Preliminary findings evaluating the listening project protocol. *Frontiers in Pediatrics*, 2, 80.

Porges, S.W. and Dana, D. (2018). *Clinical Applications of the Polyvagal Theory: The Emergence of Polyvagal-Informed Therapies*. New York, NY: W.W. Norton and Company.

Porges, S.W. and Furman, S.A. (2011). The early development of the autonomic nervous system provides a neural platform for social behaviour: A polyvagal perspective. *Infant and Child Development*, 20, 106–118.

Porges, S.W. and Lewis, G.F. (2010). The polyvagal hypothesis: Common mechanisms mediating autonomic regulation, vocalisations and listening. *Handbook of Behavioural Neuroscience*, 19, 255–264.

Porges, S.W., Macellaio, M., Stanfill, S.D., McCue, K. *et al.* (2013). Respiratory sinus arrhythmia and auditory processing in autism: Modifiable deficits of an integrated social engagement system? *International Journal of Psychophysiology*, 88, 261–270.

Tronick, E., Als, H., Adamson, L., Wise, S. and Brazelton, T.B. (1978). The infant's response to entrapment between contradictory messages in face-to-face interaction. *Journal of the American Academy of Child Psychiatry*, 17, 1–13.

van der Kolk, B.A. (2015). *The Body Keeps the Score: Brain, Mind, and Body in the Healing of Trauma*. New York, NY: Penguin Books.

Williamson, J.B., Heilman, K.M., Porges, E., Lamb, D. and Porges, S.W. (2013). A possible mechanism for PTSD symptoms in patients with traumatic brain injury: Central autonomic network disruption. *Frontiers in Neuroengineering*, 6, 13.

Williamson, J.B., Porges, E.C., Lamb, D.G. and Porges, S.W. (2015). Maladaptive autonomic regulation in PTSD accelerates physiological aging. *Frontiers in Psychology*, 5, 1571.

Wundt, W.M. and Judd, C.H. (1902). *Outlines of Psychology*. London: W. Engelmann.

References for Knowledge and Practice Reflection

Atkinson, J. (2002). *Trauma Trails: The Transgenerational Effects of Trauma in Indigenous Australia*. North Melbourne: Spinifex Press.

Bamblett, L. (2013). *Our Stories Are Our Survival*. Canberra: Aboriginal Studies Press.

Bamblett, M., Harrison, J. and Lewis, P. (2010). Proving culture and voice works: Towards creating the evidence base for resilient Aboriginal and Torres Strait Islander children in Australia. *International Journal of Child and Family Welfare*, 13(1–2), 98–113.

Dana, D. (2021). *Anchored: How to Befriend Your Nervous System Using Polyvagal Theory*. Sydney: Pan MacMillan.

Harris, M. and Fallot, R.D. (2001). Envisioning a trauma-informed service system: A vital paradigm shift. *New Directions for Mental Health Services*, 2001(89), 3–22.

Kickett, G., Chandran, S. and Mitchell, J. (2020). Dabakan Kooyliny Go Slowly, Walk Slowly, Walk Together: Culturally Strong Therapeutic Care for Aboriginal and Torres Strait Islander Children, Families and Communities. In J. Mitchell, J. Tucci and E. Tronick (eds), *The Handbook of Therapeutic Care for Children: Evidence Informed Approaches to Working with Traumatised Children and Adolescents in Foster, Kinship and Adoptive Care* (pp.159–184). London: Jessica Kingsley Publishers.

Kim, I, and Ashmore, T. (2019). The Trauma-Informed Inpatient Facility. In R. Benjamin, J. Haliburn and S. King (eds), *Humanising Mental Health Care in Australia: A Guide to Trauma-informed Approaches* (pp.342–354). London: Routledge.

Kontio, R., Joffe, G., Putkonen, H., Kuosmanen, L. *et al.* (2012). Seclusion and restraint in psychiatry: Patients' experiences and practical suggestions on how to improve practices and use alternatives. *Perspectives in Psychiatric Care*, 48(1), 16–−24.

Substance Abuse and Mental Health Services Administration (SAMHSA) (2014). *Trauma-Informed Care in Behavioural Health Services – Treatment Improvement Protocol (TIP) Series 57* (HHS Publication no. (SMA) 13-4801).

Tucci, J., Mitchell, J., Holmes, D., Hemsworth, C. and Hemsworth, L. (2015). Constructing a child protection policy to support a safeguarding children culture in organizations and institutions. *Children Australia*, 39, 45–64.

Tucci, J., Weller, A and Mitchell, J. (2018). Realizing 'Deep' Safety for Children who have Experienced Abuse: Application of Polyvagal Theory in Therapeutic Work with Traumatized Children and Young People. In S. Porges and D. Dana (eds), *Clinical Applications of the Polyvagal Theory: The Emergence of Polyvagal-Informed Therapies* (pp.89–105). New York, NY: W.W. Norton.

Watson, S., Thorburn, K., Everett, M. and Fisher, K.R. (2014). Care without coercion—mental health rights, personal recovery and trauma-informed care. *Australian Journal of Social Issues*, 49(4), 529–549.

CHAPTER 3

The Social Brain

Louis Cozolino, Chloe Drulis and Carly Samuelson

As social organs of adaptation, our brains are shaped and reshaped by the nature and quality of our relationships. Within a matrix of care, communication, challenge and struggle, our social interactions determine the growth of neurons, the production of neurochemicals and trigger genetic expression. In essence, early caretaking and all intimate relationships are evolution's way of shaping each human brain. Without mutually stimulating interactions, people (and neurons for that matter) wither and die. In neurons, this process is called apoptosis (programmed cell death); in humans, it is called failure to thrive, anaclitic depression, or dying of a broken heart. Regardless of age, it is vital for us to feel a part of, participate in, and contribute to our communities. The inability to connect with others results in alienation, anxiety and depression. As scientific discoveries shed light on the translation of relationships into the structures and functions of our brains, we are gaining insight into both the impact of developmental trauma and new possibilities of healing.

In this chapter, we explore this concept of the brain as a social organ and how it informs our understanding of mental health, suffering and healing. We will look back to our common tribal histories to see how the values and strategies of our ancestors provide clues about the social instincts which still live within us. We will also consider what can be learned about mental health and the treatment of mental distress from what we have understood from the fields of evolution and neuroscience. Finally, and most importantly, we will explore how this knowledge can be applied to our work as therapists.

The social brain

The recognition of the brain as a social organ suggests that humans have evolved to link together to create super-organisms that we call families, tribes and nations. Our brains have evolved many systems dedicated to receiving, processing and sending social information to others. For example, we have a specific neural system dedicated to the recognition of right-side-up faces that allows us to immediately distinguish familiar from unfamiliar others (Gauthier *et al.*, 2000; Halgren *et al.*, 1999). When faces are turned upside-down, processing gets transferred to our object recognition systems, which is why we find it harder to recognize inverted faces. Another neural network connecting the prefrontal cortex and the amygdala is dedicated to the regulation of emotion and the construction of attachment schema.

Humans have also evolved to automatically send and receive messages about our emotions, bodily states and states of mind via mirror neurons. Mirror neurons exist within neural systems designed to support the creation of an internal representation of the actions, expressions and emotions of others within our own bodies. This allows us to be able to feel our own version of what others are feeling, especially strong emotions like pain, fear, disgust, love and joy. This is especially important for the parents of young children who need to read the primitive expressions of comfort and distress acted out by their children. Research has shown that our internal organs are automatically linked to our facial expressions to provide others with a real-time readout of our internal biological state (Porges, 2011).

Most neural systems dedicated to social connectedness are built via an interaction between our genetic inheritance and our lived experience. The complex wiring of our cortex is largely shaped by our particular set of interpersonal experiences early in life. As social animals, this adaptation strategy most likely maximizes the survival of both the individual and the tribe. Of course, this is not without its problems. The brains of many children are shaped by people and situations that may not be good models for survival outside the family and thus, poorly suited to long-term adaptation. This certainly describes many of the clients who come to us seeking help. Our challenge is to make their unconscious adaptational patterns conscious, and then modify them in ways more in line with their present situation and long-term goals.

Human infants are born into the most abject dependency of any living creature. Because of this basic fact, connection equals survival. It takes many years for us to be able to survive without parents or caretakers. Because of this, a human's first order of business is to attach to our parents and trigger the bonding instincts in them so they take care of us. We stare into their eyes, grab their fingers, smile and coo, and cry when they leave us alone. For at least the first decade of life, our caretakers and immediate family are our entire world. These interactions teach us about the safety and dangers of the world, how to connect with others, regulate our anxieties, and give us a sense of what the future will bring.

The genes we inherit from our parents serve to organize the brain while experience orchestrates ongoing genetic transcription (epigenetics) that allows experience to shape the brain. When we play peek-a-boo with a child we hide our face with our hands, then expose our face, and say 'peek a boo' with wide eyes, an exaggerated smile, and a high-pitched voice. The baby's eyes and mouth open wide and then they give us a big smile and maybe even an open mouth laugh. What just happened in our brains? First, the surprise and big smile stimulated metabolic activity in both the baby's and the parent's brain, delivering extra glucose and oxygen to support learning. We both experience surges of oxytocin, dopamine and serotonin triggered by our mutual enjoyment, making us feel good and want to do it again (Again! Again!) (Schore, 1997). Epigenetic processes within the baby's brain trigger neuroanatomic growth that supports a sense of joy and creates the building blocks of long-term well-being.

A good example of this is the epigenetic translation of pleasurable experiences into the building of endorphin receptors on the baby's amygdala. The more of these receptors we build, the more endorphins we have in our nervous system to keep the amygdala downregulated, decreasing our vulnerability to stress, anxiety and fear. This is one of the many physiological variables related to things like ego-strength, grit and resilience. In stark contrast to this situation are the many children who lack quality caretakers, attentive others, or positive stimulation. Within the brains of these children, opposite biochemical and neuroanatomic processes occur that lead them to be more vulnerable to stress. This is why children with a greater number of adverse social experiences during childhood (e.g. parental psychopathology, exposure to domestic violence) are far more likely to experience psychological, physical and adaptational difficulties later in life (Felitti *et al.*, 1998). Our social experiences are translated, for better and worse, into the structure of our brains and tend to stabilize over time.

Our conceptual challenge

In Eurocentric cultures, we are taught to cherish our individuality and encouraged to experience the world from the perspective of a separate self. This naturally leads us to see ourselves and others as isolated beings rather than a part of the larger whole. Another consequence of this separation is that we tend to search for technical solutions to human problems and imagine that our brains function like computers. Take, for example, the way in which physicians responded to the high mortality rates of children in orphanages early in the last century. Assuming that micro-organisms were to blame, they isolated children from caretakers and one another. Despite these interventions, children continued to die at alarming rates until attachment researchers suggested that they be allowed to interact with one another and nurtured by consistent caretakers (Blum, 2002).

This is powerful evidence for the fact that our brains are social organs and that human contact and attunement are vital to survival and healthy development. John Bowlby and his colleagues provided us with the insight that the mother-child dyad is also a complex adaptive organism (Bowlby, 1969). Attachment schema, although interpreted as existing within the child, are actually expressions of the adaptational patterns of the mother-child interactions. This is why children can have different attachment schema with each parent and others outside the family. Once the definition of 'a living system' is liberated from the individual, we are free to consider two or more interconnected people as a living system that needs to be understood for its unique properties.

Early experiences have a disproportionately powerful role in sculpting the networks of attachment and affect regulation due to the strength of learning during these sensitive periods (Ainsworth *et al.*, 1978). The child's first reality is the parents' unconscious, transferred via right-hemisphere-to-right-hemisphere attunement, well before self-awareness and the emergence of a separate identity (Enlow *et al.*, 2013). Because it is encoded in early implicit memory, it is never experienced as anything other than the self. Just as positive experiences equip us with feelings of self-assurance and optimism, suboptimal bonding experiences become stored within implicit memory, carried into adulthood, and become woven into our adult relationships.

The view that the human brain is a social organ is supported by thousands of studies in social psychology as well as many other scientific disciplines. Going back to the middle of the last century, the field of psychoneuroimmunology had been exploring the connections between relationship quality and our physical health. Many family therapists also see the family as a biological organism that they use to understand and address the symptomatology of an individual member. The idea that the brain functions as a social organ emerged in neuroscience during the 1970s when researchers began to discover links between the individual biochemistry of primates and the behaviour of entire troops (Kling and Steklis, 1976). Since then, the fields of social and affective neuroscience have been charting the neural terrain dedicated to social and emotional interactions which allow us to form, maintain and sustain interpersonal relationships. Despite all the evidence, it remains a struggle to think of the social interdependency of the brain because the idea is in such stark contradiction to the dominant philosophical and political theories that organize Western thought.

The evolution of the social brain

To understand how the brain evolved into a social organ, we begin with the assumption that our highly social brains have been shaped by natural selection to enhance survival via cooperation. Cooperation-based survival is seen across many species from beehives, to herds of impala, to penguin colonies. We can witness the fact that our surviving primate ancestors, such as bonobos, chimps and apes, are highly social beings. The best evidence suggests that anatomically modern humans evolved over the last 100,000 years in tribal communities of between 75 and 125 individuals. These interdependent groups, held together by kinship, cooperation and shared culture, were the environment in which the human brain was shaped for its survival. As brains became increasingly sophisticated, tribes became even more interdependent and adaptive super-organisms.

While Western culture has changed a great deal during just the last five thousand years, our brains changed at a much slower rate. Our instincts, physiology, biochemistry and the neural networks that evolved in the context of tribal life are essentially unchanged. It is possible that a good deal of the anxiety and depression so common in modern society may be partly explained by the alienation of our tribal brains. There is also considerable evidence supporting the idea that those who become a member of one or more 'tribes' tend to struggle less with the isolated nature of modern culture. From church-goers to sports fans to gang members, the drive to join some version of a tribe and the benefits derived from membership are undeniable. It appears that at this point in our evolution, we have a strong instinct to keep one foot firmly planted in our tribal past.

In contrast to tribal life, the relatively recent emergence of industrial society is characterized by larger groups, division of labour, and constant contact with strangers. Equality and cooperation are replaced with dominance hierarchies, competition, and a decreasing concern for fairness. If you have not already noticed, these changes cause stress for our essentially Paleolithic brains organized by our more primitive social instincts. This appears to contribute to the difficulties encountered by indigenous groups during attempts at assimilation with their colonial conquerors. It is also central to the challenges of mental health workers of the dominant culture to understand and assist those whom their culture has conquered and continues to marginalize. Some of the basic differences between tribal and industrial societies include:

The tribe	Industrial society
Small groups	Large groups
Cooperation	Individualism
Equality/Fairness	Dominance hierarchy
Democratic decision making	Imposed and enforced rules
Cohesiveness	Competition
Shared responsibilities	Unequal division of labour

If these tribal values shaped the evolution of our social brains for most of our history, then we can expect that they continue to exist at the core of our primitive social instincts. It is likely that the most viable tribes were egalitarian, flexible and inclusive, thus maximizing the contribution of all of their members. On the other hand, tribes that exhibited coercive social control were less likely to succeed. This may be why we are not able to tolerate more than minimal coercion or injustice within groups of familiars and need to find scientific and religious rationalizations to objectify and denigrate those whom we oppress. Perhaps contemporary humans have such a low tolerance for inequality because we were programmed long ago to champ at the bit of unjust social control that had come to be associated with tribal failure. To this day, highly functional and long-lived countries and institutions manage to create a sense of living under generally accepted customs and fair laws.

Sociostasis

Each of us is a slightly more complex version of a neuron – we all receive, process and transmit information and are a small part of a larger whole. Like neurons, we also transmit information across the space which separates us – the social synapse. In addition, we activate, inhibit and influence each other through our interactions via sociostasis. Each neuron and every brain is a matrix of chemical, electrical and genetic information, which serves our survival and the survival of those in our tribe.

The basic principle is that brains connect, attune and regulate one another just like ensembles of neurons within a functional neural network. In functional relationships, this serves the goal of mutual regulation and positive group coordination. The same abilities also allow for the transmission of trauma in dysfunctional families and the negative phenomena of groupthink, group hysteria and the destructive behaviour of mobs. Our brains are also filled with images, emotions and incessant internal dialogues which guide our moment-to-moment experience. We are clearly wired to function as individuals embedded within multiple groups, balancing our own needs with the needs of those around us. Think about all of those spontaneous voices you hear in your head that remind you of the perceptions of others and the rules of the group. The endless 'shoulds' that go around in our heads that can make us feel that we are not good enough likely served to improve tribal coordination back into prehistory. The judge and jury we carry around in our heads keeps us in line via guilt and shame, constantly reminding us to stay in line and worry about the concerns of the herd.

The notion that the family is a complex biological organism (as proposed by Murray Bowen, 1978) is supported by the discovery that we regulate each other's arousal, mood and immunological functioning. This is why we see many health benefits and risks of being in either good or bad relationships. This process of 'sociostasis' is the mechanism by which a family's behaviour

becomes organized around the regulation of anxiety. The role of the identified patient, the breakdown of open communication and the formation
of dysfunctional alliances are all attempts to regulate both the anxiety of
the more powerful memories of the family. The common adult experience
of going back home and regressing to old patterns of thoughts, behaviours
and feelings clearly reflects this process.

The term 'placebo effect' is generally thought of as a person's ability
to feel better after taking a sugar pill. This effect is so powerful that any
good research study must have a placebo or contrast group to be considered solid science. The word 'placebo' is Latin for 'I shall please', reflecting
the patient's desire to live up to their doctor's expectations. This desire
to please can be amplified by the doctor's status, bearing and reputation.
The optimism of the healer parallels that of the encouraging parent who
has dreams of her children's success and supports their unfolding in the
process. Ongoing neuroplasticity and neurogenesis provide us with a solid
foundation for ongoing optimism with any client at any time regardless of
their struggle. In essence, the placebo effect is a sociostatic mechanism that
impacts our biochemistry, neuroanatomy and conscious experience. It has
been suggested that a better term for this sociostatic process is a 'meaning
response' that can be applied to the power of social beliefs on an individual
(Moerman and Jonas, 2002).

Chinese Americans born during inauspicious years have been found
to have significantly shorter lifespans, an effect that is proportional to
how strongly they hold to traditional cultural beliefs (Phillips, Ruth, and
Wagner, 1993). In another important example, drugs usually have the
strongest results just after they are released, when doctors and patients are
expecting positive results. Drugs become less effective over time as negative
reports, side-effects, and doubts about the drug become public. Research
in classrooms has shown that when teachers were given false IQ results
and told which children in their classroom were about to bloom over the
next academic year, the randomly chosen bloomers showed greater gains in
total IQ and reasoning compared to the control group. These students were
also rated by their teachers as more intellectually curious, better adjusted,
happier and less needy of approval than the students in the control group.
The power of relationships to change lives, and the sociostatic mechanisms
which drive them, are powerful and undeniable.

The social synapse

As you probably already know, individual neurons are separated by small
gaps called synapses. Although the word gap implies emptiness, these tiny
gaps are filled to capacity with a wide array of chemical substances that
carry out highly sophisticated communication. Commonly called neural

transmission, this relentless trans-synaptic gossip allows each neuron to live, grow and build functional relationships with one another. Over vast expanses of evolutionary time, synaptic transmission has grown increasingly intricate to meet the needs of more complex brains. There is no such thing as an individual neuron. Neurons that are unable to connect with and develop a functional relationship with other neurons die. The surviving neurons work together to create the functional neural networks which we depend on for everything, from breathing to consciousness.

The social synapse is the space between us, the medium through which we communicate with and link to one another, and it is anything but empty space. When we smile, wave and say hello, our behaviours are converted into sights and sounds which are transferred across the social synapse to the sense organs of others – their cell surface, if you will. Receptors in the sense organs of the receiver convert these electrical and mechanical messages into electrochemical impulses within their brains. These signals stimulate internal biochemical changes, new behaviours, and the sending of messages back across the social synapse. From the moment we are born, our survival depends on connecting to those around us through touch, smell, sights and sounds. If we are able to connect with available and nurturing others, we will usually bond, attach and survive.

Growing up as a member of a marginalized or oppressed group will be converted into neural structures in these same ways. Given that our self-concept is infused with our place in the family, neighbourhood and the general culture, prejudice becomes woven into our brains, minds and our developing sense of self. Racial disadvantages within a society, which accrue over generations, result in compounding negative psychological, social and biological effects (Geronimus, 1992; Mays, Cochran and Barnes, 2007).

The social synapse has an exceedingly broad bandwidth, ranging from the conscious communication of words, sustained facial expressions and touch, to unconscious messages via pupil dilation, scent and fleeting facial expressions. Dilated pupils signal to others that we see them as trustworthy and that it is safe to approach, while blushing lets others know we are aware that we have committed a social faux pas and feel embarrassed by our transgression (Hess, 1975; Lynch, 1985). Both of these reactions are not under conscious control but evolved as automatic and unconscious forms of social communication. Scientists continue to uncover new ways in which we are linked, imitate each other, coordinate our behaviours and build each other's brains.

The biochemistry of attachment

Mother-child bonding is the cradle of the evolution of the human social brain. For young children, survival does not depend on how fast we can run, climb a tree, or tell the difference between edible and poisonous mush-rooms. Rather, we survive based on our abilities to bond with our parents and become woven into the social world around us. One aspect of the building of attachment schema is the linking of good feelings (elevated lev-els of oxytocin/dopamine/serotonin) with proximity to good attachment figures, and associating bad feelings (lower levels of these biochemicals) with separation from them (Feldman, 2012).

Experiencing a positive and supportive connection with another acti-vates soothing biochemistry, supporting greater affect regulation and amyg-dala inhibition. In turn, these changes allow for greater protein synthesis, upregulated immunological functioning and increased neuroplasticity necessary for learning. These basic changes drive the neurodynamics of the brain in ways that allow for better executive functioning and problem-solv-ing abilities. They also bring the changes that occur in the consulting room into our client's lives.

A prime mechanism of evolutionary change occurs via changes in the biochemistry within areas of our cortex and limbic system which drive our social behaviours. Oxytocin, vasopressin and endorphins, which initially shaped the experience of reward and reaction to physical pain, were later leveraged to make us feel better when with our loved ones and anxious when apart. These neurochemicals are involved with everything from parental instincts, attachment and pair bonding, to empathy, compassion and altruistic behaviour. Oxytocin and vasopressin modulate bonding, social behaviour and anxiety in humans and a wide range of other species. Oxytocin has also been found to be generated and released in the amygdala and the heart, reflecting their central role in both anxiety and attachment.

The effects of oxytocin are to direct a child's attention towards their mother while driving maternal behaviour and inhibiting irritability and aggressiveness. For example, when an infant suckles at their mother's breast, the nipple triggers the hypothalamus to release oxytocin into the bloodstream, triggering a sense of well-being in the mother and contrac-tions of the muscles of her breasts to force milk to the nipples (Carter, 1990, 1998; Panksepp et al., 1998; Ross and Young, 2009). Vasopressin, the male equivalent to oxytocin, facilitates pair bonding, attachment, and the main-tenance of monogamy. Its antagonistic relationship with testosterone leads to decreased aggression and sexual behaviour in males while in caretaking relationships (Delville, Mansour and Ferris, 1996). The growth of oxytocin receptors is stimulated early in life via epigenetic expression triggered by maternal attention.

The touch, pressure and warmth of another increases oxytocin and decreases blood pressure, which may explain why intimate relationships and massage correlate with physical and emotional well-being (Bartz and Hollander, 2006; Uvnas-Moberg, 1997). Oxytocin and vasopressin also support the protein synthesis necessary for neuroplastic processes involved in learning, which is why positive emotional connections with teachers result in better educational outcomes (Insel, 1997; Ostrowski, 1998). With higher levels of oxytocin, we pay more attention to faces, movements and social cues from others. Increasing oxytocin levels has been shown to promote trust and empathy, increase perspective taking of others, and enhance communication during conflict. This is probably why a little oxytocin will increase generosity, charitable contributions and prosocial behaviour in people with autism (Green *et al.*, 2001).

Individual healing

While evolution has burdened us with ample sources of mental distress, it has also provided us with social brains that we can use to heal one another. It is no secret that the most powerful lever of positive change across psychotherapy, education and counselling is the quality of the human connection we are able to establish with those we work with. By utilizing the basic Rogerian principles of warmth, congruence and positive regard, therapists leverage their connection with their clients' social brains. This process supports emotional regulation and neuroplasticity in the service of positive change. Therapists who see therapy as a technical intervention that they perform on a client, as opposed to a human journey they take with a client, can easily miss the power of sociostasis to drive positive therapeutic change. Techniques, clinical knowledge and experience are all important, but it is the quality of the relationship that creates the state of brain and mind that allows us to benefit from our therapists, guides and teachers.

During early periods of exuberant neural growth, our experiences are converted into neural infrastructures that either make us more resilient or more vulnerable to mental and physical illness later in life. A basic assumption is that loving connections and secure attachments build healthy and resilient brains, while neglectful and insecure attachments can result in brains that are vulnerable to stress, dysregulation and illness. Some good news is that attachment circuits remain plastic throughout life as evidenced by how much grandparents are capable of loving their grandchildren, despite meeting them later in life (Vaillant, 2002). By treating clients as worthy of our attention and care, we activate mirror neuron systems that allow for learning through imitation, support plasticity and boost their courage to try new ways of being. There are many ways in which psychotherapy parallels re-parenting. Through the therapeutic relationship, we are attempting to modify the same circuits of attachment, emotional regulation and autobiographical memory as those shaped during childhood. We also use the same attentive and nurturing sociostatic processes to help our clients regulate their anxiety, provide them with challenges at the edge of their capabilities and help them to articulate their thoughts, feelings and experiences. All of these aspects of psychotherapy are central to positive parenting, secure attachment and building resilience.

From a neuroscience perspective, what we may experience as resistance is the reflection of a complex network of implicit emotional, somatic, motor and sensory memories programmed earlier in life. They are the brain-mind's best guess about what is necessary to survive today, based on what happened long ago. Our primitive brain works on a strict assumption that past experience is the best predictor of what we should do in the present. The more stressed or frightened we become, the more likely we will regress to old, familiar patterns of interacting with the world. We see this all the time in children who develop new skills, only to see them disappear in the face of anxiety and trauma.

Therefore, resistance is not something that we have to wait out; instead, the focus on and resolution of resistance is a central component of therapy. A core aspect of successful therapy is embracing resistance as a past accomplishment that allowed a client to survive stressful and dangerous circumstances. By embracing resistance, you take away their need to employ it, which allows them to be less anxious, less defensive and more open to change. This was Carl Roger's secret weapon – a sophisticated method usually missed by those without experience.

The transference a client brings to therapy is another part of the resistance they bring in which is based on past learning. Transference is another part of resistance that is based on past learning and often arises in therapy. While sometimes difficult to navigate, the transference brings past struggles with parents and other figures into the therapeutic relationship, allowing a client to be seen, understood and worked with. Transference and attachment schema always become activated during therapy relationships, and they are generally interconnected. Both are forms of implicit memory systems that are based on early relationships and can be triggered, positively or negatively, in the context of current relationships. Negative transference can be more distressing but positive transference is usually more difficult to uncover and process.

Group healing

The mismatch of values between indigenous and dominant groups has left a trail of suffering back into prehistory. Unlike Western culture, indigenous cultures most often approach generativity through cooperation toward a common goal. Each member shares responsibility and motivation to meet the collective needs of the group. This synergy is reflected in many facets of tribal life. Important processes, such as educating the younger generation, are approached collaboratively through hands-on experience, relationships and storytelling. These practices appear to optimize mental and physical health, immunological functioning and the neuroplasticity required for learning and adaptation.

We survive by attuning to, imitating and learning from our caretakers and others in our family. Analysts often say that a child's first reality is their mother's unconscious. As such, it is also a matrix for the transfer of parental psychopathology, intergenerational trauma, cultural prejudice and oppression. Colonization, marginalization and genocide jeopardize the mental and physical health of survivors, their children and the entire community for many generations (Menzies, 2019). The collateral damage manifests in insecure attachment, more adverse experiences, and the difficulties involved with integrating into a society without place or purpose (Milroy, 2005).

Many victims of violence and abuse have been additionally traumatized because of their membership in one or more marginalized group. The impact of these experiences can only be appreciated in the context of their race, class, gender, sexual orientation or particular challenges. The complexity of this intersectionality denies any simple diagnosis, theory or treatment. It also points to the necessity of our participation in the work of social justice, diversity and inclusion if we are to be taken seriously in the consulting room. Psychotherapy, especially with those victimized by social trauma, is by definition a politically subversive act.

Indigenous practices such as storytelling, using somatosensory experiences, and social bonding are powerful tools for rebuilding communities after trauma. Storytelling of loss, hardship and of better times to come is a powerful means of processing and healing from trauma. Crafting a cohesive narrative allows victims to tether painful memories to a historical timeline that cannot be controlled and distorted by others. Somatosensory experiences, such as physical touch, song and dance, tap into neural pathways that promote healing (Perry, 2008). Despite our cultural differences, we all have similar underlying biochemistry which drives our connectivity, learning, immunological functioning and well-being. The goal in all of these modalities is to create and foster a sense of connection, a recognition of what has been lost, a vision of rebirth and possibilities for tomorrow. But, more importantly, if we are to facilitate healing, we must understand and respect the basic principles of tribal life, listen to and learn from members of other societies and enthusiastically support the kinds of programmes our clients feel are necessary for healing. As 'healers', we need to participate in these rituals and incorporate them into our understanding and appreciation of our clients.

It is clear that our social brains require supportive and cohesive communities to provide us with a sense of structure, security and meaning. So how does a group cope with a 'blow to the basic tissues of social life that damages the bonds attaching people together and impairs the prevailing sense of community' (Erikson, 1976)? How does a group grapple with being subjugated, displaced and fragmented, while forced to navigate a dominant society that is antithetical to its core values and basic social instincts? Further, how does a group deal with a cultural trauma that has been internalized, normalized and passed down to the next generations (Duran and Duran, 1995)? The healing process needs to include reclaiming one's cultural history, exorcizing internalized prejudice, working actively for change and developing a positive personal narrative for the future. At the same time, those in the dominant culture, often the therapists trying to be of assistance, need to engage in an exploration of their own biases and prejudices, work actively for social justice and participate in the necessary reparation required for their own healing.

Diversity and inclusion is much more than a heterogeneous headcount – it should also be reflected in an openness to concepts and worldviews that may be unfamiliar or unaligned with our own. As one example, what if poor health is better understood and treated as a loss of connection between the family, the land and our ancestors (Krieg, 2009)? For those with a deeply historical and intimate connection with the land, there are likely forms of secure and insecure attachment to environment that have yet to be studied. This type of attachment may serve identity development and self-esteem in ways never conceived of within Western psychology. There may be ways in which it serves affect regulation that John Bowlby never conceived of from the perspective of his analytic chair. Those of us who are attempting to be of service need to be wary of superimposing our worldview onto others. Perhaps the greatest gift we can offer our clients is to be quiet, listen deeply and open our minds to new learning. Rather than approaching our clients only as mental health professionals, what if we worked together to create spaces for increased understanding and appreciation? What if we worked together as equals for mutual healing? We suspect this is when we would discover the true healing power of our social brains.

KNOWLEDGE AND PRACTICE REFLECTION

Joe Tucci, Janise Mitchell, Ed Tronick and Stephen W. Porges

This chapter by Cozolino, Drulis and Samuelson affirms the significance of relationships in the evolution of the human species. We are meant to connect. Our survival depends on it. Our capacity to develop is totally reliant on it. Our neurobiology is hardwired to belong to a family, a community, a network of people for whom we care and who care for us. Importantly, it explores beyond the individual to the group.

It is why interpersonal violence has such a poisonous impact on our beings. Trauma blocks and distorts the social synapse, as Cozolino has defined here and in his earlier work (Cozolino, 2012, 2020). It permeates our physiological states. It affects our memory. It shapes the way we view ourselves and our identity as it relates to others. It sets up preferred ways of responding to threat and danger. It reorganizes our need and drive to be connected, amplifying the ongoing consequences of the violation over the life course. Where relationships should nurture, mend and heal, after violence, they become sites of terror, fear and confusion.

Critically, Cozolino and colleagues refer more broadly to violation that occurs because power structures in society serve to oppress specific groups, which experience such power differences as marginalization based on age, race, sex, gender, socio-economic status, cultural identification, disability and history. So trauma is not only the interpersonal violence from one individual to another, but also the outcome of members of one group's discrimination and prejudice expressed in attitude, language and behaviour towards another group's members. This forms a background pastiche of disadvantage and adversity through which individual acts of violence become more pronounced, reinforcing the powerlessness of those individuals in relation to others.

Cozolino, Drulis and Samuelson maintain that:

> The healing process needs to include reclaiming one's cultural history, exorcising internalized prejudice, working actively for change, and developing a positive personal narrative for the future. At the same time, those in the dominant culture, often the therapists trying to be of assistance, need to engage in an exploration of their own biases and prejudices, work actively for social justice and participate in the necessary reparation required for their own healing.

Trauma-transformative practice needs to consider the matrix of power within which it sits. Such critique of power has not traditionally been located with trauma knowledge. It has been more the purview of authors who emphasize justice and accountability (Friere, 1972; Reynolds, 2010, 2013), narrative and community development based work (Waldergrave *et al.*, 2003, 2012; White and Epston, 1990; White, 2006; Denborough, 2006) and compassion-oriented interventions (Gilbert, 2009, 2010, 2020a, 2020b).

But the integration of other frames of reference about the ways in which violence is an expression of oppression means that a richer vein of interpretive resources becomes available for practitioners and organizations. As Tucci and Mitchell take up in Chapter 17, it is the small acts of resistance against violence that need to be listened to, attended to and supported to grow and that challenge the influence that oppression holds in communities. This is not a means through which victims and survivors come to execute their lost sense of personal agency. Personal agency is a fraught construct in the trauma field. It is not simple. If individuals are designed along sociostatic principles, then collaboration and cooperation are the logical conclusions. Individual agency is more in keeping with Western views about the self as contained within a non-permeable boundary with individual motivations, intentions and action. Instead, in keeping with other traditions of thought, the self is far less rigid – always expressed in union with others and drawing on the physical, cultural and spiritual environment that it relates to.

Trauma-transformative practitioners, organizations and systems recognize the influence of the social context from which victims and survivors emerge to seek out support. They are clear that inclusion and diversity are essential in relation to themselves, other personnel and service users, ensuring that there are non-discriminatory policies in place. But more than that, trauma-transformative practice holds a pluralistic view of knowledge, resisting the temptation to give more weight and authority to one form of knowledge over another. The knowledge domains that trauma-transformative practitioners, organizations and systems should at the very least hold are: the deep explanatory frames stemming from neuroscience, research and evidence-based knowledge, cultural wisdom (especially that derived from the knowledge of First Nations peoples), insights drawn from those with lived and living experience of trauma, and knowledge that comes from the reflections of practitioners as they undertake their roles in supporting victims and survivors. It is important that the knowledge architecture of a trauma-transformative framework as it is applied is explicitly articulated and the underlying value base and philosophy underpinning it is analysed for congruency.

Pluralist practitioners, organizations and systems that are willing to remain open to new knowledge from different sources serve their community of service users and stakeholders effectively, ensuring that the referencing of certain knowledge over other knoweldge does not replicate the discursive practices of power that lead to the subjugation and oppression of some groups in society. It keeps open the willingness of practitioners, organizations and systems to being challenged by knowledge that cannot be dismissed because it is viewed as more inferior in form and substance.

Even more critically, as will be evidenced, in subsequent chapters, trauma-transformative practice will need to ensure that its design is explicitly geared towards anti-oppressive and decolonizing ways of working. Commitment to such practice is critical in recognizing the corrosive effects of colonizing and discrimination-based forms of trauma in the present and over time, transgenerationally.

References
References for chapter

Ainsworth, M.D.S., Blehar, M.C., Waters, E. and Wall, S. (1978). *Patterns of Attachment: A Psychological Study of the Strange Situation.* Hillsdale, NJ: Erlbaum.

Bartz, J.A. and Hollander, E. (2006). The neuroscience of affiliation: Forging links between basic and clinical research on neuropeptides and social behaviour. *Hormones and Behaviour*, 50, 518–528.

Blum, D. (2002). *Love at Goon Park.* Cambridge: Perseus.

Bowen, M. (1978). *Family Therapy in Clinical Practice.* Northvale, NJ: Jason Aronson.

Bowlby, J. (1969). *Attachment.* New York, NY: Basic Books.

Carter, C.S. (1998). Neuroendocrine perspectives on social attachment and love. *Psychoneuroendocrinology*, 23, 779–818.

Delville, Y., Mansour, K.M. and Ferris, C.F. (1996). Testosterone facilitates aggression by modulating vasopressin receptors in the hypothalamus. *Physiology and Behaviour*, 60, 25–29.

Duran, E. and Duran, B. (1995). *Native American Post-Colonial Psychology.* Albany, NY: State University of New York Press.

Enlow, M., Egeland, B., Carlson, E., Blood, E. and Wright, R. (2013). Mother-infant attachment and the intergenerational transmission of post-traumatic stress disorder. *Development and Psychopathology*, 26(1), 41–65.

Erikson, K.T. (1976). Disaster at Buffalo Creek. Loss of communality at Buffalo Creek. *The American Journal of Psychiatry*, 133(3), 302–305.

Feldman, R. (2012). Oxytocin and social affiliation in humans. *Hormones and Behaviour*, 61(3), 380–391.

Felitti, V.J., Anda, R.F., Nordenberg, D., Williamson, D.F. *et al.* (1998). Relationship of childhood abuse and household dysfunction to many of the leading causes of death in adults: The Adverse Childhood Experiences (ACE) Study. *American Journal of Preventive Medicine*, 14(4), 245–258.

Gauthier, I., Tarr, M.J., Moylan, J., Skudlarski, P., Gore, J.C. and Anderson, A.W. (2000). The fusiform 'face area' is part of a network that processes faces at the individual level. *Journal of Cognitive Neuroscience*, 12(3), 495–504.

Geronimus A.T. (1992). The weathering hypothesis and the health of African-American women and infants: Evidence and speculations. *Ethnicity and Disease*, 2(3), 207–221.

Green, L., Fein, D., Modahl, C., Feinstein, C., Waterhouse L. and Morris M. (2001). Oxytocin and autistic disorder: Alterations in peptide forms. *Biological Psychiatry*, 50(8), 609–613.

Halgren, E., Dale, A.M., Sereno, M.I., Tootelll, R.B., Marinkovic, K. and Rosen B.R. (1999). Location of human face-selective cortex with respect to retinotopic areas. *Human Brain Mapping*, 7, 29–37.

Hess, E.H. (1975). The role of pupil size in communication. *Scientific American*, 233, 110–119.

Insel, T.R. (1997). A neurobiological basis of social attachment. *American Journal of Psychiatry*, 154, 726–735.

Kling. A. and Steklis, H.D. (1976). A neural substrate for affiliative behaviour in nonhuman primates. *Brain Behaviours and Evolution*, 13, 216–238.

Krieg, A. (2009). The experience of collective trauma in Australian Indigenous communities. *Australasian Psychiatry*, 17(S1), 28–32.

Lynch, J.J. (1985). *The Language of the Heart: The Body's Response to Human Dialogue.* New York, NY: Basic Books.

Mays, V.M., Cochran, S.D. and Barnes, N.W. (2007). Race, race-based discrimination, and health outcomes among African Americans. *Annual Review of Psychology*, 58, 201–225.

Menzies, K. (2019). Understanding the Australian Aboriginal experience of collective, historical and intergenerational trauma. *International Social Work*, 62.

Milroy, H. (2005). Preface. In S.R. Zubrick, S.R. Silburn, D.M. Lawrence, E.G. Mitrou, R.B., Dalby E.M. and Blair (eds), *The Western Australian Aboriginal Child Health Survey: The Social and Emotional Wellbeing of Aboriginal Children and Young People* (pp.xiii–xxviii). Perth: Curtin University of Technology and Telethon Institute for Child Health Research.

Moerman, D.E. and Jonas, W.B. (2002). Deconstructing the placebo effect and finding the meaning response. *Annals of Internal Medicine*, 136(6), 471–476.

Ostrowski, N.L. (1998). Oxytocin receptor mRNA expression in rat brain: Implications for behavioural integration and reproductive success. *Psychoneuroendocrinology*, 23, 989–1004.

Panksepp, J., Normansell, L., Herman, B., Bishop, P. and Crepeau, L. (1998). Neural and Neurochemical Control of the Separation Distress Call. In. J.D. Newman (ed.), *The Physiological Control of Mammalian Vocalisations* (pp.263–300). New York, NY: Plenum Press.

Perry, B. (2008). Foreword. In C. Malchiodi (ed.), *Creative Interventions with Traumatised Children* (pp.ix–xi). New York, NY: Guilford Press.

Phillips, D.P., Ruth, T.E. and Wagner, L.M. (1993). Psychology and survival. *Lancet*, 342(8800), 1142–1145.

Porges, S. (2011). *The Polyvagal Theory: Neurophysiological Foundations of Emotions, Attachment, Communication, Self-Regulation.* New York, NY: W.W. Norton & Company.

Ross, H.E. and Young, L.J. (2009). Oxytocin and the neural mechanisms regulation social cognition and affiliative behaviour. *Frontiers in Neuroendocrinology*, 30(4), 534–547.

Schore, A.N. (1997). Early organization of the nonlinear right brain and development of a predisposition to psychiatric disorders. *Development and Psychopathology*, 9, 595–631.

Uvnas-Moberg, K. (1997). Oxytocin linked to anti stress effects: The relaxation and growth response. *Acta Physiologica Scandinavica*, 640, 38–42.

Vaillant, G.E. (2002). *Aging Well.* New York, NY: Little, Brown and Company.

References for Knowledge and Practice Reflection

Cozolino, L. (2012). *The Neuroscience of Human Relationships: Attachment and the Developing Social Brain* (second edition). New York, NY: W.W. Norton & Company.

Cozolino, L. (2020). *The Pocket Guide to Neuroscience for Clinicians.* New York, NY: W.W. Norton & Company.

Denborough, D. (2006). Stories from Robben Island: A Report from a Journey of Healing. In D. Denborough (ed.), *Trauma: Narrative Responses to Traumatic Experience* (pp.205–226). Adelaide: Dulwich Centre Publications.

Friere, P. (1972). *Pedagogy of the Oppressed.* London: Penguin Books.

Gilbert, P. (2009). *The Compassionate Mind: A New Approach to the Challenge of Life.* Constable and Robinson.

Gilbert, P. (2010). *Compassion Focused Therapy: The CBT Distinctive Features Series.* London: Routledge.

Gilbert, P. (2020a). Compassion: From its evolution to a psychotherapy. *Frontiers in Psychology*, 11, 3123.

Gilbert, P. (2020b). Evolutionary Functional Analysis: The Study of Social Mentalities, Social Rank and Caring-Compassion. In J.N. Kirby and P. Gilbert (eds), *Making an Impact on Mental Health* (pp.4–42). London: Routledge.

Reynolds, V. (2010). *Doing Justice as a Path to Sustainability in Community Work.* www.taosinstitute.net/education/taos-phd-program/completed-dissertations/vikki-reynolds-dissertation. Accessed 19 July 2023.

Reynolds, V. (2013). *Justice-Doing at The Intersections of Power: Community Work, Therapy and Supervision.* Adelaide: Dulwich Centre Publications.

Waldegrave, C. (2012). Developing a 'Just Therapy': Context and the Ascription of Meaning. In A. Lock and T. Strong (eds), *Discursive Perspectives in Therapeutic Practice.* Oxford: Oxford University Press.

Waldegrave, C., Tamasese, K., Tuhaka, F. and Campbell, W. (2003). *Just Therapy – a Journey: A Collection of Papers from the Just Therapy Team New Zealand.* Adelaide: Dulwich Centre Publications.

White, M. and Epston, D. (1990). *Narrative Means to Therapeutic Ends*. New York, NY: W.W. Norton & Company.

White, M. (2006). Working with People who are Suffering the Consequences of Multiple Trauma: A Narrative Perspective. In D. Denborough (ed.), *Trauma: Narrative Responses to Traumatic Experience* (pp.25–86). Adelaide: Dulwich Centre Publications.

CHAPTER 4

Oxytocin and the Healing Power of Love

C. Sue Carter

Introduction

Over the last century, biomedical research has focused on the consequences of illness and disease. However, it is now clear that perceived social support and psychological safety are also critical to human well-being (Ryff *et al.*, 2004). Humans experience secure attachments as 'love'. Although there are many definitions of love, selective relationships and attachments are typically used in most attempts to characterize love (Carter, 1998). Love and secure attachments are foundational and protecting, helping to restore the body in the face of threats or danger (Bowlby, 1982). As we understand love more deeply, we also can begin to optimize the healing power of love and psychological safety.

The evolution of 'love' and oxytocin began over 600 million years ago during the emergence on Earth of multicellular organisms (Carter and Kingsbury, 2022). This biology is powerful in coping with stress, and depends on ancient structures that have often been overlooked. For example, the causes and consequences of sociality and specifically social attachments are grounded in a biological system that operates largely below the level of human consciousness and which I am calling 'sociostasis'. Examining the causes and consequences of sociostasis also provides an expanded perspective on the biology that can restore and heal, even after experiences of chronic stress and trauma.

Despite the generally accepted importance of love, the consequences of positive experiences can go relatively unrecognized, except during periods of stress or loss (Carter, 2017a; Carter, 2017b). For humans, 'love lost' is one of the most powerful forms of distress and trauma (Bowlby, 1982). Losing a loved one can literally be deadly. The same biological systems that are the underpinnings of love's capacity to heal, probably help to explain the consequences of social deprivation and loss. Although the specific nature of the biology of loss is only now becoming apparent, the same sociostatic systems that are necessary to form relationships become dysregulated when mammals experience isolation (Grippo *et al.*, 2009; Pohl *et al.*, 2018). The biology of both love and loss is not yet well identified but involves changes in oxytocin and hormones of the hypothalamic-pituitary-adrenal (HPA) axis, immune system, inflammatory processes, mitochondria and perhaps even the microbiome.

Awareness of cultural and developmental context also is important, especially as clinicians seek to optimize outcomes in children with a history of adversity. It is important to understand that in humans, as in other mammals, the sociostatic system is fine-tuned during early life to predict later demands (Ellis and Del Giudice, 2019). The oxytocin receptors can be epigenetically adjusted by early nurture or neglect (Danoff *et al.*, 2021a; Perkeybile et al., 2019). However, the directionality of the effects of early life experiences must be assessed in what has been termed a context of 'adaptive calibration' (Ellis and Del Giudice, 2019). Behavioural strategies that work in one context might be disastrous in others. Awareness of the capacity of oxytocin and its receptors to be tuned by early experience and social context provides an adaptive mechanism through which individual differences can occur (Ellis et al., 2021; Danoff *et al.*, 2021b).

In this narrative review, I have described adaptive functions of the ancient peptide molecule known as oxytocin. Oxytocin is central to a clinical understanding of the benefits of positive experiences, as well as the mechanisms through which mammals deal with stress and adversity (Carter *et al.*, 2020; Carter and Kingsbury, 2022). A combination of physiological and behavioural processes allows us to anticipate and cope with various challenges across the lifespan. Oxytocin, through effects on the autonomic nervous system and other biological systems, regulates the emotional experiences that we described as 'safety' (Porges, 2021). By narrowing our focus to the oxytocin system and its role in sociostasis, we can begin to detect patterns in physiology and behaviour through which love and social bonds support a sense of safety. These systems can protect the mammalian body from all forms of stress and restore us after trauma. Awareness of the nature of these is crucial to understanding the biology of health and well-being.

Oxytocin as a biological metaphor for safety

The behavioural biology of oxytocin is described in detail elsewhere (Hurlemann and Grinevich, 2018; Jurek and Neumann, 2018; Carter *et al.*, 2020; Carter, 2022a). Oxytocin links us socially to other humans and is an essential part of an autonomic and biochemical buffer against stress and threats. Oxytocin allows social co-regulation and loving relationships to exist and to be beneficial by protecting against biological and behavioural overreactions in threat and fear systems, including acting as a buffer against 'shutting down' in the face of isolation (Grippo *et al.*, 2009) or other traumas (Porges, 2021).

Threats and fear are adaptive, at least when danger is real, and these have always been part of the human experience. Because fear and stress are rooted in an interactive biology that also supports sociality and love, it can be difficult to experimentally disentangle the physiology of positive versus negative experiences (Carter, 2017a). Nonetheless, it is clear that when feelings of threat or anxiety continue past the time of the actual danger and become chronic, these are potentially damaging. Chronic stress can lead to depression, emotional shutdown, addiction or, in extreme cases, suicide. It also promotes chronic inflammatory conditions that directly harm the brain and body (Furman *et al.*, 2019).

The same chemical features that make oxytocin biologically active also made it difficult to study, helping to stir controversy around the molecule (Alvares *et al.*, 2017) and concern over the value of measuring oxytocin, especially in bodily fluids (MacLean *et al.*, 2019). Understanding the importance of this system at the biological level is relatively recent, but depends on interactions of oxytocin with other molecules and their receptors, including vasopressin and molecules in the HPA axis such as corticotropin-releasing hormone (CRH) (Carter *et al.*, 2020). The effects of oxytocin depend not just on the availability of oxytocin itself, but also on its receptors. Oxytocin receptors are located on cell membranes throughout the body and especially in the brain, and these can be influenced by a variety of other molecules. Stimulation of G-protein-coupled receptors for oxytocin triggers subcellular cascades, allowing these neuropeptides to have multiple functions. Further complicating this story, oxytocin receptor expression and binding are context dependent, sexually dimorphic, and altered by experiences, especially those around the time of birth. Oxytocin can also act on other types of receptors besides those called 'oxytocin receptors'. Among other functions, oxytocin confers neuroprotection for the developing brain and upregulates and protects mitochondrial function, supporting the availability of energy across the lifecycle (Bordt *et al.*, 2019; Carter *et al.*, 2020), and regulates the microbiome, with broad health consequences (Sherwin *et al.*, 2019).

Oxytocin: Not just a female hormone

Research on oxytocin initially faced several obstacles. Oxytocin as a psychologically relevant molecule was ignored because it was believed to be a hormone only relevant to women and acting only during childbirth and lactation. Oxytocin is indeed of special importance for women. However, it affects men as well, and across the lifespan. Further complicating this story, sex differences are often reported in response to different kinds of early experiences or chronic stressors across the lifespan. The exact mechanisms for sex differences are not well understood, but arise in part through interactions of oxytocin with other systems regulated by vasopressin, CRH and sex steroids (Carter, 2007; Carter and Perkeybile, 2018).

Another factor that slowed the understanding of oxytocin arose because the protective effects of oxytocin are most easily detected only in the face of stressors, traumas and other forms of adversity (Carter, 2022a, 2022b). Oxytocin binds to other molecules when it is active and can dampen threat, but it usually will not stop the body from responding to genuine danger.

Oxytocin and stimulation of the oxytocin receptor generally support patterns of growth, resilience and healing. For example, oxytocin plays a role in the programming of stem cells into neurons and cardiomyocytes, with the capacity to heal damaged tissues in the brain and heart (Gutkowska and Jankowski, 2012). Oxytocin's action may help to explain the female advantage in longevity (Horn and Carter, 2021). Oxytocin is truly 'Nature's medicine', and for this reason it is critical to discover and optimize oxytocin's natural protective properties (Carter et al., 2020).

There is increasing interest in the use of oxytocin as a 'drug'. However, the characteristics of oxytocin that present challenges to its use as an exogenous medicine are only now being recognized (Alvares et al., 2017). For these reasons, it is important whenever possible to understand and to take advantage of the body's own capacity to create and maximize the functions of the endogenous oxytocin system, rather than depending on pharmaceuticals.

The healing power of love and oxytocin

Good relationships are powerful medicine with health benefits that are recognized throughout most cultures. Epidemiological studies searching for secrets to extend longevity showed that individuals, especially men, living in psychological isolation were more likely to die after a heart attack than those with companions. After the death of a partner, especially in the elderly, the second member of the pair may become vulnerable to disease (Ryff et al., 2004). Correlational studies such as these do not prove that oxytocin is the magic that explains social support. However, oxytocin does facilitate social engagement and may increase a psychological sense of safety. The cardio-protective effects of the autonomic nervous system, and especially the parasympathetic nervous system, are regulated by oxytocin (Carter et al., 2020). This integrated system allows a dynamic balance between growth and restoration, while enabling the body to respond quickly and adaptively to acute stress. Oxytocin also may help to overcome chronic diseases, especially those associated with excessive inflammation.

Experimental studies support the importance of oxytocin in the cardiovascular systems. Oxytocin is part of the mechanism guiding normal heart development. Mice that are genetically deficient in oxytocin develop abnormal hearts (Gutkowska and Jankowski, 2012). In tissue culture (and thus even in the absence of a central nervous system), oxytocin acts on undifferentiated stem cells, transforming these into clusters of miniature hearts beating in synchrony. Furthermore, in laboratory models of atherosclerotic plaques, oxytocin reduces inflammation. Through processes such as these, oxytocin might be able to prevent or even reverse the effects of heart disease, with some of the benefits occurring locally at the site of damage.

Many other beneficial practices are associated with oxytocin. For example, exercise is one of the most reliable ways to both protect against disease and to release oxytocin (Jong *et al.*, 2015). Oxytocin in turn helps to restore heart rate and blood pressure to normal, with potential benefits to the cardiovascular system. Heart disease is only one of many disorders that may benefit from the healing power of both exercise and oxytocin. It has been shown in animal models that exercise is beneficial in slowing the growth of breast cancer. Remarkably, these studies have suggested that this effect of exercise also is mediated by oxytocin (Liu *et al.*, 2020).

Oxytocin is a central component of the immune system. The thymus is a source of oxytocin and expresses an abundance of oxytocin receptors. Early experiences 'educate' the immune system through functions that require the presence of oxytocin (Geenen *et al.*, 2013). In a group of volunteers deliberately exposed to a treatment that causes inflammation, a concurrent exposure to oxytocin blocked symptoms such as fever. The capacity of oxytocin to reduce inflammation is likely to be a factor in the beneficial effects of healthy relationships.

Sociostasis

As a general concept, sociostasis recognizes the fact that, especially in social mammals, the capacity to deal with challenge, stress and trauma is typically coordinated with the presence or absence of others. There is increasing evidence that this dependence of mammals on others is based on specific neural and chemical pathways that require others or a 'mental representation' of others (Bowlby, 1982). These systems form biobehavioural mechanisms that coordinate health, wellness and survival with the social environment. This is possible in part through the unique properties of oxytocin (Carter *et al.*, 2020), including its capacity to regulate the parasympathetic system (Porges, 2021). I have described the internal system formed by these mechanisms as 'sociostasis' (Carter, 2022b).

The concept of sociostasis exists within the historical context of homeostasis and allostasis, models that have been used to describe the internal physiology through which vertebrate organisms deal with challenge and stress. Homeostasis, as defined by Cannon in the early 20th century (Goldstein, 2009), refers to the tendency of physiological processes to maintain stability around a set point. The concept of homeostasis was later extended to include active processes necessary to adapt to change and also to predict future stressors. As commonly used, the concept of allostasis involves active adaptation to stressors and 'achieving stability through change' (Sterling, 2014; McEwen and Wingfield, 2003).

Historically, homeostasis and allostasis focused on hormones in the HPA axis, including cortisol, as well as metabolic hormones and molecules in the immune system. Homeostasis and allostasis are also regulated by the autonomic nervous system (Sterling, 2014), but both were focused on processes within an individual and failed to acknowledge the important role of others. However, especially in mammals, the processes described as foundational to homeostasis and allostasis function differently when mammals are alone from when they are living in pairs or social groups. Furthermore, a vast array of biological processes are in place to encourage social engagement, including the distress or motivation to reunite with companions that arises during social isolation (Bowlby, 1982).

Cozolino previously used the term sociostasis to describe the reciprocal influence individuals have on one another as they regulate each other's biology, psychology and states of mind across what he termed the 'social synapse' (Cozolino, 2021). The role of relationships in emotional homeostasis is one example among many of the importance of sociality in homeostasis and allostasis. This awareness is now well accepted in psychology but was historically absent from most 'stress' research as well as medical theories in general. Consistent with Cozolino, I have suggested that 'sociostasis' be used more broadly to draw attention to the central role of social interactions in physiological and behavioural homeostasis and allostasis.

Oxytocin and sociostasis

Oxytocin sits at the centre of sociostasis. Oxytocin also functions through complex interactions with other protective systems. Key among these are neuroendocrine pathways that involve vasopressin and the HPA axis, including corticotropin-releasing factors (CRF1 and CRF2) and their receptors (Vuppaladhadiam et al., 2020). Fully appreciating the importance of sociality and oxytocin requires awareness of the consequences of both for the regulation of immune and autonomic processes (Carter, 2017a; Carter et al., 2020; Porges, 2021; Carter and Kingsbury, 2022). Interactions among these systems help to explain how and why oxytocin and sociality are repeatedly implicated in dealing with what Cannon described as 'homeostasis' (Goldstein and Kopin, 2007), Selye (1956) called the 'stress of life' and others have called 'allostasis' (Sterling, 2014; McEwen and Wingfield, 2003).

Survival depends on the capacity to respond to acute challenges and also chronic conditions. The physiology of acute versus chronic defences is often different (Bangasser *et al.*, 2019). For example, systems dependent on vasopressin, CRF, glucocorticoids and other classical stress hormones have benefits in the face of an immediate threat or danger. These molecules may act quickly and are associated with acute stressors and individual defence strategies. Acute responses to behavioural and physiological threats may be essential to survival (Quintana and Guastella, 2020). In contrast, chronic exposure to threats and 'stress' hormones and over-activity of the immune system are damaging (Carter and Kingsbury, 2022). Social buffering and oxytocin may be of particular importance during chronic conditions. Furthermore, time matters in the management of challenge. By calibrating physiological and behavioural responses in anticipation of future demands (Janeček and Dabrowska, 2019), it has been shown in animal models that oxytocin facilitates an accurate sense of safety and reduces over-reactivity to irrelevant stressors.

There are many stressful periods in the mammalian life course during which oxytocin is particularly beneficial. Among these are the need to make a safe transition from intrauterine to extrauterine life during birth (Kingsbury and Bilbo, 2019; Carter *et al.*, 2020). Oxytocin also allows a slow reproductive strategy, including in humans the eventual development of a massive cortex, permitting cognition and language, supported by breast-feeding and extended parental behaviour (Carter, 2014). Embedded in the success of human evolution is the capacity to develop selective and lasting social attachments and trust – essential components of love. A sense of safety also is of importance to survival and longevity across time. As one example, in isolated social rodents, telomeres tend to shorten, a process that can be reversed by treatment with exogenous oxytocin (Stevenson *et al.*, 2019). Species, including primates and bats, that invest heavily in their offspring, allowing their young to be dependent on parents in early life, also tend to have greater longevity (Horn and Carter, 2021). The biological properties of oxytocin help to explain the long-term physical and emotional benefits of secure relationships (Porges, 2021).

Evolution and oxytocin

Understanding the biological properties of oxytocin provides a novel perspective on mammalian evolution. Over the course of mammalian evolution a set of biological solutions to the stresses of life emerged (Carter and Kingsbury, 2022). The specific biology of those solutions is especially obvious in social mammals, including humans, that are capable of experiencing the benefits of selective sociality and sociostasis.

Oxytocin evolved from biological mechanisms that allowed mammals to feed their young on milk. In placental mammals, which includes humans, oxytocin also facilitates uterine contractions and milk ejection.

However, oxytocin receptors are found in the brainstem as well as in tissues that are regulated by the autonomic nervous system, including the heart and digestive system. Because oxytocin regulates the autonomic nervous system it has indirect consequences throughout the body. Oxytocin is also found in the immune system, including the thymus, and supports the protective aspects of that system. Oxytocin functions throughout the body as a stress-coping molecule that is both an anti-inflammatory and anti-oxidant. Oxytocin also regulates the mitochondria (power plants of each cell) (Bordt *et al.*, 2019) and the intestinal microbiota (Sherwin *et al.*, 2019).

Oxytocin helped to create a biochemical bridge from our premammalian (reptilian) ancestors to modern humans. At the centre of human evolution are the extensive interactions of oxytocin throughout the body, mediated in part by the wide-ranging effects of the vagus nerve (Porges, 2021). Although oxytocin-like molecules and some components of the parasympathetic nervous system are found in non-mammalian vertebrates, the presence of oxytocin and the ventral vagal complex of the parasympathetic nervous system were essential to human evolution, development of a large brain and eventually consciousness (Carter, 2014).

The ancient evolution of co-regulation and love

Oxytocin and the more primitive molecule, vasopressin, originated from ancestral peptides that helped animals successfully move from life in the sea to dry land. Vasopressin is at least 100 million years older than oxytocin and has functions that are more primitive than oxytocin. Vasopressin protects against dehydration, regulates blood pressure and increases reactivity to other threats. Vasopressin is associated with the neurobiology of anxiety, fear and avoidance learning. Although oxytocin and vasopressin were derived from a common ancestor, depending on context, their physiological functions can appear to be strikingly different. For example, under some conditions, vasopressin seems to promote 'anxiety' while under other conditions it may increase 'bravery'. Both males and females synthesize vasopressin. However, in areas of the brain implicated in defensiveness, vasopressin production is increased by androgens, which may help to explain sex and context differences in the expression of aggression.

It is difficult to separate the functions of oxytocin and vasopressin even in animal research. Under conditions of safety, either oxytocin or vasopressin may promote social engagement (Cho *et al.*, 1999; Bales *et al.*, 2004). Vasopressin may be of particular importance under conditions of extreme or chronic stress and in males when the neuroendocrine system seem to default to more primitive pathways (Zuloaga *et al.*, 2020). However, in a context of heightened anxiety or fear, it is possible that oxytocin functions more like vasopressin, possibly by binding to and stimulating vasopressin receptors.

Further complicating this story, the oxytocin-vasopressin system is constantly changing across the life cycle. Oxytocin can directly affect the development of the brain and cardiovascular system (Carter, 2003), and it also programmes the immune system (Geenen *et al.*, 2013). The genes for the oxytocin receptor in voles are 'epigenetically' tuned by early experience. In the presence of sensitive parenting, the genes in a baby that regulate the oxytocin receptor are more likely to be available for stimulation, and at least in rodents, we find that these changes can last for a lifetime (Perkey-bile *et al.*, 2019).

What have we learned from non-human mammals about oxytocin and 'love'?

The origins of much of our current understanding of the science of social attachment and pair bond formation began in studies conducted in small field mice known as prairie voles. Beginning in the late 1970s, my colleagues and I discovered that both in nature and in the laboratory, prairie voles were capable of forming lifelong pair bonds. These small rodents lived together until one or both members of the pair died (Getz *et al.*, 1981).

Prairie voles also showed other traits of monogamy. Both parents nurtured the young, with fathers carrying out all aspects of infant care except nursing. Older siblings also baby sat for younger siblings. Juvenile prairie voles moved out of the family to find mates and scrupulously avoided incest. Prairie voles exhibited the traits that humans associate with extended families, constructed around an apparently monogamous pair (Carter and Getz, 1993). But, we soon discovered that monogamy, like love, can be a paradox. In the 1980s, in the early days of our studies, DNA fingerprints became possible. DNA revealed that prairie voles were having sex outside the pair bond. Monogamy, or at least the traits associated with monogamy, were real and they were based in biology. However, monogamy was not simply about sexual exclusivity. In fact, sexual preferences were not the defining feature of monogamy. We did find that sexual interactions could facilitate pair bonding. But at the core of the prairie vole family were invisible social bonds and what we were observing was more accurately called 'social monogamy' (Carter *et al.*, 1995). But awareness that selective social behaviours were the central feature of social monogamy, and apparently more important than sexual monogamy also opened avenues to understanding the physiological basis of social attachments.

Over the decades that followed we, and then many others, conducted experiments showing that the capacity for pair bond formation was regulated by emotional states, and these depended on physiology. Nature is conservative and reuses neural and endocrine systems. We now know that the neurobiology of pair bonding in voles indeed had parallels with what humans call love. Furthermore, we found that prairie voles, like humans, had high levels of oxytocin. Prairie voles also had heart rate patterns similar to those found in humans. The parasympathetic branch of the autonomic nervous system is regulated in part by oxytocin and both are associated with the capacity to sustain safe relationships (Grippo *et al.*, 2007). Prairie voles also were exquisitely sensitive to the effects of early nurture, another process that was influenced by oxytocin (Perkeybile *et al.*, 2019). The basic neurobiology of social bonding was centred around oxytocin and shared by humans and prairie voles. Through good luck and with help from many brilliant collaborators, we had stumbled on a rodent model that allowed us to examine the chemistry of love (Carter, 2022b).

As these stories became public, oxytocin was termed by the media 'the hormone of love'. It certainly would have been easier to understand the neurobiology of love if oxytocin were acting alone. Of course, that is not the case. Many molecules and neural systems work behind the scenes to support love. We were able to show that among the other factors essential for selective social attachments as well as male parental behaviour was vasopressin.

Pair bonding required a pair of hormones. Bonding in voles, as in humans, also occurred in the context of other physiological processes, including those associated with a sense of safety or reductions in fear (Carter, 2022b). These are basic and very old emotions and the story of love has its biochemical origins long before the existence of humans or even primitive mammals.

Biological prototypes for love

The evolutionary and biochemical prototype for love and social bonds is the mother-child interaction. Processes that help to define mammals, including lactation and parental care of their young, are facilitated by oxytocin. The same physiological pathways that permit social bonds are shared with maternal behaviour, birth and lactation. Oxytocin is generally associated with positive social behaviours, including social engagement and bonding. Oxytocin also may induce a sense of safety, reduce reactivity to stressors, block fear and increase trust. But even in maternal behaviour, oxytocin does not work alone (Carter, 2022a).

Vasopressin also is important to normal birth, parenting and care of the young, especially in males (Bales *et al.*, 2004). Vasopressin can increase protective behaviours and aggression, which in some cases benefits the family. Although generally directed toward intruders, the emotional states that lead to aggression may escalate and spill over into violence within the family.

Vasopressin is made primarily in the brain and is a classic 'stress hormone', with receptors in the cardiovascular system, kidneys and throughout the body. States of chronic arousal or stress are especially dangerous. Medical disorders such as pre-eclampsia, in which pregnant women retain water, have high blood pressure and sometimes premature labour, have been linked to excessive emotional stress and to vasopressin. Furthermore, excess stress or fear-induced release of vasopressin or hypersensitivity of the vasopressin receptors may help to explain premature birth – among the world's most serious medical mysteries (Fill Malfertheiner *et al.*, 2021).

Generally, oxytocin tempers fear and increases both trust and social behaviour. But in individuals who have a history of neglect, trauma or extreme stress, oxytocin's actions may paradoxically trigger the vasopressin system, enhancing fear. The unique properties of the oxytocin and vasopressin systems allow these two molecules to be highly adaptive and to dynamically support individual survival, as well as emotions that are associated with love. However, stimulating the vasopressin receptors may induce the dark side of love including jealousy, territoriality and aggression (Carter, 2022a).

Biochemical magic beneath the power of love?

Oxytocin was essential to human evolution and the development of the massive human cortex (Carter, 2014). Even in modern humans, oxytocin continues to facilitate the birth, growth and nurture of immature babies. Oxytocin helps, directly and indirectly, to promote healing and restoration. For example, oxytocin has anti-inflammatory properties (Carter and Kingsbury, 2022). Oxytocin influences both the immune system and the generally protective vagal branch of the autonomic nervous system. Vagal pathways, regulated by oxytocin, are necessary for social communication and engagement through actions on the muscles of the face and head (Porges, 2021). Oxytocin is secreted in the presence of extreme stressors and may protect against 'shutdown' responses to trauma. Furthermore, the autonomic nervous system regulates all of our internal organs, as well as the distribution of blood and nutrients throughout the body. Through effects on the autonomic nervous system, oxytocin regulates oxygen to the brain, thus supporting human cognition, culture and eventually civilization (Carter, 2014).

The autonomic nervous system consists of bidirectional pathways through which peptide systems, including oxytocin and vasopressin, may be accessed and influenced. In a context of safety, oxytocin's action on the autonomic nervous system is a critical component of the healing power of love. In a context of fear, trauma or chronic stress, the outcome of exposure to oxytocin, especially when given as a drug, is less predictable (Carter *et al.*, 2020). This topic deserves additional study as we seek ways to better understand the epigenetic role of social experiences in human well-being.

Love is one of nature's most rewarding experiences. But what happens when love is absent or lost? Behaviourally, the effects are well documented. The absence of love or a loving relationship, especially in early life, is associated in later life with patterns of self-defence and a sense of threat (Harlow and Harlow, 1966). If not repaired, this loss can inhibit the later capacity for love. With knowledge of the mechanisms beneath either the presence or absence of love, there is an opportunity to inform optimal relationships and parenting. Because of the evolved and conserved nature of love, awareness of mechanisms through which negative or positive experiences across the lifespan affect this system will help us understand, predict and possibly heal the consequences of neglect or trauma.

Love is intrinsically beautiful, but also complex and mysterious. Although love can be difficult to define, the list of love's functions is long (Carter, 1998). Love influences all aspects of human existence. Love is powerful medicine. (Carter *et al.*, 2020). However, the mechanisms through which love protects and heals are only now being discovered. Throughout life, oxytocin influences sociality, and social experiences influence oxytocin. Knowledge of the neurobiology of love and oxytocin may help to explain the exceptional reproductive success of humans and also our resilience in the face of fear and aggression. The emotional and physical health and longevity of our species, and perhaps our planet, depends on our capacity to understand and apply our knowledge of the biology of the love, especially in times of adversity and trauma.

KNOWLEDGE AND PRACTICE REFLECTION

Janise Mitchell, Joe Tucci, Ed Tronick and Stephen W. Porges

Sue Carter has devoted her career to understanding the neurobiology of love. In her chapter, she carefully explains the evolution and function oxytocin as one of the key hormones that promote the experiences of love and its physiological consequences.

In it, she associates love and loss – identifying how the pathways of the two experiences are intertwined. Loss is a critical dimension of the trauma experience. For example, children who are forced to live with family and domestic violence suffer significant losses even as those around them seek to protect them. Tucci (2019) noted that:

> If children have to move to escape violence, they lose their home, their friends and their neighborhood. Their routines change beyond their

control. They leave behind everything they have known. They are forced to start again. If they have had to move a number of times, they will find it difficult to settle into a new place and make friends again, learn new rules at school, and remember the names of their new friends. They will expect to move again. It will be painful to become too attached to anything or anyone. Family violence causes the loss of predictability and familiarity for children.

Children lose what has been. They lose a part of themselves that liked the way it was. It is not a loss that they can easily overcome. Experiences of family violence serve to disconnect children from their culture. They lose the meanings associated with the beliefs of their family and community. They find it difficult to understand and fulfill the responsibilities they have as a part of their community. The importance of their traditions decay. They lose the principles that their culture offers them about what is right and wrong, what is respectful and disrespectful, what it means to belong to a way of seeing the world that is so vital to the way they see themselves and their relationships. With a loss of culture comes a loss of identity. Children affected by family violence live in-between worlds. They are not fully part of their own culture – it feels alien to them. Yet, they are not totally accepted into the community that sees them as outsiders. In this world, their culture sets them apart. Neither feels secure… (p.21)

As Carter writes 'love lost' can often be deadly. She offers a strong argument to consider how the approach to loss should be part of the way a trauma-transformative practitioner and organization operates.

As well as an awareness that trauma-based behaviours serve a survival function for victims and survivors of violation, an understanding of the significance of loss in the lives of victims and survivors may be just as important. Loss comes in many forms. It is the loss of a continuous sense of self, the narrative that carries with it the meaning of what the individual and community held as hope for the way life would turn out. It is the restructuring of relationships, with certain people falling out of the network that a victim and survivor can rely on. It is the reduction in relationships around which the social qualities of living are experienced and resourced. It is the tangible loss of employment or education, with very real consequences for daily living. It is the disruption to routines that help to offer constancy as change whirls around us at times of transition and crises. It is the loss of home, of belonging and safety. It is loss of connection to the ways in which community shares meanings about living, ancestry, culture. It is the interruption of the sensory experience of the elements and the environment.

Echoing Carter's reflections about the neurobiology of loss and love, David Kessler (2019) has written so beautifully, 'life gives us pain. Our job is to experience it when it gets handed to us. Avoidance of loss has a cost' (p.34).

Kessler, reflecting on his decades of experience in tending the bereavement of so many people, including his own, points to acts of making meaning as the ways in which grief is experienced. Such meaning is individual and relationally contextualized. It comes from having grief seen and acknowledged. It involves engaging in what Carter (and Cozolino and colleagues in the previous chapter) has called 'sociostasis' – the moment-by-moment changes in stress relating to the experience of another. It emphasizes the ways in which reciprocal calibration of our physiology mirrors and underpins the way our mind-body responds to the meaning that we come to hold of stressful moments, such as loss of a loved one or place.

One perspective of such relational meaning making is posited by McAdams and Jones (2017):

> ...to make sense and meaning out of personal experiences...is a deeply and complexly social process, strongly shaped by cultural norms...we are coauthors of our own life stories at best, and shameless plagiarists... (p.12)

At multiple levels then, the grief process occurs through active interpersonal organization that has as one possible outcome the experience of the loss being recognized. The loss is allowed to be experienced and mourned and the ongoing connection to the loss is validated and shared within a community of relationships that are supportive, synchronized and continuous.

Carter also argues that 'love is a powerful medicine'. The concept of love in human services practice has been taboo, stemming from its traditions in the medical model. As we referenced in our opening chapter, the privileging of this approach denies the potential for 'therapeutic intent' that can arise in environments, networks of relationships and communities, that can be found in the therapeutic milieu of living within a well-resourced and supported network of relationships. Discourses about boundaries, and not getting 'too involved' within the therapeutic process stem from traditions of one-to-one therapy. But how does this translate to the work of building an attuned network of relationships argued for by Tronick in Chapter 5 and explored in the context of therapeutic care by Mitchell and Macnamara in Chapter 16? What then is the role of love?

In all the trauma-informed literature, neither love or loss makes it into the list of qualities that are required for a practitioner or an organization to take into account in the way they approach service users, and, more importantly, victims and survivors of violation. Two sides of the same coin, love and loss offer a map for appreciating how those affected by trauma express their needs, seek out comfort, and call out for humanity from the important people in their lives, including the institutions which set themselves up to offer such hope.

Trauma-transformative practice would encompass a greater emphasis on loss and the grieving that accompanies it. This loss may be related to the felt absence of people and relationships which have been destroyed by violation. It can be the loss associated with damage to connection to community, belonging and culture. It can be the loss arising from an edited history that no longer holds ancestral links to land and place. It can be the experience of loss of a pet, a friendship circle, a network of others who offered attuned care and love. It may be the loss of a sense of what the future may offer, a goal and an ambition and wish that will no longer be fulfilled. The process of grieving is a collective act of humanity. The process of grieving as it relates to the sense of loss forced on an individual or group arising from violation carries with it multiple needs for safety and integration. Trauma-transformative practitioners, organizations and systems appreciate the experience of loss that accompanies trauma and are not shy to explore it and build into systems and processes a commitment to the time and relationships that can softly and respectfully sit alongside grief so that over time its meaning is significant but not always as acutely painful.

References
References for chapter

Alvares, G.A., Quintana, D.S. and Whitehouse, A.J.O. (2017). Beyond the hype and hope: Critical considerations for intranasal oxytocin research in autism spectrum disorder. *Autism Research*, 10(1), 25–41.

Bales, K.L., Kim, A.J., Lewis-Reese, A.D. and Carter, C.S. (2004). Both oxytocin and vasopressin may influence alloparental behaviour in male prairie voles. *Hormones and Behaviour*, 45(5), 354–361.

Bangasser, D.A., Eck, S.R. and Ordoñes Sanchez, E. (2019). Sex differences in stress reactivity in arousal and attention systems. *Neuropsychopharmacology: Official Publication of the American College of Neuropsychopharmacology*, 44(1), 129–139.

Bordt, E.A., Smith, C.J., Demarest, T.G., Bilbo, S.D. and Kingsbury, M.A. (2019). Mitochondria, oxytocin, and vasopressin: Unfolding the inflammatory protein response. *Neurotoxicity Research*, 36(2), 239–256.

Bowlby, J. (1982). Attachment and loss: Retrospect and prospect. *The American Journal of Orthopsychiatry*, 52(4), 664–678.

Carter, C.S. (1998). Neuroendocrine perspectives on social attachment and love. *Psychoneuroendocrinology*, 23(8), 779–818.

Carter, C.S. (2003). Developmental consequences of oxytocin. *Physiology and Behaviour*, 79(3), 383–397.

Carter, C.S. (2007). Sex differences in oxytocin and vasopressin: Implications for autism spectrum disorders? *Behavioural Brain Research*, 176(1), 170–186.

Carter, C.S. (2014). Oxytocin pathways and the evolution of human behaviour. *Annual Review of Psychology*, 65, 17–39.

Carter, C.S. (2017a). The oxytocin-vasopressin pathway in the context of love and fear. *Frontiers in Endocrinology*, 8, 356.

Carter, C.S. (2017b). The role of oxytocin and vasopressin in attachment. *Psychodynamic Psychiatry*, 45(4), 499–517.

Carter, C.S. (2022a). Oxytocin and love: Myths, metaphors and mysteries. *Comprehensive Psychoneuroendocrinology*, 9, 100107.

Carter, C.S. (2022b). Sex, love and oxytocin: Two metaphors and a molecule. *Neuroscience and Biobehavioural Reviews*, 104948.

Carter, C.S., DeVries, A.C. and Getz, L.L. (1995). Physiological substrates of mammalian monogamy: The prairie vole model. *Neuroscience and Biobehavioural Review*, 19(2), 303–314.

Carter, C.S. and Getz, L.L. (1993). Monogamy and the prairie vole. *Scientific American*, 268(6), 100–106.

Carter, C.S., Kenkel, W.M., MacLean, E.L., Wilson, S.R. *et al.* (2020). Is oxytocin 'Nature's medicine'? *Pharmacological Reviews*, 72(4), 829–861.

Carter, C.S. and Kingsbury, M.A. (2022). Oxytocin and oxygen: The evolution of a solution to the 'stress of life'. *Philosophical Transactions of the Royal Society of London. Series B, Biological Sciences*, 377(1858), 20210054.

Carter, C.S. and Perkeybile, A.M. (2018). The monogamy paradox: What do love and sex have to do with it? *Frontiers in Ecology and Evolution*, 6(202).

Cho, M.M. DeVries, A.C., Williams, J.R. and Carter, C.S. (1999). The effects of oxytocin and vasopressin on partner preferences in male and female prairie voles (Microtus ochrogaster). *Behavioural Neuroscience*, 113(5), 1071–1079.

Cozolino, L. (2021). *The Making of a Therapist: A Practical Guide for the Inner Journey*. New York: W.W. Norton and Company.

Danoff, J.S., Connelly, J.J., Morris, J.P. and Perkeybile, A.M. (2021a). An epigenetic rheostat of experience: DNA methylation of OXTR as a mechanism of early life allostasis. *Comprehensive Psychoneuroendocrinology*, 8, 100098.

Danoff, J.S., Wroblewski, K.L., Graves, A.J., Quinn, G.C. *et al.* (2021b). Genetic, epigenetic, and environmental factors controlling oxytocin receptor gene expression. *Clinical Epigenetics*, 13(1), 23.

Ellis, B.J. and Del Giudice, M. (2019). Developmental adaptation to stress: An evolutionary perspective. *Annual Review of Psychology*, 70, 111–139.

Ellis, B.J., Horn, A.J., Carter, C.S., van Ijzendoorn, M.H. and Bakermans-Kranenburg, M.J. (2021). Developmental programming of oxytocin through variation in early-life stress: Four meta-analyses and a theoretical reinterpretation. *Clinical Psychology Review*, 86, 101985.

Fill Malfertheiner, S., Bataiosu-Zimmer, E., Michel, H., Fouzas, S. *et al.* (2021). Vasopressin but not oxytocin responds to birth stress in infants. *Frontiers in Neuroscience*, 15, 718056.

Furman, D., Campisi, J., Verdin, E., Carrera-Bastos, P. *et al.* (2019). Chronic inflammation in the etiology of disease across the life span. *Nature Medicine*, 25(12), 1822–1832.

Geenen, V., Bodart, G., Henry, S., Michaux, H. *et al.* (2013). Programming of neuroendocrine self in the thymus and its defect in the development of neuroendocrine autoimmunity. *Frontiers in Neuroscience*, 7, 187.

Getz, L.L., Carter, C.S. and Gavish, L. (1981). The mating system of the prairie vole, Microtus ochrogaster: Field and laboratory evidence for pair-bonding. *Behavioural Ecology and Sociobiology*, 189–194.

Goldstein, D. (2009). Walter Cannon: Homeostasis, the fight-or-flight response, the sympathoadrenal system, and the wisdom of the body. *BrainImmune*. https://brainimmune.com/walter-cannon-homeostasis-the-fight-or-flight-response-the-sympathoadrenal-system-and-the-wisdom-of-the-body.

Goldstein, D.S. and Kopin, I.J. (2007). Evolution of concepts of stress. *Stress*, 10(2), 109–120.

Grippo, A.J., Lamb, D.G., Carter, C.S. and Porges, S.W. (2007). Cardiac regulation in the socially monogamous prairie vole. *Physiology and Behaviour*, 90(2–3), 386–393.

Grippo, A.J., Trahanas, D.M., Zimmerman, R.R., Porges, S.W. and Carter, C.S. (2009). Oxytocin protects against negative behavioural and autonomic consequences of long-term social isolation. *Psychoneuroendocrinology*, 34(10), 1542–1553.

Gutkowska, J. and Jankowski, M. (2012). Oxytocin revisited: Its role in cardiovascular regulation. *Journal of Neuroendocrinology*, 24(4), 599–608.

Harlow, H.F. and Harlow, M. (1966). Learning to love. *American Scientist*, 54(3), 244–272.

Horn, A.J. and Carter, C.S. (2021). Love and longevity: A social dependency hypothesis. *Comprehensive Psychoneuroendocrinology*, 8, 100088.

Hurlemann, R. and Grinevich, V. (2018). *Behavioural Pharmacology of Neuropeptides: Oxytocin*. New York, NY: Springer.

Janeček, M. and Dabrowska, J. (2019). Oxytocin facilitates adaptive fear and attenuates anxiety responses in animal models and human studies-potential interaction with the corticotropin-releasing factor (CRF) system in the bed nucleus of the stria terminalis (BNST). *Cell and Tissue Research*, 375(1), 143–172.

Jong, T.R. de, Menon, R., Bludau, A., Grund, T. *et al.* (2015). Salivary oxytocin concentrations in response to running, sexual self-stimulation, breastfeeding and the TSST: The Regensburg Oxytocin Challenge (ROC) study. *Psychoneuroendocrinology*, 62, 381–388.

Jurek, B. and Neumann, I.D. (2018). The oxytocin receptor: From intracellular signaling to behaviour. *Physiological Reviews*, 98(3), 1805–1908.

Kingsbury, M.A. and Bilbo, S.D. (2019). The inflammatory event of birth: How oxytocin signaling may guide the development of the brain and gastrointestinal system. *Frontiers in Neuroendocrinology*, 55, 100794.

Liu, H., Gruber, C.W., Alewood, P.F., Möller, A. and Muttenthaler, M. (2020). The oxytocin receptor signalling system and breast cancer: A critical review. *Oncogene*, 39(37), 5917–5932.

MacLean, E.L., Wilson, S.R., Martin, W.L., Davis, J.M., Nazarloo, H.P. and Carter, C.S. (2019). Challenges for measuring oxytocin: The blind men and the elephant? *Psychoneuroendocrinology*, 107, 225–231.

McEwen, B.S. and Wingfield, J.C. (2003). The concept of allostasis in biology and biomedicine. *Hormones and Behaviour*, 43(1), 2–15.

Perkeybile, A.M., Carter, C.S., Wroblewski, K.L., Puglia, M.H. *et al.* (2019). Early nurture epigenetically tunes the oxytocin receptor. *Psychoneuroendocrinology*, 99, 128–136.

Pohl, T.T., Young, L.J. and Bosch, O.J. (2018). Lost connections: Oxytocin and the neural, physiological, and behavioural consequences of disrupted relationships. *International Journal of Psychophysiology*, 136, 54–63.

Porges, S.W. (2021). Polyvagal Theory: A biobehavioural journey to sociality. *Comprehensive Psychoneuroendocrinology*, 7, 1–7, 100069.

Quintana, D.S. and Guastella, A.J. (2020). An allostatic theory of oxytocin. *Trends in Cognitive Sciences*, 24(7), 515–528.

Ryff, C.D., Singer, B.H. and Dienberg Love, G. (2004). Positive health: Connecting well-being with biology. *Philosophical Transactions of the Royal Society of London. Series B, Biological Sciences*, 359(1449), 1383–1394.

Selye, H. (1956). *The Stress of Life*. New York, NY: McGraw-Hill.

Sherwin, E., Bordenstein, S.R., Quinn, J.L., Dinan, T.G. and Cryan, J.F. (2019). Microbiota and the social brain. *Science*, 366 (6465).

Sterling, P. (2014). Homeostasis vs allostasis: Implications for brain function and mental disorders. *JAMA Psychiatry*, 71(10), 1192–1193.

Stevenson, J.R., McMahon, E.K., Boner, W. and Haussmann, M.F. (2019). Oxytocin administration prevents cellular aging caused by social isolation. *Psychoneuroendocrinology*, 103, 52–60.

Tucci, J. (2019). *What really is safety for traumatised children and young people*. Australian Childhood Foundation, Abbotsford, Victoria.

Vuppaladhadiam, L., Ehsan, C., Akkati, M. and Bhargava, A. (2020). Corticotropin-releasing factor family: A stress hormone-receptor system's emerging role in mediating sex-specific signaling. *Cells*, 9(4), E839.

Zuloaga, D.G., Heck, A.L., De Guzman, R.M. and Handa, R.J. (2020). Roles for androgens in mediating the sex differences of neuroendocrine and behavioural stress responses. *Biology of Sex Differences*, 11(1), 44.

References for Knowledge and Practice Reflection

Kessler, D. (2019). *Finding Meaning: The Sixth Stage of Grief*. New York, NY: Scribner.

McAdams, D.P. and B.K. Jones. (2017), Making Meaning in the Wake of Trauma – Resilience and Redemption. In E.M. Altmaier (eds), *Reconstructing Meaning After Trauma. Theory, Research and Practice* (pp.3–16). London: Academic Press.

CHAPTER 5

Trauma Never Occurs Only Once: Being Traumatized by a Hit is Like Making Meaning of the Game of Peek-a-Boo

Ed Tronick

I am not a trauma theorist, and worse still I do not see trauma as *the* mechanism driving dysfunction or psychopathology. Rather, I am a developmentalist who sees developmental and lifelong dysfunction emerge from chronic repeated experiences and processes, primarily external interpersonal relational experiences and internal somatic and brain – neurosomatic – processes. Beyond development, I adhere to open systems as influenced by psychodynamic frameworks (Tronick, 1998; Sander, 1977; Harrison, 2003). For me, the lack of a normal developmental perspective, along with a dominant psychopathological perspective framing our thinking about trauma, limits our understanding of trauma, the value of trauma theory and trauma-informed practices. Were I smart enough, I would not use the term trauma at all. For me it is a bulge in a landscape that we note in our language and diagnoses as if it was the only feature of the landscape, but it is in fact just a more severe outcropping on many small and large bumps making up a desolate toxic landscape. Moreover, it is a constantly changing landscape. Nonetheless, for now I am stuck with the term. So, you see already that I take a jaundiced view of what is typically thought to be trauma and I would like to think I will provide a different view of trauma.

To put it bluntly and to overstate it, even though it is rare in cases of abuse and neglect, a purported traumatic event that in fact physically happens only once is never experienced only once. Repetition of it occurs because of the individual's ongoing, endogenous, reiterated, neurosomatic meaning-making processes of the meaning made of it. And while becoming traumatized is hardly a game, the process of making meaning of it and of a game, such as peek-a-boo, are much the same. At the heart of the similarity is the repetition of endogenous meaning-making processes which most often, but not always because there are single occurrence events, travel with the event's exogenous re-occurrence. The repetition instantiates the trauma and the game into the individual's way of experiencing and being in the world.

One more thing: the focus of my clinical and research work is on infants and young children, and their parents, and this chapter will draw on that work (Tronick, 2007). I think it is quite relevant to adults. However, I am not an attachment theorist (Tronick, 2003). While useful, even powerful, it is too static and a-developmental a conceptualization. It is time to move on from it to the domain of ongoing processes and experience. I will not be providing you with a new technique, but perhaps a challenging framework. In fact, I will challenge the notion of trauma as it is wedded to attachment and the trauma-informed zeitgeist as they are typically framed.

My thinking focuses on the formulation by Bruner (1990) that humans are makers of meaning. The term *makers* is critical. It emphasizes that humans are actively engaged in the process of making meaning. I see meaning making about one's self in relation to the world of people and things, and to one's own self, as a core organizing concept in therapeutic approaches, as varied and contentious as body psychotherapies, psychoanalysis, psychodynamic, cognitive behavioral therapy, dialectical cognitive therapies, dyadic therapies, attachment, relational therapies and others (Tronick, 2007; Harrison, 2003; Ogden, 1997; Modell, 1993). Meaning is central to the phenomenon of trauma, but the focus is typically on the event itself (e.g. sexual abuse), as if an event is always a trauma to all individuals, rather than on the meaning made of the event by an individual, its context, its effects on the meaning of other events, and critically how it changes over time.

Meanings are made continuously and simultaneously, in real time, at multiple levels, and by multiple somatic and neurologic systems – what I call neurosomatic meaning-making systems. Loss of any of these meanings – the meaning about oneself to oneself, or the relation of one's self to the world, results in serious psychological dysfunction and psychopathology. Modell (1993) said that the failure to 'make meaning' is a psychic catastrophe, what is typically labelled a trauma. From a developmental perspective, however, more common than failures to make meaning are the meanings made about more mundane events that distort one's sense of the world and sense of one's self. The sneering mocking look from a parent when a child somehow fails to fulfill the parent's unspecified desire that leads to the child making the meaning that she is defective and ineffective and her world is filled with contempt. And keep in mind that the process is not just of the moment. It is not one-and-done. The experience is sticky. Neurosomatic meaning-making processes are endogenous and continuously operating. They keep on going and going, affecting the meanings made as life moves on. Worse still, the initial meaning made goes on to affect the next meanings made. Those later emerging meanings generate further distortions and increasingly insidious debilitations, which indeed may be far more derailing than the initial meaning made of the experience.

The continuous process of meaning making conforms to the larger framework of open systems (Tronick and Beeghly, 2011; Tronick, 2003). A first principle of the ways in which all biological organisms grow and develop is that systems must gain resources – energy and information – to maintain their organization, to grow, and to develop. Failing to gain energy leads to dissipation of organization, and death. A child consuming milk thrives, builds muscles, increases brain cell number, and energizes growth promoting bodily processes. A child consuming chips builds fat, diminishes brain cells, and energizes short and long-term debilitating bodily processes. So too with the child's mental development and growing understanding of their world. Of course, nutrients are necessary, but the nutrients that grow mental development and understanding of the world are not physical nutrients. Rather, the nutrients are the information appropriated during the individual's engagement with the world, which meaning-making processes make meaning of that increases the individual's sense of self in the world. Think only of the primate deprivation studies or the human sensory deprivation studies to understand how a poverty of information distorts and disrupts development. In the context of trauma, think about the effects of neglect, a form of deprivation of relational information.

A consequence of the first principle of an open system demands that an individual must actively and continuously engage with the world in order to gain necessary resources. The active appropriation of resources allows the individual to integrate the new meaning with past meaning into their current and yet evolving meaning of the relation of self to the world.

Again, keep in mind that meaning making is neurosomatic. Neurosomatic meaning making is highlighted by infants' meaning makings. In infants, meanings about the world, such as this person is a stranger and scary, are made without language and advanced cognitive processes, with an immature brain, and still developing regulatory systems. Or think of a five-year-old child whose autonomic nervous system's set point for threat is low, such that small stressors lead to full-fledged fear reactions. As a result, the ambient meaning of the world is that it is dangerous and threatening. And the lulls in fearfulness are likely to be short lived because the process is ongoing and the meaning lingers and affects the meaning of even benign events. The process of making sense of the world and one's relation to it inherently involves the whole individual in an endless and continuous process.

A developmental open systems perspective holds to a view that *all* current experience affects the meaning made by an individual and to the extent possible the individual should – must – have *agency* to determine their engagement with the world and with others on a moment-by-moment basis (Sander, 1977). Thus, the individual can take hold of information to endogenously create new psychobiological meanings and ways of being in the world.

I see the meanings about the world and the self as assembled into a neurosomatic state of consciousness (Tronick, 1998, 2003; Tronick and Beeghly, 2011). The state of consciousness guides the individual's engagement with the world. But it is not static. For example, descriptions of my still-face paradigm refer to its 'signature' effect – the infant turning away, being distressed and fearful, yet the infant still feels effective – '*I can get you back*'– and keeps trying to elicit the mother. But that state of consciousness changes over time with longer exposure to the still face. The infant stops eliciting the mother, their posture collapses and they generate a helpless state of consciousness. An implication is that the typical view of trauma that sees it as static is incorrect. Like the meaning of the still face, the meaning of a trauma changes. The change is brought about by ongoing external and internal experience which modifies the meaning made of the experience over the course of daily living and development. And its meaning and the changes of meaning affect the meaning made of other events and of the self.

It is perhaps a bit of hyperbole to say that a developmental perspective holds to a view that *all* current experience affects the meaning made by an individual. But note first that the typical view of trauma is that it affects all experience for all time and is the primary event leading to psychopathology. Critically, and in contrast to many views of the singularity and power of trauma, the developmental perspective qualifies the *all* with the principal of reiteration: the *all* of experience that affect the meanings made by the individual are chronic reiterated experiences (Perry, 2008; Tronick, 2007). A strict definition of trauma, the typical pointing to an event as *the* traumatic event, and the static self-contained view of trauma do not consider reiteration of the event, its context, and the meaning made of those features and how the meaning changes. We will come back to this '*all*'.

What do I mean by the re-occurrence of experience? It is that events and the experience of them have their effects because of their reiterated occurrence and the individual experiences of them and their endogenous neurosomatic making of meaning of them many, many times. Not to be fatuous, events that shape an individual's meaning about the world are like learning to play peek-a-boo. How does a child come to know the game of peek-a-boo (Bruner and Sherwood, 1976; Commons *et al.*, 1998)? The game of peek-a-boo is a dynamic interplay of actions and information between a child and an adult. The game is rule-governed, but flexible in its enactment. Often there are unique individual and familial variations. Despite our saying that a four-month-old plays peek-a-boo, recognize that young infants do not actually play peek-a-boo. He has no idea what is going on, though it has some indecipherable meaning for him, after all he reacts to the adult's actions. It is played 'at' the infant by an adult, who initially plays *all* the sides of the game. The infant makes a large number and variety of behaviors, and has lots of varying intentions and apprehensions of what is going on, many of which are unrelated to the adult's game-playing actions. The infant looks away when she 'should' be looking toward, or she raises her shoe, or looks at her hand. What she is doing is messy – variable, unstable, disorganized. Yet, with re-occurrence, the infant attends, and begins to anticipate the coming 'boo' and some of the messiness is repaired and pared away. With more re-occurrences and development, the infant begins to become agenic and to control some of the elements and the pace of the game. She comes to signal the timing of the 'boo' and her reactions become more coherent and contingent. As the game is acquired, the infant begins to learn pieces of how to be the 'surprisee' and then the 'peek-a-booer'. Sequences and rhythms emerge.

While all that is going on for the infant, the adult continuously makes adjustments (e.g. holding positions longer) in relation to the infant's actions and her intent – what Bruner calls scaffolding (Bruner, 1990). Such scaffolding is intuitive and implicit. The selective assembling of the infant's self-organized actions and intentions, *and* her apprehension of the adult's actions and intentions, *and* the adult's reciprocal apprehension become incrementally more coherent. Their mismatches get repaired. And so on, through endless repetitions, until the game is fully 'within' the child and at the same time fully within the child-adult dyad. Simply put, coming to know peek-a-boo is a messy process that is slowly sculpted over repetitions by repairs of the messiness. Moreover, its meaning for the child changes from (perhaps) something exciting and fun, to something done with the carer, to a game done with others, to (finally) a boring game: 'I don't want to play anymore.' And none of this knowing is explicit until the second year, but before that it is simultaneously embodied in multiple psychobiological systems.

A few points about the process of acquiring the game: the acquisition of a game depends on the infant being with someone who knows the game and who must be willing to 'teach' her the game. Infants cannot teach themselves the game. At any age, the learning of the game is dependent on the repetition of the game and the development of different capacities at multiple levels (neurologic, regulatory, motor, emotional) that make the acquisition of a game possible. A three-month-old does not have the capacities to learn the game no matter how often its re-occurrence. The game is individualized. The adult who is playing it with the infant plays the game in a unique way, and the infant acquires that unique way. Better said, they co-create a unique way of doing the game together. In an important sense, they co-create a unique game of their own. Co-creation is critical for understanding the other games children learn (Tronick, 2017). The game, like all children's games, is arbitrary, in the sense that it has a history in a cultural context. It is not built-in by evolution. It is a canonical cultural artifact, played in the way it is played in a particular culture (Bruner, 1990). Other cultures play other games in their own cultural form.

More generally and importantly, we see the acquisition of a game by an infant as no different than the infant coming to know any other cultural form of behavior, or any form of procedural knowing which involves spontaneous – 'natural' – interaction; that is their way of being with others. The infant comes to know the 'game' of cuddling, the 'game' of feeding, and the 'game' of greeting a stranger. Infants develop the 'game' of being demanding, the 'game' of taking a bath, and the 'games' of changing, and nursing, and going to sleep. Each of these 'games' re-occurs tens, even hundreds, of times a month. Each has a form that is individualized and acculturated. Each is dynamic and changes with experience and development of new capacities. The process of acquisition is messy and requires repairs. And each involves repeated experiencing of the 'game' with another person to finally get it into the infant's state of consciousness. And the form that it takes in the infant reflects the form of the 'game' in the adult's state of consciousness, because its form is what guides how the adult plays the game. To jump ahead, the infant who comes to know the particular form of the 'game' of being abused, also comes to know the particular form of the 'game' of being an abuser that is in the abuser.

I hope that this account of normal developmental processes of learning 'games' – actually learning how to be in the world – is starting to have some link to our understanding of trauma. Let me make the link of this kind of developmental process of coming to know how to be in the world with the child coming to know the 'game' of being hit by an adult. Of course, being hit is not a game and peek-a-boo may seem far away from trauma, and it is, but for our purposes it is not. Being hit by an adult is clinically relevant as such and it is a metaphor for thinking about the trauma associated with any event.

To begin, the physicality of hits is not the same (Tronick and Perry, 2014). They vary in intensity and they vary as to the target. Think about a hit with an open palm to the face of moderate intensity. The first hit a child receives is not experienced the same way as the tenth; it is unique. It changes the child's state of consciousness about the world and meaning making. But so does the tenth hit, as it must because the child has made meaning of the nine preceding hits and the tenth has to be integrated with those that came before. Moreover, the hits are not the same, depending on the motivational state of the child. For example, a hit will be experienced differently if she is hit when she is concentrating on a game and feeling safe, or hiding and in a fearful state, or in an angry state. In the next moment after the hit, and then for succeeding moments, her state will change and with it the meaning of the hit will change. With mental and physical development, the 'same' physical hit is experienced differently at two years of age, at five, or at ten years, and different if, at ten years, it was last experienced at two years, or five years, or never experienced before. Furthermore, whatever agenic actions – fighting back, running away, freezing – the child takes will change the nature of the experience of the hit. Just imagine the difference between a three-year-old kicking the abuser or running away and hiding behind a couch. And to further complicate the picture, the context matters. Was the child in and around the abuser much of the time? Was the abuser a stranger? Was the abuser a parent, a carer, a babysitter?

And there is more. First, if the abuser is a someone who regularly cares for the child, we know that their caretaking is going to be at the very least problematic if not even continuously derailing. Carers who hit children do not parent well. They are angry and threatening, demanding, neglectful, falsely apologetic. What they are, in fact, can affect the child's experience of the hit. A hit in anger is not the same as a hit in frustration followed by an apology. As a consequence, the child is under continuous pressure from that distorted problematic caretaking. Its effects could be enough to derail the child's development even if there was no abuse. Importantly, the experience of the problematic caretaking exacerbates the effects of the abuse. Even a single hit in the context of disturbed parenting could be enough to disrupt the child's development. Moreover, when we say a particular event is traumatic – a hit – my bet is that it might not have so debilitating an effect except for the already vulnerable state of the child given the reiterated problematic caretaking they have received. So is a hit, a fast physical event taking only milliseconds really an acute singularity?

But there is more. It is not only the occurrence of the hit or the disturbing parenting that will derail the child. We all know about the triggers of trauma that are present all around the child all of the time that re-ignite the experience. They are unavoidable. But the child will trigger themselves. Saying that is not blaming the child, it is blaming how evolution has organized the way humans make meaning. The child will make meaning of the hit and the experience of her caretaking and she will keep on processing it. She will re-experience its vagal and HPA effects, memorializing it, perseverating on it, re-examining what happened, what she did. Most insidiously, she will anticipate it happening again. The self-generated reoccurrence, the self-generation of triggers, goes on and on with continuous never-ending meaning-making processes – processes that feed on themselves.

These self-generated meaning making processes with an older child or adult may be explicit and in awareness as well as in the body. In an infant or younger immature child, they will be neurosomatic processes that make meaning completely out of awareness; for example, a lower fear threshold in the amygdala that generates the experience of fear to benign events and leads to more internal fear and anxiety. We often see these physiological forms of trauma in our clients when they only have the feeling of the event but cannot provide details or a timeline. This lack of a narrative is because neurosomatic forms of memorializing do not generate timelines; your gut biome does not track dates and details of events but it does affect meaning making.

For those of you who focus on the brain, let me give a brain-oriented account of meaning making of experience with something like a hit (Tronick and Perry, 2014). The primary mechanism in meaning making by the brain is the capacity to create associations. When patterns of neural activity co-occur with sufficient frequency, intensity or pattern, these patterns become 'connected' at a synaptic level. But these synaptic connections are not 'empty', they have content. Perry's neurosequential model (Perry, 1999, 2008, 2009) makes it clear that the capacity to weave content – the complex array of sensory, somatic and cerebro-modulatory patterns of activity – into a form of coherence is one of the remarkable qualities of development. Indeed, development requires the sequential creation of associations – essentially, sequential meaning making – from body to brainstem to cortex.

Beginning *in utero*, the meaning-making systems (typically, but artificially referred to as 'body and brain', which is a linguistic dichotomy, not a physiological reality) weave together seamless multiple interactive dynamic systems through multiple molecular mechanisms. These mechanisms include the creation of 'activity-organized' synaptic nets that begin to create meaning for the developing organism. The sensory and somatic 'external' input from the intrauterine environment (warm, fluid embracing, ever beating maternal heart sounds, voice) experienced by the fetus becomes associated with the neural activation created. For the fetus, it carries the meaning of being 'safe and regulated' (i.e. not hungry, thirsty, cold or threatened). The operation of the neurosomatic systems, their re-occurring neural activation rhythms, holds the meaning.

Later in the ex-uterine environment, rhythmic rocking, for example, may have a primordial meaning of 'safe', a meaning inherent in coherent somatosensory organization. A frightened or overwhelmed child may self-soothe by rocking in the fetal position in an attempt to recapture, or actually create, that primordial meaning of 'safe'. Similarly, other meanings, such as 'the world is a dangerous place', are also held by bodily processes in conjunction with the brain, such as the immune system, the autonomic nervous system (ANS), gut biome, as much as by the brain when the child (or adult) is unable to generate coherent patterns of neural activity (Porges, 2011). And like the plasticity of the brain in response to environmental input, other neurosomatic processes are organized and sculpted by the early experiences, even though the conscious mind does not have access to the early experiences that created that meaning.

Neurosomatic meaning making indicates that even though the young child's somatic and neurophysiologic systems are far from fully developed, she can make meaning. She has states of consciousness, though with no implication of awareness. As such, the infant can fully organize a motivated and embodied state of distress, perhaps even an emotionally fearful state, or a motivated state of pleasure that organizes her actions in the world. One state leads to withdrawal and demands for regulatory support, the other to engagement and self-directed action on some object or communication with another. Thus, the process of meaning making begins with the first experience to create the primary associations (i.e. neural connections) that will organize the infant's world. And keep in mind that *all* of the neurosomatic systems continue to operate in the adult. They continue to make meaning: the wash of adrenalin after a near miss car accident when you know consciously everyone is okay. And these systems continue to bring the meaning of events in the past into the adult present: the feeling of terror with an ocean wave curling at you from an unremembered thumping by a wave when you were five years old, even though now you know you are safe.

Returning to the case of the physical abuse, the first time that the infant is hit, the image of a hand moving swiftly across the visual field has not yet been associated with pain. If the abuser is always the same person, and others never hit the child, the set of somatosensory associations may generalize to the properties of that person or the place where the hitting occurred (e.g. the bedroom). The child may begin to feel fearful at the sound of the abuser's voice, the smell of his aftershave, the image of his face, the sound of a door closing, and so on. And the child may then generalize from the abuser's hand to all hands moving quickly near her face – even if the person is a nurturing caregiver, moving to gently caress her face. These associations and the resulting threat-related behaviors are mediated by the simpler, lower somatosensory and action – motor – systems involved in stress and the threat response.

These more generalized and undifferentiated responses can be quite troubling and mystifying to an individual experiencing them, even when the formative experiences are part of the 'known but unremembered' aspects of a person's life. Though unavailable in conscious memory, they are nonetheless stored in the brain and body's operating patterns, activation preferences, set points and thresholds, throughout the body and encoded by implicit neural processes that are remarkably durable. Traditional talk therapy may not be sufficient to access these sub-cortical organizers of experience. Directing attentional processes to the body – a core feature of sensorimotor psychotherapy – can stimulate neural circuits associated with these memories, providing opportunities to encode new experiences that support a shift in meaning, and subsequently, a shift in experience

(Ogden and Fisher, 2014). Indeed, in infants, Piaget argued that their first meaning-making system was sensorimotor.

This picture of what is going on gives us a critical idea of why early experience has such long-term effects. The meaning-making process in infancy is developmentally robust, because so many meanings are connected to fundamental regulatory processes. These regulatory processes are shaped by early experience and continue to operate later in development in similar ways unless they are re-sculpted by experience or therapy. Thus, many of the associations created early in life are directly linked with neurosomatic processes – primary regulatory neural networks and primary somatic processes – that continue to shape and influence the meanings made throughout life, unless they are retuned by experience or interventions. Moreover, the infant has less capacity to modulate or shift the meaning, because the higher areas of the brain are not yet fully organized. That is, for example, the infant does not yet have complex time-telling capabilities or abstract cognition to allow her to make a more 'abstract' or differentiated meaning about the one abuser in relation to other nurturing carers. These gaps of capacity make the infant more vulnerable.

As the child becomes older and the limbic and cortical areas of the brain become more organized, the meaning of the hit, the abuser, and the toddler's potential to act in relation to the abuser with behaviors that appear to increase or decrease the probability of hitting, change and become more coherent and complex. The infant 'learns' (comes to know at an implicit pre-conscious level), for example, that crying (a 'fight-flight' stress-related behavior that should bring a carer to meet the infant's distress, such as hunger, thirst, cold, pain) will actually increase the hitting, whereas dissociating (and not crying) will decrease the hitting. As a toddler, she may also learn that overly compliant behavior will decrease hitting. And she may modify her meaning about hitting. Let's say her mother – a loving but overwhelmed, frustrated caregiver, who never hit before – hits her in frustration, when she is non-compliant (non-compliance is *not* possible for her with an actual repeated abuser but is with the mother given their history). Almost immediately, there will be a physically nurturing and intimate interaction as the guilty mother attempts to repair the empathic rupture (not an unusual dynamic with an overwhelmed mother and an abusive partner – the initial abuser). This change in meaning is now possible because of the development of neural systems previously unavailable to the infant. The 'meaning' of the hit evolves.

This process of changing and creating new associations requires plasticity of neural networks. Fortunately, neurons and neural networks are not only capable of change; they are specifically constructed to change in response to experience. This plasticity underlying both developmental and therapeutic change has conditions that will enhance, and others that inhibit, meaningful change (Kleim and Jones, 2008). Two primary principles of plasticity are specificity and pattern. Simply stated, neural networks that are not being activated with sufficient repetition in a meaningful pattern will not change. And let me add that plasticity applies to all the somatic regulatory systems that are sculpted by early and ongoing repeated experience.

And this principle brings us back to my view of trauma. To start, the principle of repetition implies that there is no such thing as an acute singular traumatic event, an event that happens only once. It is an ongoing process. Not to be difficult, the principle is both false and true. Allow me to state the point in the extreme: singular acute traumatic events are not different from repeated events. The meaning of an event is reiteratively processed by an individual over time, maybe over a lifetime; it lingers. Second, the meaning of the event is affected by and affects the meaning the individual makes of other events; its meaning is not static or fixed. Take an example other than a hit, the acute event of a never-to-be repeated one-time sexual abuse of a young girl by a stranger never to be seen again. It happens only once, it is singular, but is it really? Certainly, it is what we point to and it *can* have lifelong effects, but not in the sense that it is a 'thing', a lesion, an object deep in the psyche of the individual. From a developmental meaning-making perspective, the trauma is not singular. The occurrence of the event may be singular, but the meaning of the trauma is not anchored like a crystalized rock in the psyche. The processing of the trauma is ongoing and in that sense it is repeated and can have lifelong effects.

To start, there are internal neurosomatic meaning-making processes – autonomic nervous system, HPA axis, and brain processes of memory, rumination, perseveration, dissociation – that continue to operate on the meaning of the event. The meaning is repeatedly *re*processed. The operation of these neurosomatic meaning-making processes actually alters the meaning over time, even if the individual is not aware of the change. In the case of children, those meaning-making processes develop (e.g. cortical processes come online), further changing the meaning of the event.

Second, the meaning of the acute event affects the meaning of other experienced events. One obvious process is how the young girl's initial meaning of the event – '*I was too trusting*' – affects and is affected by future interactions. Perhaps that meaning disrupts her relations with others, which in turn makes her even more distrustful. And then those newly emerging meanings have their effects on the meaning made of subsequent events. Third, the acute event does not exist in isolation, but it is affected by '*all*' current and ongoing experience. The '*all*' includes what was going on when the event occurred, the meaning being made of other events, and the evolving context over time of the event. Perhaps the young girl's other ongoing relationships so robustly contradict the distrust and give her a sense of safety and certainty, which in turn makes her more trustful, or perhaps the stranger appeared less manipulative at first and any later sensitive contact provokes fear no matter who does it.

This account of what we refer to as a single-one-time only traumatic event when we talk about our clients should, I hope, make it clear that they are actually repeated events. Nonetheless, there are differences between the singular and repeated event. An event that is repeated triggers the host of processes again and again. Its effects are more likely to accumulate, be more intense and affect a wider range of experiences and the individual's sense of their world. But nonetheless the repeated event is in the context of other events, and there is a high likelihood that that they are distorted and pathological. As with the physical act of hitting, if the young girl is repeatedly abused, the likelihood that the rest of her world is 'normal' is vanishingly small. In fact, the distortions of the rest of her experience further exacerbate the consequences of the 'event'. Escaping their effects will be more difficult.

How does the evolution of the complex archeology of the meaning of a hit, or of peek-a-boo, or of being with another, or of any way of being, relate to therapy? For me, therapy is about changing meanings. How do we see the change process? Obviously, there are a myriad of driving forces and systems involved, that are inherent to making and changing meaning, including somatic and regulatory systems, neural systems and action systems: the list would go on. My view of therapeutics is very much Vygotskyan (1978): optimal development in any domain (e.g. neural, regulatory, motor, sensory) occurs when the individual is given opportunities and expectations, usually by, or with another person, that are neither too familiar and simple, nor too unfamiliar and complex (Perry, 2009; Tronick, 2007). The individual with a psychic dysfunction has to be allowed to select or guide the information that she is presented with, such that it fits to, and can be worked on, by her meaning-making capacities to make new meanings.

I would emphasize (Tronick and Beeghly, 2011) that therapeutic work with infants and young children must aim to understand deeply their intentions, the multi-level meanings that children are making about themselves, how they are making them within themselves, by themselves with objects, and most importantly with others. In adults, it is critical to determine where the meaning 'resides'. It may reside in the prefrontal cortex (as is presumed by cognitive therapies), but obviously I believe much of it resides lower down in the brainstem, regulatory and somatosensory processes. This multiplicity of neurosomatic processes demands forms of therapy that reorganize those processes through re-occurrent experiences, which may eventually make the distorting experience available to awareness.

One implication of multiple levels and kinds of meaning-making systems is that therapy cannot simply or solely focus on just one system or another – be it the somatic, or neural, or action, or cognitive or emotional systems. What development tells us about meaning making and change is that it involves all these systems, simultaneously operating as a messily organized ensemble. More specifically, change involves an individual who has agency to organize her engagement with the world, especially the world of people, with every level and every meaning-making system she possesses. But development also tells us that therapeutically induced change in meaning must enact the first principle of re-occurrence. The individual must have the opportunity to engage and re-engage in experiences that can change and generate new associations and new operations of regulatory systems at the core of meaning making.

The demand for enough experiences to allow for change is especially critical when we consider early meanings that are interwoven with fundamental somatic and regulatory processes. Admittedly, we do not know what 'enough' is, but we do know that seldom is there enough re-occurrent experience in the right systems (i.e. the bedrock associations created by our earliest somatosensory experiences in the lower areas of the brain). Most targeted therapeutic efforts do not adhere to the core principle of specificity; non-somatic therapies in and of themselves will not directly and repetitively activate the foundational somatosensory systems (and related associations) made in early life and localized in the lowest systems in the brain, and somatic therapies will not directly affect and repetitively activate higher order brain systems. Thus, as argued from the beginning, meaning making and therapeutic change involve systems at all levels of the hierarchical organization of the brain and body simultaneously.

More generally, our emphasis on the multi-level psychobiological nature of meaning making has a specific implication for therapeutic interventions for trauma. No single therapeutic approach, no matter how powerful, will be an adequate therapeutic intervention. Trauma therapy, as well as any therapy for any problem, must take multiple forms. Somatic, verbal, neurophysiologic, medication, drugs, relational, experiential, narrative, video, and all the therapies that are identified alphabetically (CBT, DBT, EMDR). With respect to all my colleagues, claims to the contrary about this or that therapy treating trauma are like the claims about snake oil: 'step right up folks, the elixir will cure everything'. Whether or not you accept the concept of multiple psychobiological processes making meaning, you must admit that the trauma is complicated, and simple solutions, quick solutions, will not be adequate. This is not a call for a kind of eclecticism, though eclecticism can be helpful. The frame is meaning making and our understanding of it. The challenge of a multiple-method therapeutic approach is to initially figure out what the neurosomatic form of the trauma is and to specify a therapeutic approach that gets at this, to track the dynamics of the change induced and the new neurosomatic form of the trauma, to figure out the next approach that will gain traction, and so on in an ongoing process. In some cases, multiple forms of therapy may be used simultaneously. To get at this multiple approach we need far more research and a change in training away from a one-size-fits-all approach to a multiple competence approach, or a team approach to therapy, or one that considers the whole range of experience and functioning of the individual. At the core, the challenge is to figure out what to do, when to do it, and when to change.

Adults and children live in a world where an hour of any kind of therapy can be lost in the welter of all the other hours. If the people in the child's life are not part of the process of change, then change will not occur; the same is likely true for adults. Traumatized children face the same dilution, even with weekly hours in therapy. They need an immersion with therapeutic others. Adults, at some point, may be able to do much on their own, but nonetheless additional scaffolding of their self-organized work with more contact (sessions) and 'work' will enhance their own work. Thus, what makes sense for us as a guide for therapy – for children and adults – is to take our cue from the developmental meaning: approach therapeutic change like learning peek-a-boo. Do it often, do it in multiple ways that fully engage every level of the individual, and let the individual agencically control the process.

KNOWLEDGE AND PRACTICE REFLECTION

Joe Tucci, Janise Mitchell, Ed Tronick and Stephen W. Porges

In this poetic piece, Ed Tronick delves deeply into the complex ways though which meaning is experienced in the moment of violation and in its aftermath. As Tronick has argued over the course of his career, meaning making is not merely a cognitive process, reliant on language and narrative, to decipher forms of hidden truths into expressions that can be more easily understood and then communicated. Instead, it is neurosomatic – occurring simultaneously at multiple physiological, bodily and cognitive levels, resulting in meaning-making states of consciousness.

> Neurosomatic meaning-making processes are endogenous and continuously operating. They keep on going and going, affecting the meanings made as life moves on. Worse still, the initial meaning made goes on to affect the next meanings made. Those later emerging meanings generate further distortions and increasingly insidious debilitations, that indeed may be far more derailing than the initial meaning made of the experience.

There is so much to take from this chapter with Tronick's use of words and constructs that, because at his own admission he sits slightly off to the side of trauma theory as a developmentalist, offers perspectives that may hold considerable resources.

Ambient meaning is one of these useful constructs. It is like the immersive soup of energy and information that is gleaned from the repetitive experience of interactions with others and/or the representation of others in our experiences. This surrounding internal sense of the quality of experience, reactions to experience and interpretations of experience is a neurological and physiological substrate from which an orienting meaning evolves. This orienting meaning serves to shape experience as it happens but is also further shaped by the experience and its meaning as it happens.

Meaning of 'known but unremembered' experiences is another important construct. As he identifies, though unavailable in conscious memory and awareness:

> ...they are nonetheless stored in the brain and body's operating patterns, activation preferences, set points, thresholds, throughout the body and encoded by implicit neural processes that are remarkably durable.

For those affected by trauma, such meanings are deeply held orienting reflexes that often predetermine responses to signals in their environment. Outside their awareness, victims and survivors are working from an internalized proforma of reactions that were imprinted before, during and after their experience of violation.

Tronick uses the phrase *'selective assembly of self-organized actions and reactions'* as a key process of meaning making. It is critical because it highlights that despite the young age of an infant, for example, that infant is not passive to the events and experiences around her. She has a degree of agency in the way that she engages with experiences in order for such meaning to eventually become more coherent. Her first efforts to make sense of a game of peak-a-boo is 'messy – variable, unstable, disorganized'. But with repetition and practice, the infant attends to different elements of the game, predicting and eventually influencing steps that she comes to expect, even though there is variety in the form the game itself is played. The meaning has become 'sticky', more enduring and more reliably recalled with the same state of playfulness and excitement each time it is played.

The conclusion of Tronick's essay is the critical call for reconsideration of therapeutic change as needing to adhere to the fundamental principle of *re-occurrence* – with those who are affected by trauma being given multiple and repeated opportunities to alter and develop new connections and reverberating activations of neurosomatic systems from which deep forms of meaning evolve. For Tronick, no single therapeutic or relational practice will lead to such change. He is in favour of casting the net wide to offer experiences to victims and survivors which facilitate the assembly and re-assembly of regulatory responses into new forms of meaning that are more social, promote agency and support further evolution, moving away from static outcomes as if they are finite end states that will not change any longer.

Finally, Tronick argues that 'if the people in the child's life are not part of the process of change, then change will not occur; the same is likely true for adults'. It is more than likely that the application of one hour of therapy is nowhere near enough to make a dent in the ensconced meaning states that have been shaped by the searing pain of trauma. Victims and survivors need to be immersed in relational experiences of care through which firmly held meanings are destabilized, reconfigured and re-experienced to allow for them to become the new base of neurosomatic reactions.

This is why collaboration between people (family, practitioners, friends) is so important. It is why trauma-transformative approaches need frameworks that actually achieve true cooperation and collective decision making in which power for change is shared across a network and in particular with the victims and survivors themselves.

Collaboration and power sharing of decision making with victims and survivors of interpersonal violence has been a staunchly held principle of the trauma-informed movement from its inception (Harris and Fallot, 2001a, 2001b; Prescott, 2001; SAMHSA, 2014).

Yet, to date, the trauma-informed literature has not really focused too much on interdiscipline, interagency and intracommunity ways of working that facilitate better service coordination between agencies and their networks. This has the potential to continue to leave service users affected by trauma having to dealing with siloed approaches that are determined by funding lines and service typology. For example, in *Humanising Mental Health Care in Australia* (Benjamin, Haliburn and King, 2019) – an insightful collection of chapters about trauma-informed care – of the final eight chapters which deal with organizational applications, only one chapter (Tucci and Mitchell, 2019) deals with the importance of interagency collaboration. This is replicated repeatedly in many of the articles about trauma-informed practice (Harris and Fallot, 2001a, 2001b, 2001c; Fallot and Harris, 2001; Bebout, 2001; Freeman, 2001; Prescott, 2001; Arledge and Wolfson, 2001; SAMHSA, 2014; Sweeney *et al.*, 2018).

Even in child protection and child welfare sectors, which arguably rely on interagency coordination and collaboration (e.g. between child protection, family support services, schools), trauma-informed practice has not particularly sought to integrate knowledge about trauma and collaborative practice into a unifying framework that can guide decision making (Strand, 2018a, 2018b; Brown, Hansen and Saxe, 2018). These, traditions have remained largely separate conceptually, even if they are applied in reality with varying degrees of success.

There is some attention paid to multidisciplinary collaboration within the one clinical setting (Reeves, 2015) and an interest in providing a common language across a service system in order to better aid referrals between services (Carter and Blanch, 2019).

For this reason, there needs to be far more significant effort put into enshrining collaborative forms of decision making into practice orientations that seek to transform and address trauma.

Tronick echoes the work undertaken in his earlier collaboration with Mitchell and Tucci in which they noted that the collaborative outcomes promised by improved interagency, cross-system and family centred practice had yet to be realized in many settings which claim to be trauma informed (Mitchell, Tucci and Tronick, 2020). Based in the work of Anne Edwards from the Department of Education at Oxford University, Mitchell, Tucci and Tronick (2020) integrated the need for a new competency for practitioners to develop in themselves which focused their intervention efforts on intentionally driven cooperation. *Relational agency* is the capacity to:

> ...work with others to expand the object that one is working on and trying to transform by recognising and accessing the resources that others bring to bear as they interpret and respond to the object. It is a capacity which involves recognising that another person may be a resource and that work needs to be done to elicit, recognise and negotiate the use of that resource in order to align oneself in joint action on the object... (Edwards, 2005, p.172)

As Mitchell herself pioneered with the development of one of the world's first therapeutic foster care programs 20 years ago (Mitchell, McPherson and Gatwiri, 2020; Mitchell, Tucci and Macnamara, 2020), the implementation of a therapeutic care team is an example of a network of distributed intelligence with individual and relational forms of expertise. These networks meet regularly, recognizing respective roles and coordinating their action and work across hierarchical structures within organizations (Macnamara, 2020). They are supported by therapeutic specialists with the expertise in understanding interpersonal dynamics and work to resource the collective. This network interacts at the boundaries where practice intersects and common knowledge emerges. Common knowledge itself comes to be mobilized in the way that the team members use it. The positioning of the child's needs, the clarity with which the child's trauma experiences are always aligned to explanations about their behavior, the understanding of the nature of the interaction between children and their relational and sensory environment, and the collective commitment to compassionate inquiry are experiences which all negotiated at the boundaries of practice. The relational process underlying the work of the care teams serves to bring together multiple inter-subjectivities and create new solutions for children and young people in-out-of-home care.

A more in-depth appreciation of collaborative and collective practice should be a defining principle of trauma-transformative practice undertaken by practitioners, organizations and systems.

References
References for chapter

Bruner, J. (1990). *Acts of Meaning.* Cambridge, MA: Harvard University Press.

Bruner, J. and Sherwood, V. (1976). Peek-a-boo and the Learning of Rule Structures. In J. Bruner, A. Jolly and K. Silva (eds), *Play: Its Role in Development and Evolution* (pp.13–27). London: Penguin.

Commons, M., Trudeau, E., Stein, S., Richards, F. and Krause, S. (1998). Hierarchical complexity of tasks shows the existence of developmental stages. *Developmental Review,* 18, 237–278.

Harrison, A.M. (2003). Change in psychoanalysis: Getting from A to B. *Journal of the American Psychoanalytic Association,* 51, 221–257.

Kleim, J.A. and Jones, T.A. (2008). Principles of experience-dependent neural plasticity: Implications for rehabilitation after brain damage. *Journal of Speech, Language and Hearing Research,* 51, 225–239.

Modell, A. (1993). *The Private Self.* Cambridge, MA: Harvard University Press.

Ogden, P. (1997). Inner body sensation. Part one. *Somatics,* 11(2), 40–43.

Ogden, P. and Fisher, J. (2014). *Sensorimotor Psychotherapy: Interventions for Attachment and Trauma.* New York, NY: W.W. Norton and Company.

Perry, B.D. (1999). Memories of Fear: How the Brain Stores and Retrieves Physiologic States, Feelings, Behaviours and Thoughts from Traumatic Events. In J.M. Goodwin and R. Attias (eds), *Images of the Body in Trauma* (pp.26–47). New York, NY: Basic Books.

Perry, B.D. (2008). Child Maltreatment: The Role of Abuse and Neglect in Developmental Psychopathology. In T.P. Beauchaine and S.P. Hinshaw (eds), *Textbook of Child and Adolescent Psychopathology* (pp.93–128). New York, NY: Wiley.

Perry, B.D. (2009). Examining child maltreatment through a neurodevelopmental lens: Clinical application of the Neurosequential Model of Therapeutics. *Journal of Loss and Trauma,* 14, 240–255.

Porges, S.W. (2011). *The Polyvagal Theory: Neurophysiological Foundations of Emotions, Attachment, Communication, and Self-regulation.* New York, NY: W.W. Norton and Company.

Sander, L.W. (1977). The Regulation of Exchange in Infant-Caregiver Systems and Some Aspects of the Context-Contrast Relationship. In L.A. Rosenblum (ed.), *Interaction Conversation and the Development of Language.* New York, NY: Wiley.

Tronick, E. (1998). Interactions that effect change in psychotherapy: A model based on infant research. *Infant Mental Health Journal,* 19, 1–290.

Tronick, E. (2003). Of course all relationships are unique: How co-creative processes generate unique mother-infant and patient-therapist relationships and change other relationships. *Psychological Inquiry,* 23, 3, 473–491.

Tronick, E. (2007). *Neurobehavioural and Social Emotional Development.* New York, NY: W.W. Norton and Company.

Tronick, E. (2017). A Radical Phenomenology of Gaining Meaning. In K. Brandt, S. Seligman, B. Perry and E. Tronick (eds). *Infant and Early Childhood Mental Health: Core Concepts and Clinical Practice.* Arlington, VA: American Psychiatric Press.

Tronick, E. and Beeghly, M. (2011). Meaning making and infant mental health. *American Psychologist,* 107–119.

Tronick, E. and Perry, B. (2014). The Multiple Levels of Meaning Making and the First Principles of Changing Meanings in Development and Therapy. In G. Marlock and H. Weiss, with C. Young and M. Soth, (eds), *Handbook of Somatic Psychotherapy* (pp.345–355). Berkeley, CA: North Atlantic Books.

Vygotsky, L.S. (1978). Interaction Between Learning and Development. In L.S. Vygotsky (ed.), *Mind in Society.* Cambridge, MA: Harvard University Press.

References for Knowledge and Practice Reflection

Arledge, E. and Wolfson, R. (2001). Care of the Clinician. In M. Harris, and R.D. Fallot (eds), *Using Trauma Theory to Design Service Systems* (pp.91–98). San Francisco, CA: Jossey-Bass/Wiley.

Bebout, R.R. (2001). Trauma Informed Approaches to Housing. In M. Harris, and R.D. Fallot (eds), *Using Trauma Theory to Design Service Systems* (pp.47–56). San Francisco, CA: Jossey-Bass/Wiley.

Benjamin, R., Haliburn, J. and King, S. (2019). *Humanising Mental Health Care in Australia: A Guide to Trauma-informed Approaches*. London: Routledge.

Brown, D.A., Hansen, S. and Saxe, G.N. (2018). System Change Designed to Increase Safety and Stabilisation for Traumatised Children and Families: Trauma Systems Theory. In V.C. Strand and G. Sprang (eds), *Trauma Responsive Child Welfare Systems* (pp.87–104). New York, NY: Springer.

Carter, P. and Blanch, A. (2019). A trauma lens for systems change. *Stanford Social Innovation Review*, 17(3), 48–54.

Edwards, A. (2005). Relational agency: Learning to be a resourceful practitioner. *International Journal of Educational Research*, 43, 168–182.

Fallot, R.D. and Harris, M. (2001). A Trauma Informed Approach to Screening and Assessment. In M. Harris, and R.D. Fallot (eds), *Using Trauma Theory to Design Service Systems* (pp.23–32). San Francisco, CA: Jossey-Bass/Wiley.

Freeman, D.W. (2001). Trauma Informed Services and Case Management. In M. Harris, and R.D. Fallot (eds), *Using Trauma Theory to Design Service Systems* (pp.75–82). San Francisco, CA: Jossey-Bass/Wiley.

Harris, M. and Fallot, R.D. (2001a). Envisioning a Trauma Informed Service System: A Vital Paradigm Shift. In M. Harris and R.D. Fallot (eds), *Using Trauma Theory to Design Service Systems* (pp.3–22). San Francisco, CA: Jossey-Bass/Wiley.

Harris, M. and Fallot, R.D. (2001b). Trauma Informed Inpatient Services. In M. Harris, and R.D. Fallot (eds), *Using Trauma Theory to Design Service Systems* (pp.33–46). San Francisco, CA: Jossey-Bass/Wiley.

Harris, M. and Fallot, R.D. (2001c). Designing Trauma Informed Addiction Services. In M. Harris and R.D. Fallot (eds), *Using Trauma Theory to Design Service Systems* (pp.57–74). San Francisco, CA: Jossey-Bass/Wiley.

Macnamara. N. (2020). Therapeutic Care Teams: Horizontal Teams in a Virtual World. In J. Mitchell, J. Tucci and E. Tronick (eds), *The Handbook of Therapeutic Care for Children: Evidence Informed Approaches to Working with Traumatised Children and Adolescents in Foster, Kinship and Adoptive Care* (pp.219–240). London: Jessica Kingsley Publishers.

Mitchell, J., McPherson, L. and Gatwiri, K. (2020). 'Support and Love and All that Stuff'; Evidence of Impact in the Treatment and Care for Kids Program. In J. Mitchell, J. Tucci and E. Tronick (eds), *The Handbook of Therapeutic Care for Children: Evidence Informed Approaches to Working with Traumatised Children and Adolescents in Foster, Kinship and Adoptive Care* (pp.109–136). London: Jessica Kingsley Publishers.

Mitchell, J., Tucci, J. and Macnamara, N. (2020). What are the Key Elements of Therapeutic Care? In J. Mitchell, J. Tucci and E. Tronick (eds), *The Handbook of Therapeutic Care for Children: Evidence Informed Approaches to Working with Traumatised Children and Adolescents in Foster, Kinship and Adoptive Care* (pp.21–34). London: Jessica Kingsley Publishers.

Mitchell, J., Tucci, J. and Tronick, E. (eds), *The Handbook of Therapeutic Care for Children: Evidence Informed Approaches to Working with Traumatised Children and Adolescents in Foster, Kinship and Adoptive Care*. London: Jessica Kingsley Publishers.

Prescott, L. (2001). Defining the Role of Consumer-Survivors in Trauma Informed Systems. In M. Harris, and R.D. Fallot (eds), *Using Trauma Theory to Design Service Systems* (pp.83–90). San Francisco, CA: Jossey-Bass/Wiley.

Reeves, E. (2015). A synthesis of the literature on trauma-informed care. *Issues in Mental Health Nursing*, 36(9), 698–709.

Strand, V.C. (2018a). Applying Trauma Theory to Agency Practice. In V.C. Strand and G. Sprang (eds), *Trauma Responsive Child Welfare Systems* (pp.13–18). New York, NY: Springer.

Strand, V.C. (2018b). Applying Trauma Theory to Organizational Culture. In V.C. Strand and G. Sprang (eds), *Trauma Responsive Child Welfare Systems* (pp.19–40). New York, NY: Springer.

Sweeney, A., Filson, B., Kennedy, A., Collinson, L. and Gillard, S. (2018). A paradigm shift: Relationships in trauma-informed mental health services. *British Journal of Psychiatric Advances*, 24(5), 319–333.

Substance Abuse and Mental Health Services Administration (SAMHSA) (2014). *Trauma-Informed Care in Behavioural Health Services – Treatment Improvement Protocol (TIP) Series 57* (HHS Publication no. (SMA) 13-4801).

Tucci, J. and Mitchell, J. (2019). Therapeutic Services for Traumatised Children and Young People Healing. In R. Benjamin, J. Haliburn and S. King (eds), *Humanising Mental Health Care in Australia: A Guide to Trauma-informed Approaches* (pp.319–320). London: Routledge.

CHAPTER 6

The Integrated Brain: The Neuropsychological Roots of Shame

Efrat Ginot

The experience of shame

Without a doubt, feelings of shame are among the most difficult to tolerate. The humiliation dealt to our self-esteem and the threats to our sense of self are bound together with intense visceral discomfort and self-denigrating narratives. What makes the experience of shame such a searingly painful state are the intense self-hatred and disgust and the all-consuming dark place where there is little hope for redemption or for a more positive outlook about who we are (Lewis, 2019).

When experiencing shame, we may wish to die, hide, or disappear from the face of the earth all together. At times, acute feelings of shame result in confusion, an inability to think, speak, or a sense of a true catastrophe, where the body and mind shrink away in intense self-despisal (Lewis, 2019). Shame can be experienced away from others, triggered by a spontaneous memory of an event or of one's perceived humiliating behavior. Often, shame, like embarrassment, is experienced in the presence of others, where the threats and injury to the well-being of the self are seen as inflicted by the other.

Some researchers differentiate the state of shame into two dimensions: the first, the internal dimension, is seen as the ongoing tendency to be highly self-critical and self-hating; the second, the external dimension, involves one's intense feelings of worthlessness in reaction to perceived judgments coming from others (Hiramatsu *et al.*, 2021). But in effect, regardless of the initial source or trigger, shame is unique in its ability to cause an overwhelming state of panic and self-loathing. Moreover, the two sources of shame converge to form one powerful and demoralizing feeling of being severely inferior to others or to one's expectations of oneself. A humiliating encounter can become especially devastating when it finds an echo in an internal self-loathing feeling pattern, and internally generated shame is rooted in perceived humiliation, mostly in relation to others.

Feelings of shame persist even as we move away from the acute sense of humiliation. At those times, the memories of the exposure of real or perceived mistakes and flaws feel just as painfully raw as when first they took place. The dreaded experience of shame causes many to avoid situations that may trigger it (Cibich *et al.*, 2016). Often, in conscious and unconscious efforts to avoid the painful dysregulation that shame brings, we shy away from taking risks, from pursuing desires, and from fully participating in the world.

The innate character of shame

Like other primary emotions, shame is not learned but innate (Muris *et al.*, 2018). And like all other emotion states, it has been shaped by evolutionary pressures. It is important here to view shame in the context of the new understanding of innate emotion states. This approach explores emotions as important body/mind processes that developed in order to ensure survival and optimal functioning for both the individual and the group (Adolphs and Anderson, 2018). As automatic, fast-occurring visceral sensations signified the presence of danger or impediment to survival, our ancestors learned to identify a wide range of threats and the best automatic defenses against them. The view that emotions are innate emphasizes the embodied nature of emotions – they are part of our brain circuits. Although each emotion system is unique and discernible, our primary emotions have acquired the ability to become very nuanced and to overlap with each other. For example, sexual lust is often entwined with love and caring and panic, intersecting with the fear system and negative emotions such as shame or an ongoing vulnerability.

Along the way, all emotions, both the positive (feelgood, rewarding) and the negative ones (state of distress and dysregulation, punitive), became the inner guidelines that allowed us to navigate the environment and achieve important life goals. Emotions such as sexual lust and excitement, care, and seeking push us forward to fulfill attachment and parenting goals, whereas emotions such as fear, panic, and anxiety have taught humans what to avoid (Adolphs and Anderson, 2018). As we see in the following segments, the relationship between the fear system and shame is especially noticeable.

Among the seven emotion states identified by Panksepp and Biven (2012): (1) seeking/expectancy, (2) fear/anxiety, (3) rage/anger, (4) lust/sexual excitement, (5) care/nurturance, (6) panic/grief/sadness, (7) play, fear and anxiety became indispensable in securing our ancestors' survival. As central in the struggle for actual survival, the fear system (containing both fear and anxiety) acquired a robust presence in our brains/minds/bodies. The amygdala and its related regions process many emotions but, as a host of studies have shown, it is particularly sensitive to threats of impending danger, both real and imagined. In effect, the amygdala functions as the alerting system pushing through visceral sensations to deal with danger (Fox and Shackman, 2019). Over millennia, the amygdala has become extremely successful in its mission, and as some have argued, it has done so at the cost of our stable sense of well-being (Ginot, 2022; Tottenham and Gabard-Durnam, 2017).

To enhance its efficacy and success, the amygdala, which underlies the fear system, had to recruit other circuits responsible for a wide variety of mental functions such as attention, learning and memory, prediction, habits, and expectations. All came under the influence of the amygdala. We quickly identify threats, both real and imagined, we remember them, and act defensively by fleeing, fighting, or freezing. We have acquired an increased sensitivity to anxiety and to the negative ruminations that come with it. We tend to remember and hold on to negative events as signals for future survival, and as fear and anxiety unconsciously influence automatic learning processes and habit forming, our brain/mind inevitably establishes automatic negative predictions and expectations (Ginot, 2015; Tottenham, 2014). Unsurprisingly, the fear system also influences many aspects of social functioning (Swee *et al.*, 2021); it educates us about our standing among others. With the threat of losing the support of others, it instinctively directs our behavior toward getting along with others.

At the heart of the experience of shame is indeed the dread of being inferior to others, being judged by them and exposed to be flawed and therefore deficient and disappointing. And here is where shame, fear and anxiety are inextricably entwined. One wonders whether the evolutionary function of shame is to motivate members of the group to fit in, to perform well in order to be accepted. Doing well in the group also meant a valuable contribution to the general well-being of the community, securing more food and shelter, and getting along, for example. What is so difficult to tolerate when feeling shame is the injury to the conscious sense of who we are and how we want others to see us. In extreme cases, the disapproval of others, real or imagined, can lead to intense anxieties about the intactness of our sense of self, or to the despair associated with feelings of being annihilated by those we love and depend on.

But these essential needs could not avoid becoming entwined with fears and ruminations. Throughout evolution and during our individual development, emotional circuits increasingly connected to the developing higher level cognitive functions of the prefrontal cortex and especially the default mode network. Consequently, we have become increasingly aware that a failure to satisfy the expectations of others may be harshly judged and looked down on. For our ancestors, fear of not doing as well could have increased fear (real or only imagined) about an actual denunciation by the group. Similarly, the threat about a potential rejection and thus the loss of our support system would have thrown us into a panic and the conviction that all was lost.

Indeed, we can imagine that throughout human history, the survival of a community depended on the best efforts and cooperation of its members. Obviously, the definition of 'group survival' has changed over time, but the fear of being criticized, rejected, and shunned by the group or by family and friends has not. Indeed, the visceral experiences as well as the negative self-narratives that are part of the feeling of shame also signal that a real or imagined failure has severe and irreversible consequences. During a humiliating state, the image or thought about being emotionally and interpersonally decimated takes center stage. Shame and embarrassment occur within the social and interpersonal sphere where the perceptions of others on who we are hold an unusual and devastating power. A better understanding of how we are affected by real or imagined criticism and learning to find ways to regulate our emotions to this is one of the common goals of psychotherapy.

The integrated brain

The emotion states of fear and anxiety have acquired the capacity to recruit all other mental functions. Early threats to the intactness of the self invariably influence the attention we give to threat, how readily we perceive it, how we interpret it and think about its meaning to us, and eventually what we do about it. In fact, the story of emotions, including shame, and how they are represented in our consciousness reflects the many neural layers and interconnectedness that characterize brain processes. In general, when we talk about our internal states, we use the term *feeling* more often than the term *emotion*. This is true for both clinical discussions and therapeutic practice, in literature and in the common jargon.

In essence, *feeling* is used to describe what we think of as an emotional experience, but a *feeling* describes very complex and integrated conscious and unconscious processes spanning across all our faculties (Damasio, 2010; Pessoa 2018). When we say we are feeling sad, for example, we are describing a few interdependent processes. We experience unpleasant, painful, and heavy sensations in our body, usually in our chest and around our eyes when we cry; we can articulate the thoughts that describe how we feel, words that convey the pain we feel. We can talk about feelings of loss, grief, disappointment, fear, love, attachment, sexual desire, hopes for the future, the resilient part of our personality, and much more. Often we can relate to ourselves and to others the most nuanced of feeling states.

We also communicate what we feel through body postures, facial expressions, gestures, all nonverbal communication of internal emotion/feeling states. These entwined brain/mind and body processes happen simultaneously (Pessoa and Hof, 2015). We can understand feelings, then, as the culmination and the conscious representation of all these unseen, unconscious neural processes (Adolphs and Anderson, 2018; Damasio, 2010; Panksepp and Biven, 2012). When such integrated brain-mind-body processes are activated by external or internal triggers, they reach consciousness. When we become aware of them, they signify that some important changes have taken place in our physiology and internal state (Adolphs and Anderson, 2018; Damasio, 2010). As these physiological changes in response to external or internal triggers become entwined with other mental functions, they become what we consciously recognize and identify as feelings.

The increasing discoveries regarding this interconnectedness among different brain regions underscores one of the most significant advances in recent neuroscience research. During millennia of human evolution, the brain developed (relatively) new regions, primarily the prefrontal cortex residing in the front of the brain. However, the neural activity these newer areas generate does not occur within a layered architecture; in other words, the newer additions do not lie on top of the lower ones, controlling them, as was previously thought. Instead, evolutionary development demonstrates that these new systems are embedded *within* old ones (Pessoa, 2018; Pessoa and Hof, 2015).

The amygdala and its related circuits are the brain regions that underlie the fear system. Active even prior to birth, the amygdala has vast connections to all brain regions and therefore greatly influences the emotional colors of our thoughts, beliefs, and actions. The quick and automatic reactions of the amygdala to real and perceived threats all but guarantee that most of us are vulnerable to emotional insults from a wide range of normative, run-of-the-mill events and experiences.

What may seem benign and meaningless to parents, for example, is still injurious to toddlers, children, and adolescents. From early on, children are vulnerable to anxiety-inducing experiences and to the dysregulation they cause. Inevitable interpersonal injuries or even perceived shaming situations may arouse shame. The visceral discomfort becomes totally intertwined with the negative personal meaning of such encounters and with increasingly entrenched self-denigrating thoughts. In effect, pockets of anxiety and negative self-narratives develop, even with good parenting and within a loving and supportive environment.

Whereas the amygdala's activity comes online in utero, the prefrontal cortex lags in its development. With the absence of a more reasoned perspective and understanding, dysregulating interpersonal encounters will be perceived as internally devastating to the child's self-esteem. This is often so in cases of childhood ongoing traumas and cases of physical, sexual, and verbal abuse, for example. But even within a more benign context, children will react internally to many events and interactions with intense feelings of shame and embarrassment. This result is increased anxiety and an irrational interpretation as to the source and meaning of the upsetting interpersonal situations with parents or peers. In child-centered ways, children interpret dysregulating interactions as due to their own disappointing and therefore shameful behavior.

Anxious self-states and shame

As a result of the wide interconnection among neural circuits, innate emotions, environmental events, memories, habits and learning processes result in brain-wide neural maps. Each map coalesces around a primary emotion and in effect constructs a particular self-state. These neural maps, or self-states, run the gamut from complete separation to great overlap and integration. Briefly, such self-states can be divided into negative or positive ones; those suffused and underpinned by anxiety, sadness, anger, self-denigration, shame, and negative memories to mention a few; and those characterized by more prevalent positive outlooks, memories, motivation, self-acceptance and contentment, for example. Most of us are familiar with the experience of entirely and involuntarily sinking into a negative feeling state, 'forgetting' the existence of the other more resilient and optimistic one.

Most significantly, the inseparable mixture of emotions and cognitions explains how during our early years such neuropsychological processes shape and establish our narratives about the self and others. In this context, the influence of the fear system on other mental functions is significant in its outsize influence. In effect, as the amygdala's influence is quite inevitable throughout development and beyond, most of us develop a self-state that is more fearful, anxious, vulnerable, and prone to feel shame (Ginot, 2015). This process is, of course, the result of the interacting forces of both innate tendencies and environmental pressures. As (innate) very unpleasant visceral discomfort signals a threat of being negatively judged for a disappointing performance, this experience becomes enmeshed with intense self-loathing thoughts, and the state of shame takes over. In the process, if we cannot successfully enough regulate the triggered state of shame we will fully identify with the negative judgment of others, believing it to be a true assessment of who we are.

In order to better understand the upsetting power of shame, we need to remember a few additional features of self-states in general. To ensure survival, the brain/mind's ability to learn, remember, and form habits of all kinds became central. The affect-based acquired lessons which make maps or self-states can become rigid and narrow our ability to perceive things through a fresh, unbiased lens. If an anxious self-state has 'learned' to become overly sensitized to a particular negative threat or experience it will tend to predict and expect a particular threat even when unwarranted. Again, we recall the importance of a vigilant fear system to survival. For the vigilant amygdala to be successful, it was important to err on the side of caution rather than careless inattention. The feeling of shame, whether triggered by internal moods or memories or by the judgment of others, can also become habituated, reflecting an exaggerated preoccupation with its projected pain.

Consequently, quick reaction to perceived danger to the self's well-being, whether real or projected, became entwined with the system of shame as well. This has created, for example, anxiety and worries about being shamed and the feeling that it could be totally intolerable, and even annihilating to the sense of self. A habitual certainty about being shamed regardless of one's actual behavior, or perceiving judgment where none is expressed, only intensifies shame and the anxious feelings enmeshed with it.

It is not surprising, then, that several studies found connections between the feelings of shame and symptoms of social anxiety. This association was found among patients diagnosed as suffering from social anxiety as well as among adolescents who were not formally diagnosed with this form of anxiety (Muris *et al.*, 2018). Shame was also present among adults who were diagnosed with generalized anxiety disorder, excess worry, and rumination (Fergus *et al.*, 2010; Levinson *et al.*, 2014). Similarly, shame was associated with the sense of inadequacy, excess vulnerability, and avoiding participation in the world (Cibich *et al.*, 2016; Gouva *et al.*, 2015).

An important aspect that these studies highlight is the fact that, like all other feelings and traits, shame is strongly influenced by temperamental factors. Young adults with a predisposition for anxiety and shyness experience shame more intensely and in more areas of their lives (Kagan, 1998; Levinson *et al.*, 2014). This may explain why some children who were raised in dysregulated homes do not grow into excessively anxious and shy adults. An innate shy and anxious temperament will render toddlers, children, and adolescents more sensitive to shaming interactions. Unwittingly, loving but critical parents, a rejection from one's peer group, and continuous insults from verbally abusive siblings may further sensitize states of anxiety entwined with shame.

At the same time, shame seems to be present among individuals who even without a formal diagnosis of anxiety still show clear patterns of interpersonal anxiety such as vulnerability, a sense of inadequacy, and fear of fully participating in the world. As the presence of vulnerable self-states is pervasive and inevitable (Ginot, 2022), the dread of being shamed is almost universal (Oexle *et al.*, 2017).

The developmental processes of self-conscious feelings

Self-conscious feelings, especially the emerging consciousness of shame, begin approximately between 18 and 24 months. These feelings are linked to toddlers' nascent sense of competence, their need to gain approval from those close to them, and the increasing demands from attachment figures (Lewis, 2019; Schore, 2012). Feelings of shame and embarrassment require a more sophisticated set of cognitive skills, especially the ability to evaluate oneself in relation to others and 'conclude' that one has succeeded or failed.

Such self-evaluative processes depend on a learned sense of right and wrong as well as on a basic understanding of what *good* and *bad* mean to those caring for the young child (Lewis, 2019). Similarly, an understanding of adults' expectations, and of the spoken and unspoken rules that determine good behavior and acceptance by others, is part of this growing process of self-evaluation. The awareness of disappointing attachment figures begins to arouse fears about losing a caregiver's love, support, and validation (Muris *et al.*, 2018).

Although such processes may appear to be too advanced or sophisticated for a toddler or a young child, they happen within the context of a very rapid development of social understanding and language. We can see how anxiety about how we are judged by others is an inextricable part of feelings of shame and embarrassment. We remember the evolutionary roots of shame. Indeed, as adolescents and adults, we find that one of the significant features that accompanies shame is our internal conviction that if we are exposed as 'deficient', presumed consequences are catastrophic. The irrationality of such ingrained beliefs does not make them less convincing.

Ever ready to avoid the anxieties that such perceived deficiencies arouse, we consciously and unconsciously gauge our looks, social standing, prestige, competence, success, and much more. In addition, fears of shaming oneself through words or deeds in the future, and thus losing respect and acceptance, are part of this state of rumination as well. The results of these comparisons are usually informed by our entrenched denigrating self-narratives, adding a sense of inevitability to feelings of inferiority, shame, and increasing anxiety.

Most of all, I think, we dread the visceral sensations of shame and the extremely unpleasant and painful cognitive convictions that are part of it. In our fertile imagination, failures or awkward interactions with others provide an indisputable proof that, indeed, we are fundamentally flawed. This anxiety and painful feelings of shame are often enacted in private, away from others. We may mull over how we presented ourselves or communicated in a group; for example, we may ruminate about things we said, actions we took, and beat ourselves up for being inadequate. Although such emotion states are that intense only temporarily, they still exact their toll in heightened negative feelings that make us feel hopeless about ourselves.

Developmental processes: Intersubjectivity

Our feelings of shame and their self-denigrating narratives are rooted in the child's earliest emotional experiences within their intersubjective environments. States of anxious dysregulation will shape many of the child's encoded memories, forming the earliest network representations of visceral and emotional states of well-being or frustration and stress. It's important to emphasize that early-forming networks influence subsequent experiences. The neural strength of early negative learning and expectations will impact how future experiences are perceived, experienced, and understood.

Intersubjectivity can be defined as these pervasive and ongoing mutual experiences driven by conscious and unconscious, verbal and nonverbal communication. In particular, the child's need for resonance and empathic attunement and a caregiver's own ability to mirror this need are central to intersubjective interactions. As a result of the need for attunement, alongside the child's essential separateness and inherent temperament, there are also self-states that are utterly attuned to the caregiver's physical presence, emotions, and vocal communications.

This lack of differentiation is not simply a result of the child's supposed non-existent subjectivity. Rather, this deep attentiveness of the child to the parent's state of mind and behaviors is due to an active, evolutionarily determined psychobiological need. This ongoing attentiveness is an aspect of the all-important attachment needs a young child has. Paying close attention to the caregiver ensures the child's sense of togetherness and, thus, security (Beebe and Lachmann, 2002; Braten and Trevarthen, 2007; Cozolino, 2006; Schore, 2012; Stern, 1985; Tronick, 2007).

But although an interactional model of understanding development changes with the child's progress, it still has one enduring feature: the child's other-centered focus (Braten, 2007; Braten and Trevarthen, 2007). The primary phase of intersubjectivity emphasizes verbal and nonverbal exchanges between parents and infants, and their mutual mirroring of each other's emotional states. Infants and toddlers have shown particular sensitivity to their caregiver's expressions and vocal tones. Infants' brain circuits actually change in response to inter-parental fights, enhancing their amygdala's reactivity to threat. Infants also display a tendency to detect and pay more attention to facial expressions.

The strong attention paid to the adults around them and the identification and learning processes make infants especially vulnerable to anxiety-inducing intersubjective interactions and especially those involving misattuned parental behavior. Although infants may not experience shame as toddlers and older children do, an accumulative lack of attunement and empathic relating may form the foundation for greater sensitivity to upsetting interactions. When underpinned by the amygdala and its brain-wide influence, such sensitivity may later distort how we interpret what shaming interactions are. We may unconsciously exaggerate the shaming intents of others, misinterpret what they mean, and easily fall into a state of shame without the more reality-bound perspective.

In the secondary intersubjective phase, toddlers and their caregivers progress to a different mode of attunement. Here, toddlers seek and find shared intentions and interests with their caregivers. The need for shared emotions, thoughts, and behaviors becomes the foundation for the child's sense of self. During this phase, a shared agreement about the toddler's sense of competency and accomplishments is especially important. Toddlers often seek confirmations and emotional echoes to their exuberance and exploratory behaviors. During this period, toddlers are especially animated by feelings of pride and a quest for autonomy. Conversely, they are also sensitive to disapproving and overly harsh communications that arouse feelings of shame, disappointment, and a sense of deflation; these feelings are a primary focus for toddlers around 18 months of age (Braten and Trevarthen, 2007; Schore, 2003).

In addition, developing verbal skills enable toddlers to acquire new forms of intersubjectivity and modes of interaction as well as internal ways of interpreting these emotions. A toddler's ongoing attention to and involvement in the emotions, language, and behaviors of caretakers become more nuanced and sophisticated. At the same time, the automatic learning and identification processes that encode these complex processes virtually guarantee an unavoidable internalization of the many facets of the parent's feeling states and behaviors.

In effect, the child is exposed to two kinds of communications which they encode and make their own: the direct communications directed toward the child on the one hand, and the parents' verbal and nonverbal communication about their own internal feeling states and ways of coping with them, on the other. As we often witness in patients and in ourselves, when tracing the effects of parents' personality characteristics, their own shame about their perceived failures and shortcomings is transmitted to their children, who unavoidably internalize it as their own.

Tertiary intersubjective participation occurs between three and six years of age; it is defined by an even greater understanding of, and absorption in, the thoughts and emotions of others. As a child's cognitive skills expand, they become increasingly entangled with their caregivers' emotional, cognitive, and behavioral personality traits. During this phase, there is a significant increase in children's ability to ruminate, think of themselves in autobiographical mode, utilize their imaginations, and give meaning to emotional events. These growing abilities lead to a web of interpretations that may distort the meaning of actual interactions and events (Gazzaniga, 2008; Gazzaniga et al., 2014). Within this context, the state of shame may be further triggered by the already reinforced unconscious pattern that predicts and expects being judged, demeaned, and shamed.

Studies that examined the degree to which children identify with adults' ideas, feelings, and actions have shown that during play, children often repeat whole conversations that they have been exposed to in interactions with their parents. In these observations, a caregiver's verbal comments and actions became part of the children's conversations and a way of act-ing with their playmates (Braten, 2007). Throughout these developmental intersubjective periods there are increasing opportunities for children to learn from and imitate parental attitudes. The criticism verbalized by car-egivers, even if infrequent or just carelessly given, may still lead to feelings of shame. Insults from teachers, peers, and others in the child's life will have similar effects.

As some researchers have found, children largely understand things in a literal way; a parent's statements, in the child's mind, describe things as they really are (Richardson and Saxe, 2020a, 2020b; Saxe, 2010; Saxe and Houlihan, 2017). Parental anger and disapproval of the child, for example, are perceived by the child as a true assessment of who they are. Children have no ability to see a parent's negative outbursts as an expression of their own personal turmoil, agitation, or limitations, not an accurate assessment of the child's character. The attentiveness to a parent's opinions and the power such opinions carry inevitably result in an immature and distorted interpretation about the source of emotional difficulties. The source of a child's injury is unconsciously seen by the child as coming from themselves – their own actions, feelings, and thoughts. When such experiences are put into words in a ruminative internal monologue, they become negative self-narratives (Braten, 2007; Ginot, 2015; Grawe, 2007; Lewis and Todd, 2004, 2007; Lyons-Ruth, 2003; Olds, 2006).

Furthermore, parental internal emotional states and behaviors that have nothing to do with the child will also be co-opted by the child as if they were their own. The child may come to believe they are the source of the feelings and behaviors emanating from the parents; examples include a parent's own tendencies to become irritated or impatient, episodes of depression or chronic low mood, frustration with a job or marriage, anxiety, self-denigration, and frequent parental fighting. As higher-order development continues, children increasingly see themselves as responsi-ble co-authors of anything they feel or think, even though the experiences they are immersed in and ruminate about originate from a parent (Braten and Traverthan, 2007; Hermans, 2004).

On a neuropsychological level, as was already mentioned, children believe that their parents' words reflect reality as it is (Saxe, 2010; Saxe and Houlihan, 2017). Before the age of four or five years, children do not yet understand that their parents' words are just opinion that does not actually reflect who the child is. A parent's criticism is perceived as a true evalua-tion as to the child's 'flaws.' The innate tendency to feel shame when being criticized or diminished readily takes hold and becomes part of the child's internalized experience of themselves. Only when a particular region comes online, the right temporo-parietal junction, do they start to recognize that the actions and opinions of others may only convey their own particular 'truth.'

Unfortunately, however, for many of us, those early emotional states of shame and their convincing veracity become the foundation of brain-mind-body emotional habits and irrefutable beliefs. As we know, early encoded and learned perceptions, feelings and behaviors tend to be very influential on subsequent experiences, co-opting them and integrating them within existing shame states. Consequently, the tendency to feel shame can become increasingly reinforced and therefore easily triggered, repeated, and emotionally devastating. Unless we become aware of the ori-gin and meaning of our tendency to experience shame and learn to 'tame' its effects with the help of psychotherapy and mindfulness, it will continue to consciously and unconsciously influence how we experience ourselves.

The mirror neuron system and the neural default mode system

Research on the mirror neuron system further demonstrates the child's susceptibility to negative states of shame and the development of nega-tive narratives. The mirror neuron system has been shown to establish a neuropsychological link between interacting subjectivities that observe or relate to each other. Specifically, this system, found in the premotor cortex, imitates and predicts the actions of others. When studied, the observer's brain activity resembles that of the observed. This phenomenon is medi-ated by a neuropsychological process of embodied simulation, creating in our own brains the actions, affects, and intentions of those we observe or interact with. These processes constitute the roots of empathy and inter-subjectivity (Gallese, 2006, 2008, 2009; Iacoboni, 2008; Ramachandran, 2011; Rizzolati et al., 2002).

The mirror neuron system, then, supports the intersubjective building blocks of attachment and identification. At the same time, however, chil-dren may identify with the negative ideas and attitudes parents have about them. Recalling the child's vulnerability to a parent's emotional states, the mirror neuron system mediates not just a nonverbal understanding of action and intention. Through our ability to get absorbed in the other's emotional state, the mirror neuron system also enables the important functions of unconscious imitation and learning. This, of course, leads to the child's resonance with a parent's pain and anxiety, their own shameful beliefs about themselves.

These intersubjective processes affect both parents and children. But as young children are the vulnerable ones, their absorption in, imitation of, and learning from their parents clearly shape and determine their developing self-narratives.

Narrative patterns and the integrated brain-mind-body

As continually stressed in this chapter, similar to other emotion states, the experience of shame is complex and blended. Intertwined with raw emotional states are the verbal assessments, interpretations, and sensations that give meaning to a particular internal state. To quote Panksepp and Biven (2012), 'In humans these [affective states] are always accompanied by cognitive changes, such as emotionally entangled attributions, ruminations, all sort of plans and worries' (p.451).

In the case of shame, these thoughts and narratives are often inseparable parts of the painful and dread-inducing situations. When triggered in response to shaming situations (again, whether real, perceived or, most often, a mix of both), familiar internal monologues and ruminations attack us with the demeaning, self-hating and anger-filled self-assessments.

As we have already seen, this process starts early on and is shaped by both innate and environmental factors. But as a result of our limited reality-bound perspective as young children, the self-blaming, embarrassed negative interpretations of our anxious and dysregulated feeling states tend to be distorted. As language increasingly becomes the symbolic carrier of emotions, narratives provide a link to the embodied, painful experience of shame. A loss of self-confidence and self-value simultaneously gives rise to the wish to 'disappear,' to escape the intense anxiety about the severe injury to one's self-worth.

In this way, feelings of shame develop their own language within each individual. Importantly, early and distorted self-denigrating narratives are often enhanced and made even more destructive by the slower-developing left hemisphere (i.e. the explainer) and the prefrontal cortex as a whole (Gazzaniga, 2008; Gazzaniga et al., 2014; Lewis and Todd, 2004, 2007). This immaturity adds to the self-centric meaning given to an emotional state. In the midst of traumatic, painful, or shaming experiences, children have no choice but to arrive at distorted conclusions about their self-worth, competency, and importance to the parent and later on to their peers. As a result, as adults, the meaning of a shaming or injurious experience echoes already entrenched unconscious convictions of their badness and inferiority. When triggered, these unconscious brain-mind-body circuits of shame become conscious, leading to the intense experience of shame.

Indeed, listening to adult patients of all ages, one can often feel, hear, and connect with the old, pained, and immature childhood part – a part that still experiences itself and others through the distorting lens of a developing brain-mind. For many of us, negative self-narratives are easily triggered during dysregulated feelings reminiscent of the states that gave rise to the familiar self-derogatory beliefs.

In a broad sense, self-narratives are another important example of how brain-mind processes are integrated; visceral physiology, emotion, cognition, and action tendencies are intertwined within the brain-mind, even if we are not aware of this unity. In other words, narratives are the verbal expressions of all these entwined processes. We typically think of each of these as separate entities, holding on to the somewhat intuitive notion that in our felt experience, as well as within the brain, emotion, thoughts, and actions are different and distinct phenomena.

But as we know now, subjectively felt experiences such as anxiety, shame, and embarrassment integrate and convey all of our mental functions. Cognition and emotions overlap in most areas of the brain and there are no brain regions in which those functions reside as separate entities. In addition, functions such as attention, expectations, and behavior are also integrated with emotions and cognition. In effect, enacted behaviors such as attention and defensive behaviors such as avoidance, for example, are closely enmeshed with them (Okon-Singer, 2018; Lewis and Todd, 2004, 2007; Pessoa, 2016, 2018; Todd *et al.*, 2012, 2013, 2018, 2020). Neurally, and therefore experientially, the state of shame is constructed of emotions, attention, perceptions, thoughts, and enacted behaviors, all intertwined into a brain-mind-body map.

Self-narratives enmeshed with the feelings of shame often contain strong beliefs that there is nothing worse to the sense of self than being 'found out' as a fraud or an imposter. This sense of dread, and in severe cases a fear of imminent psychic annihilation, is particularly overwhelming when old negative feelings, defensive behaviors and narratives are a pervasive and strong part of a 'shame pattern.' In that case, there tends to be a fast, unconscious and automatic identification with the judgment of others and to see it as the legitimate and true assessment of one's actions. Recalling that among young children this tendency to unquestionably 'believe' the adults in their life is a developmental phase, we can appreciate the strength of early patterns that are especially sensitive to being shamed.

As the quick action and the outsize influence of the fear system go on to influence other emotions, cognitive functions, and defensive behaviors, feelings of shame and embarrassment become woven into a dysregulated self-state. Most of these interconnected processes occur out of our awareness. This is especially true of events and situations that took place during the first years, prior to the full development of the memory system. What is significant during these years and well into adolescence is the propensity of all children to give meaning to their experiences. But this meaning, as we saw, is highly shaped by already existing neural maps and their conscious expressions as self-states or patterns. In very context-dependent and unique fashion, children are prone to understand negative emotions as emanating from them (Braten and Trevarthen, 2007) and therefore they are interpreted as their fault. Within the enmeshed neural maps, the innate painful experience of shame is particularly sensitive to distorted interpretations about what is happening. As a result, shame often becomes entwined with exceedingly negative ideas about self-worth as well as feelings of dread in anticipation of its occurrence. Internal processes and temperament are always interacting with the interpersonal environment. As the following section discusses, external life circumstances can aggravate states of shame as well.

Some inevitable precursors of shame

The more we realize how prone the brain-mind is to experience anxiety and other innate dysregulated feelings, the more we can appreciate how vulnerable we are as children to interpersonal situations that may increase feelings of anxious self-consciousness. Even within the most loving and supportive family environments there are many opportunities inside the family but also among peers to feel the sting of judgment, disapproval, and real or perceived insults. Often, in spite of their best intents, parents are also occasionally under the influence of various unconscious and conscious patterns; they may be stressed, impatient, moody or frequently distracted by outside crises, career or internal pressures. All these can lead to unconscious acts of rejection, invalidation, critical words, diminishing and impatient behaviors or excessive need to control and direct a child's personality.

Just as important, is the child's developing sense of their competence and success. Often, for example, when children struggle in school because of undiagnosed learning and attention challenges they develop intense ongoing fears and shame about failing. Consciously and unconsciously comparing themselves to others increasingly colors their narratives about their abilities. In the absence of parental support, teachers' understanding and actual remedial help, many children become increasingly and secretly convinced that something is very deficient about them.

Other factors that unwittingly and indirectly can lead to feelings of shame and embarrassment extend to the child's emotional resonance with the emotional atmosphere at home. The quality of the parents' relationship as partners, for example, seems to be a central factor that may raise a child's anxiety levels and heighten shame reactions throughout childhood. Between 6 and 14 months of age, babies become highly disturbed by inter-parental conflicts, paying more attention to negative emotions and displaying fewer play-like behaviors (Du Rocher Schudlich et al., 2011;

Graham *et al.*, 2015). Temperamentally anxious and reactive infants and children seem to be especially vulnerable to conflicts and hostile verbal exchanges in their environment (Mammen *et al.*, 2017). Similarly, fights and conflicts between parents or a difficult divorce have been found to contribute to a child's sensitivity to negative states including shame (Graham *et al.*, 2013, 2015). Children who are exposed to ongoing inter-parental conflicts may experience feelings of panic over a possible divorce and its immediate consequences for their sense of safety and belonging. Children may feel shame about how inter-parental fights indicate a painful failure of their family to thrive and their parents' inability to get along. Remembering children's tendencies to co-opt their parental feelings, words, and behaviors, the parents' inability to keep the family unit together may be internalized by the child as their own failure and therefore a source of shame.

Frequent shaming or bullying experiences from one's peers, for example, may coalesce into shameful perspectives through which we see ourselves as adults. What we perceive to be shaming experiences later in life may easily consciously and unconsciously trigger vulnerable states – in this case, a state of shame. For example, frequent negative attitudes about a child or adolescent's appearance and particularly weight have been found to lead to eating disorders as a way to unconsciously deal with feelings of shame (Kelly and Tasca, 2016; Troop and Redshaw, 2012). Ongoing verbal abuse, frequent undermining and insulting comments, and the use of excessive violent control, sexual and physical abuse are all traumatic experiences strongly tied to shame. Across development, but especially during the early years, such traumatic experiences severely damage the child's self-esteem and how much more they unconsciously see themselves relative to others.

Other external circumstances that have been shown to contribute to elevated levels of anxiety and self-conscious feelings are socially determined conditions such as poverty and racial discrimination. Growing psychological and neuropsychological data increasingly provides important knowledge about the pernicious effects of such conditions on generations of children (Callaghan and Richardson, 2012; Callaghan and Tottenham, 2016). Parents' heightened stress due to difficult external situations over which they have little control can also influence the child's growing sense of themselves; in addition to identifying with the parent's own shame and anxiety about their struggles, children may also develop self-conscious feelings about their situations (Brown *et al.*, 2009; Rachel *et al.*, 2017). Life factors such as lower financial and racial discrimination, however, do not always result in self-conscious feelings of shame among children. And importantly, attuned parents can do a great deal to offset the negative narratives that may lead to shame.

As these factors interact with parents' own psychological histories, they may exacerbate existing interpersonal and internal difficulties. A wide range of destabilizing factors such as immigration, racial discrimination, and financial worries may contribute heavily to children's increased feelings of anxiety, insecurity, and shame if they compare themselves to others. Watching parents struggle to survive and provide for the family and being aware of their frustrations and difficulties may cause children to unconsciously internalize the emotional states of stress and fear, and often the parent's shame at falling short despite their efforts to provide. In addition, as children themselves experience aspects of deprivation they may interpret such situations as reflecting on who they are and on their self-worth. Again, as young children they do not have the ability to realize that they have no control over their difficult circumstances; the entangled emotions of anxiety and internalized shame seem the only reality available to them.

Shame, defenses, and therapy

Keeping in mind that the brain's primary purpose is to learn about the environment in order to survive, and that this learning is greatly influenced by the amygdala, we can assume that each one of these parental behaviors and situational difficulties, from the more benign to the traumatizing, can result in the development of vulnerable, anxious, and shame-infused patterns in us all.

As we often see in patients, as well as in ourselves, an ongoing preoccupation with anxieties about failing, being judged as deficient, and finally being found out as worthless imposters, can take up a great deal of our psychological life, both conscious and unconscious. Simultaneously, these fears of failing and being shamed unconsciously recruit unconscious defences, whose main function is to avoid any situations that may hold the potential for failures, real or imagined.

The innate and automatic inclination to avoid the entangled state of anxiety and shame can become generalized. The tendency to predict and expect future experiences based on the past, which often results in unconscious expectations of failure and therefore shame, does not allow us to learn from reality. Avoiding challenges, we do not test our existing abilities, strengths, and limitations; therefore, we do not give ourselves the opportunity to develop new ideas about our many attributes, nor do we learn to better regulate the experience of shame and reconstruct a new, less threatening view of it. Entrenched avoidant behaviors do not allow us to learn and relearn how to deal with difficult situations and failures in real time, meaning, how to interpret them with a more reality-bound perspective.

Conversely, quite a few of us may develop cognitive strategies that in their dedication to protect us from the pain and dysregulation of shame, from feeling worthless or deeply insecure, create extreme compensatory defenses. Such defenses, in essence, construe one's narcissistic qualities.

Often, such people unconsciously oscillate between two internal structures, both quite removed from a more reality-bound perspective. In one extreme pole, an unconscious early neural map harbors intense fears and convictions about oneself as worthless and, furthermore, doomed to be found out and shamed. In the other pole, in the effort to soothe these fears, ideations and narratives of grandiose abilities take center stage.

People may need to frequently be validated, feel superior to others, and display an indelible façade of greatness. Mostly what gets enacted among others is the grandiose defense; it is much harder for people to get a glimpse of their pained internal fears and convictions about being deficient and become aware of the dread of shame. Caught between these two opposing forces, neither of which reflect one's actual capability, a wide swathe of more nuanced personality attributes is lost; the middle does not exist. Mostly, such a patten does not work, especially when because of fear, one's grandiosity remains in the form of wishes and fantasies alone. Regardless of the defenses utilized against experiencing projected failure and shame, people still suffer the debilitating consequences of both the feelings of shame and the defenses against them. Often, people start therapy not understanding why they suffer and why their lives are so limited or do not reflect any of their more conscious desires.

In effect, psychotherapy can be very useful in helping people to become aware of and better understand their suffering. Patients may learn the source of their intense shame and how it has held them back from trying new things. Therapy can help patients to better tolerate experiences of failure, and through acquiring a mindful perspective regulate the feelings of shame. An important goal of therapy is to unpack the entangled emotions, narratives, and behaviors that automatically repeat themselves in the context of familiar triggers. The general goal is to help others and ourselves to better lives with inevitable innate states, which although beneficial in our distant past have left us vulnerable to fears, anxiety and dysregulating shame, among others. Although mindfulness, through therapy or meditation, cannot eliminate feelings of shame and the dread about them, it can most certainly lessen and better regulate their painful effects.

Lastly but no less important, therapy and other avenues of psychological education can contribute a great deal to children's emotional health. Understanding the great vulnerability of a young and growing brain may help parents, teachers, and other caretakers become more mindful about the power of their words and actions. In particular, parents' emotional influence on the child's implicit memories needs to be acknowledged. Similarly, being mindful that in search of meaning of their internal states children often interpret even careless put-downs as justified and a source for shame.

Obviously, occasionally all parents make mistakes; parents, like all human beings, have no choice but to enact and express their personalities and vulnerabilities. Parents carry their past with them and, like all people, succumb to personal and environmental pressures. Nevertheless, we cannot underestimate the power of mindfulness and its clear relationship to greater empathy toward a child (Fonagy and Bateman, 2006; Fonagy *et al.*, 2002). An insight into and empathy for what children may experience can provide parents with the tools for mindful attitudes toward children, especially those who are more sensitive, anxious, and shy (Burke, 2010; Kabat-Zinn, 2005). A mindful openness toward their own behavioral tendencies will help the adults in the child's life consider their immeasurable influence on their emotional well-being in regard to the outsize dread of shame as well as all other feelings.

KNOWLEDGE AND PRACTICE REFLECTION

Janise Mitchell, Joe Tucci, Ed Tronick and Stephen W. Porges

Efrat Ginot's chapter on shame is not specifically about trauma. But the parallels between the two experiences are compelling. As she highlights, shame plays a part at the intersection of many brain-body systems which share their evolution with the need to defend against physical threat and danger. Shame is the manifestation of a disruption experienced at an emotional level. It is a long-standing interpersonal feedback loop that aimed, from an evolutionary perspective, to reinforce community norms, reflecting to the individual that they had stepped outside a moral or socially held value. The experience of that feedback was instantaneous and painful.

However, over time, shame has become much more than that. It is an intrinsically recorded regulatory dynamic that combines a number of emotions – all perceived as threats to the well-being of the self. It is marked by deep experiences of humiliation, degradation, embarrassment, mortification. As Ginot points out so eloquently:

> …we dread the visceral sensations of shame and the extremely unpleasant and painful cognitive convictions that are part of it. In our fertile imagination, failures or awkward interactions with others provide an indisputable proof that, indeed, we are fundamentally flawed. This anxiety and painful feelings of shame are often enacted in private, away from others. We may mull over how we presented ourselves or communicated in a group; for example, we may ruminate about things we said, actions we took, and beat ourselves up for being inadequate.

It is the private dimension of shame that correlates to interpersonal violence so easily. Abuse and violence often occur in the family, or similar contexts, by perpetrators who are known to individuals, especially women and children. It occurs away from the public gaze. It is built on pretense and deceit. Shame follows, with victims and survivors being manipulated into believing that the abuse was their fault. They are to blame for their own pain.

The reactions they receive from others only serve to reinforce the shame, which at a broader level turns into the negative attribution of qualities afforded to all victims and survivors, and itself becomes a stigma. This community narrative communicates that they are not trustworthy enough to be believed, that they have some other agenda, that they are on a mission to prove their innocence. They hear voices of criticism that tell them that they should get over the trauma, that they are too weak to manage what others have always just put up with. These external provocations turn into the inner self beliefs that victims and survivors carry with them. They set up expectancies of meaning making that serve to prove these inner critiques, making the shame even more powerful and painful.

It makes it almost impossible for victims and survivors to talk to someone about it – they often test reactions with innocuous descriptions about hypothetical situations before trying to open up about their own experiences. They are frightened that they will not be believed or their experiences will not be validated. Even more critically, there is the real possibility that family or institutional loyalty may interfere with their experience being acknowledged and acted on. This can leave them in a vulnerable position.

Shame becomes a default frame of reference for many victims and survivors of interpersonal violence, unless of course they are able to find others with whom they can experience a shared sense of solidarity. In this context, often with the normalizing impact of hearing similar stories of violation and realizing that they are not on their own, they begin the process of engaging with resources that enable them to listen to more influential but edited versions of life narratives that speak to them of their inherent qualities of resistance or compassion. They learn that their actions of internalizing the messages accompanying violence intended by the perpetrator may have served to protect them or others (their mother, their siblings, their pets) from further violation. The guilt that had been made true via distorted versions of the truth is unsettled, allowing for other explanations and realizations to be made.

In most trauma-informed literature to date, very little has been mentioned about shame. Where it has, it is described as a byproduct of the trauma and related to its consequences. However, an understanding of shame is essential to the way practitioners and organizations interact with victims and survivors. There needs to be a real and embedded appreciation of how the content of the communication from all personnel can activate and reinforce destructive narratives associated with shame, in its many emotional forms. Such personnel can be trained to be active in promoting counter-messages to demonstrate to victims and survivors that there is a dignity and courage in coming forward to seek out support.

Shame sits at the heart of trauma. It extends the social wound that interpersonal violation inflicts. And as such, it is a core element of what needs to be attended to by trauma-transformative practitioners, organizations, and systems.

References

References for chapter

Adolphs, R. and Anderson, D. J. (2018). *The Neuroscience of Emotion: A New Synthesis*. Princeton, NJ: Princeton University Press.

Beebe, B. and Lachmann, F. (2002). Organizing principles of interaction from infant research and the lifespan prediction of attachment: Application to adult treatment. *Journal of Infant, Child and Adolescent Psychotherapy*, 2(4), 61–89.

Braten, S. (2007). Altercentric Infants and Adults: On the Origin and Manifestation of Participant Perception of Others' Acts and Utterances. In S. Braten (ed.), *On Being Moved: From Mirror Neurons to Empathy* (pp. 111–136). Amsterdam: Benjamins.

Braten, S. and Trevarthen, C. (2007). Prologue: From Infant Intersubjectivity and Participant Movements to Simulation and Conversation in Cultural Common Sense. In S. Braten (ed.), *On Being Moved: From Mirror Neurons to Empathy* (pp.21–34). Amsterdam: Benjamins.

Brown, R., Copeland W.E., Costello, J., Erkani., A. and Worthman, M. (2009). Family and community influences on educational outcomes among Appalachian youth. *Journal of Community Psychology*, 37(7), 295–808.

Burke, C.A. (2010). Mindfulness-based approaches with children and adolescents: A preliminary review of current research in an emergent field. *Journal of Child and Family Studies*, 19(2), 133–144.

Callaghan, B.L. and Richardson, R. (2012). The effect of adverse rearing environments on persistent memories in young rats: Removing the brakes on infant fear memories. *Translational Psychiatry*, 2(7), e138–e138.

Callaghan, B.L. and Tottenham, N. (2016). The stress acceleration hypothesis: Effects of early-life adversity on emotion circuits and behaviour. *Current Opinion in Behavioural Sciences*, 7, 76.

Cibich, M., Woodyatt, L. and Wenzel, M. (2016). Moving beyond 'shame is bad': How a functional emotion can become problematic. *Social and Personality Psychology Compass*, 10(9), 471–483.

Cozolino, L. (2006). *The Neuroscience of Human Relationships: Attachment and the Developing Brain*. New York, NY: W.W. Norton and Company.

Damasio, A.R. (2010). *Self Comes to Mind: Constructing the Conscious Brain*. New York, NY: Vintage Books.

Du Rocher Schudlich, T.D., White, C.R., Fleischhauer, E.A. and Fitzgerald, K.A. (2011). Observed infant reactions during live interparental conflict. *Journal of Marriage and Family*, 73(1), 221–235.

Fergus, T.A., Valentiner, D.P., McGrath, P.B. and Jencius, S. (2010). Shame- and guilt-proneness: Relationships with anxiety disorder symptoms in a clinical sample. *Journal of Anxiety Disorders*, 24(8), 811–815.

Fonagy, P. and Bateman, A. (2006). Progress in the treatment of borderline personality disorder. *British Journal of Psychiatry*, 188(1), 1–3.

Fonagy, P., Gergely, G., Jurist, E.L. and Target, M. (2002). *Affect Regulation, Mentalisation and the Development of the Self*. New York, NY: Other Press.

Fox, A.S. and Shackman, A.J. (2019). The central extended amygdala in fear and anxiety: Closing the gap between mechanistic and neuroimaging research. *Neuroscience Letters*, 693, 58–67.

Gallese, V. (2006). Intentional Attunement: Embodied Simulation and its Role in Social Cognition. In M. Mancia (ed.), *Psychoanalysis and Neuroscience* (pp.269–301). New York, NY: Springer.

Gallese, V. (2008). Mirror neurons and the social nature of language: The neural exploitation hypothesis. *Social Neuroscience*, 3, 317–333.

Gallese, V. (2009). Mirror neurons, embodied simulation, and the neural basis of social identification. *Psychoanalytic Dialogues*, 19, 519–536.

Gazzaniga, M.S. (2008). *Human: The Science Behind What Makes Us Unique*. New York, NY: Harper Collins.

Gazzaniga, M.S., Ivry, R.B., and Mangum, G.R. (2014). *Cognitive Neuroscience: The Biology of the Mind* (fourth edition). New York, NY: W.W. Norton and Company.

Ginot, E. (2015). *The Neuropsychology of the Unconscious: Integrating Brain and Mind in Psychotherapy*. New York, NY: W.W. Norton and Company.

Ginot, E. (2022). *Our Anxious Selves: Neuropsychological Processes and Their Enduring Influence on Who We Are*. New York, NY: W.W. Norton and Company.

Gouva, M., Mentis, M., Kotrotsiou, S., Paralikas, T. and Kotrotsiou, E. (2015). Shame and anxiety feelings of a Roma population in Greece. *Journal of Immigrant and Minority Health*, 17(6), 1765–1770.

Graham, A.M., Fisher, P.A. and Pfeifer, J.H. (2013). What sleeping babies hear: A functional MRI study of interparental conflict and infants' emotion processing. *Psychological Science*, 24(5), 782–789.

Graham, A.M., Pfeifer, J.H., Fisher, P.A., Carpenter, S. and Fair, D.A. (2015). Early life stress is associated with default system integrity and emotionality during infancy. *Journal of Child Psychology and Psychiatry*, 56(11), 1212–1222.

Grawe, K. (2007). *Neuropsychotherapy: How the Neurosciences Inform Effective Psychotherapy*. Burlingame, CA: Analytic Press.

Hermans, H.J.M. (2004). The Dialogical Self: Between Exchange and Power. In H.J.M. Hermans and G. Dimaggio (eds), *The Dialogical Self in Psychotherapy* (pp.13–28). New York, NY: Brunner-Routlege.

Hiramatsu, Y., Asano, K., Kotera, Y., Endo, A., Shimizu, E. and Matos, M. (2021). Development of the external and internal shame scale: Japanese version. *BMC Research Notes*, 14, 297.

Iacoboni, M. (2008). *Mirroring People: The New Science of How We Connect with Others*. New York, NY: Picador.

Kabat-Zinn, J. (2005). Bringing mindfulness to medicine: An interview with Jon Kabat-Zinn, PhD. Interview by Karolyn Gazella. *Advances in Mind-Body Medicine*, 21(2), 22–27.

Kagan, J. (1998). Biology and the Child. In W. Damon and N. Eisenberg (eds), *Handbook of Child Psychology: Social, Emotional and Personality Development* (pp.177–235). New York, NY: Wiley.

Kelly, A.C. and Tasca, G.A. (2016). Within-persons predictors of change during eating disorders treatment: An examination of self-compassion, self-criticism, shame, and eating disorder symptom. *International Journal of Eating Disorders*, 49(7), 716–722.

Levinson, C.A., Kaplan, S.C. and Rodebaugh, T.L. (2014). *Personality: Understanding the Socially Anxious Temperament*. New York, NY: Wiley.

Lewis, M. (2019). The Self-Conscious Emotions and the Role of Shame in Psychopathology. In V. LoBue, K. Pérez-Edgar, and K. Buss (eds), *Handbook of Emotional Development* (pp.311–350). New York, NY: Springer.

Lewis, M.D. and Todd, R. (2004). Toward a Neuropsychological Model of Internal Dialogue: Implications for Theory and Clinical Practice. In H.J.M. Hermans and G. Dimaggio (eds), *The Dialogical Self in Psychotherapy* (pp.43–59). New York, NY: Brunner-Routledge.

Lewis, M.D. and Todd, M. (2007). The development of self-regulation: Toward the integration of cognition and emotion. *Cognitive Development*, 22, 405–430.

Lyons-Ruth, K. (2003). Dissociation and the parent-infant dialogue: A longitudinal perspective from attachment research. *Journal of the American Psychoanalytic Association*, 51, 883–911.

Mammen, M.A., Busuito, A., Moore, G.A., Quigley, K.M. and Doheny, K.K. (2017). Physiological functioning moderates infants' sensory sensitivity in higher conflict families. *Developmental Psychobiology*, 59(5), 628–638.

Muris, P., Meesters, C. and van Asseldonk, M. (2018). Shame on me! Self-conscious emotions and big five personality traits and their relations to anxiety disorder symptoms in young, non-clinical adolescents. *Child Psychiatry and Human Development*, 49(2), 268–278.

Oexle, N., Rüsch, N., Viering, S., Wyss, C. *et al.* (2017). Self-stigma and suicidality: A longitudinal study. *European Archives of Psychiatry and Clinical Neuroscience*, 267(4), 359–361.

Okon-Singer, H. (2018). The role of attention bias to threat in anxiety: Mechanisms, modulators and open questions. *Current Opinion in Behavioural Sciences*, 19, 26–30.

Olds, D.D. (2006). Identification: Biological and perspectives. *Journal of the American Psychoanalytic Association*, 54, 17–46.

Panksepp, J. and Biven, L. (2012). *Archeology of Mind: The Neuroevolutionary Origins of Human Emotion*. New York, NY: W.W. Norton and Company.

Pessoa, L. (2016). Beyond disjoint brain networks: Overlapping networks for cognition and emotion. *Behavioural and Brain Sciences*, 39, e129.

Pessoa, L. (2018). Understanding emotion with brain networks. *Current Opinion in Behavioural Sciences*, 19, 19–25.

Pessoa, L. and Hof, P. (2015). From Paul Broca's great limbic lobe to the limbic system. *Comparative Neurobiology*, 523(17), 2495–2500.

Rachel, J., Mazza S.E., Lambert, J. Zunzunegui, M.V. *et al.* (2017). Early adolescence behaviour problems and timing of poverty during childhood: A comparison of life course models. *Social Science and Medicine*, 177, 35–42.

Richardson, H. and Saxe, R. (2020a). Development of predictive responses in theory of mind brain regions. *Developmental Science*, 23(1), e12863.

Richardson, H. and Saxe, R. (2020b). Early Signatures of and Developmental Change in Brain Regions for Theory of Mind. In B. Chen and K.Y. Kwan (eds), *Neural Circuit and Cognitive Development* (pp.467–484). New York, NY: Academic Press.

Ramachandran, V.S. (2011). *The Tell-Tale Brain: Unlocking the Mystery of Human Nature*. New York, NY: W.W. Norton and Company.

Rizzolati, G., Fogassi, L. and Gallese, V. (2002). Motor and cognitive functions of the ventral premotor cortex. *Current Opinion in Neurobiology*, 12, 149–154.

Saxe, R. (2010). The Right Temporo-Parietal Junction: A Specific Brain Region for Thinking about Thoughts. In G. Leslie (ed.), *Handbook of Theory of Mind* (pp.1–35). London: Taylor and Francis.

Saxe, R. and Houlihan, S.D. (2017). Formalising emotion concepts within a Bayesian model of theory of mind. *Current Opinion in Psychology*, 17, 15–21.

Schore, A.N. (2003). *Affect Regulation and the Repair of the Self*. New York, NY: W.W. Norton and Company.

Schore, A.N. (2012). *The Science of the Art of Psychotherapy*. New York, NY: W.W. Norton and Company.

Stern, D.N. (1985). *The Interpersonal World of the Infant: A View from Psychoanalysis and Developmental Psychology*. New York, NY: Basic Books.

Swee, M.B., Hudson, C.C. and Heimberg, R.G. (2021). Examining the relationship between shame and social anxiety: A systematic review. *Clinical Psychology Review*, 90, December 2021.

Todd, R.M. and Anderson, A.K. (2013). Salience, State, and Expression: The Influence of Specific Aspects of Emotion on Attention and Perception. In K.N. Ochsner and S. Kosslyn (eds), *The Oxford Handbook of Cognitive Neuroscience* (Vol. 2, pp.11–31). Oxford: Oxford University Press.

Todd, R.M., Cunningham, W.A., Anderson, A.K. and Thompson, E. (2012). Affect-biased attention as emotion regulation. *Trends in Cognitive Sciences*, 16(7), 365–372.

Todd, R.M. and Manaligod, M.G. (2018). Implicit guidance of attention: The priority state space framework. *Cortex*, 102, 121–138.

Todd, R.M., Miskovic, V., Chikazoe, J. and Anderson, A.K. (2020). Emotional objectivity: Neural representations of emotions and their interaction with cognition. *Annual Review of Psychology*, 71, 25–48.

Tottenham, N. (2014). The Importance of Early Experiences for Neuro-Affective Development. In S.L. Andersen and D.S. Pine (eds), *The Neurobiology of Childhood* (pp.109–129). London: Springer-Verlag Publishing/Springer Nature.

Tottenham, N. and Gabard-Durnam, L.J. (2017). The developing amygdala: A student of the world and a teacher of the cortex. *Current Opinions in Psychology*, 17, 55–60.

Tronick, E. (2007). *The Neurobehavioural and Social-emotional Development of Infants and Children*. New York, NY: W.W. Norton and Company.

Troop, N. A. and Redshaw, C. (2012). General shame and bodily shame in eating disorders: A 2.5 year longitudinal study. *European Eating Disorder Review*, 20,(5), 373–378.

CHAPTER 7

An Evolution-Informed Biopsychosocial Approach to the Integration of Compassion Focused Therapy for Childhood Trauma

Paul Gilbert, Deborah Lee and Marcela Matos

Introduction

This chapter is in four sections. First, we outline an evolution-informed biopsychosocial approach to mental health problems, compassion and trauma. This focuses on four basic functions of the mind: motives, emotions, competencies and behaviours. Second, we explore the nature of compassion as an evolved motive and social mentality, supported by context-appropriate emotions, complex cognitive competencies and specific behaviours. These create brain states that orientate individuals to prosocial behaviour towards themselves and others, and harness important psychophysiological systems for the regulation of threat and well-being. Here we also explore the relationship between attachment and the care-focused social mentalities and compassion. Key to this process is the recognition that the evolution of caring and attachment introduced a second (oxytocin-vagal) system for threat regulation, forms of social connectedness and sources of positive affect. Third, we explore the impacts of trauma on a range of threat and care-focused psychophysiological systems and development linked to the four psychological functions outlined in Section 1. Fourth, we explore how trauma disrupts a number of different social mentalities linked to caring, cooperating, competing and sexuality. Finally, we outline some of the key processes of compassion focused therapy (CFT) and how stimulating the psychophysiological systems of care and compassion acts as a corrective psychophysiological intervention that re-orientates individuals to more helpful, threat-regulation strategies, with abilities for creating caring and helpful relationships with themselves and others.

Section 1: Contextualizing trauma and compassion in basic evolved functions of the mind

Compassion focused therapy is rooted in the basic sciences of psychological functioning (Gilbert, 1984, 1989, 1993, 2014, 2022a). Using traditional psychological science, as found in typical textbooks, the basic functions of the mind can be identified as: motives, emotions, (cognitive) competencies and behaviours (Davey, 2018). There are other ways we can classify the functions of the mind but these are the ones CFT works with. The nature and processes of compassion relate to all four domains, and trauma can affect all of these (Gilbert, 2014, 2022bc; Lee, 2022). Figure 7.1 presents a brief outline of these core functions, how they interact with each other, and how they can (later) be affected by experiences of trauma.

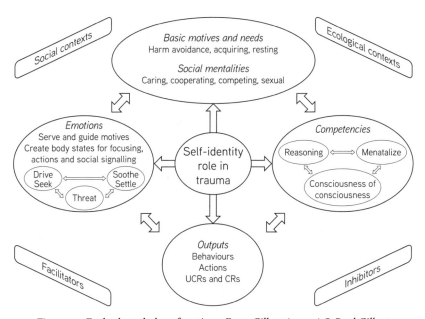

Figure 7.1: Evolved psychology functions. From Gilbert (2022a) © Paul Gilbert

Motives

Motives are regarded as the main 'drivers' of the mind because they guide all other processes (Davey, 2018). Three major evolved motives give rise to three basic life tasks which all living things must pursue for survival and reproduction:

- Harm avoidance motives: these evolve with 'feature detectors for threat' that enable threat sensitivity and detection that triggers defensive and protective behaviours. All species need to be motivated to, and have ways to, detect threat and defend themselves.

- Resource-seeking and acquiring motives: these evolve with 'feature detectors for resources' that enable the seeking, detecting and acquiring of resources (food/shelter/mates), in order for species to continue to survive and pursue reproduction goals. Again, this is species wide.
- Rest and digest motives: these evolve with 'feature detectors for safeness' that enable the deactivation of threat and resource-seeking behavioural systems and facilitate recuperation and replenishment when not under threat and when basic needs are met. The brain and body are organized differently under conditions of sufficiency, no threat and safeness.

Trauma can impact all these motivational systems in different ways. For example, there is extensive evidence that trauma sensitizes the motive to be threat and harm avoidant (Dunkley *et al.*, 2018) linked to the amygdala (Stevens *et al.*, 2017) and other neurocircuits (Terpou *et al.*, 2019). Traumatized people can startle easily and identify threat from ambiguous cues. Trauma also disrupts motives for resource and reward seeking and in the extreme results in forms of anhedonia, a loss of interest in seeking or acquiring resources (Fan *et al.*, 2021). Although anhedonia is often seen as an emotion-based problem, it can also reflect a motive-based difficulty of loss of 'desire', which explains why it can be pervasive rather than episodic.

Music (2022) highlights how neglected children who are not stimulated into rewarding, playful, joyful, mirroring or interesting activities can fail to have their explorative and resource-/reward-seeking systems stimulated. They may show little interest in play and do not express strong reward-focused preferences; they have 'lost their spark' (Music, 2022). In addition, although not specifically tested, trauma and neglect can create fear of having positive or pursuing positive 'desires' (Gilbert *et al.*, 2014). Different from anhedonia is psychological *numbing*, where individuals want to close down because they feel overwhelmed by painful feelings and emotions. This is brilliantly captured in the Pet Shop Boys song called 'Numb'. Numbness can be something people pursue through drugs and other means to stop feeling pain. It can be associated with disengagement and loss of interest in social relationships, which are experienced as overwhelming or threatening. Numbing has also been linked to dissociation (Frewen and Lanius, 2006).

Depressive anhedonia, in contrast, is where individuals would very much like to be able to feel positive emotions and reconnect, but experience an inner deadness, with a loss of positive affect, and can suffer from psychomotor retardation or agitation. Both of these differ from alexithymia and also the withdrawal seen with intense grief (see Gilbert, 2022a, p.50 for further discussion). These distinctions are important for therapy (Gilbert, 2022a). Trauma can also affect people's abilities to experience states of rest and digest, of contentment, and of feeling safe. This can be because as children they did not experience states of safeness, where one might lose oneself in joyful play or curiosity. Hence, the psychophysiological infrastructures for safeness and open curiosity, such as the vagal nerve, have not matured to enable them. Also, threat in the home may have been highly unpredictable, and even short periods of feeling safe could be suddenly disrupted. It follows, therefore, that any therapy will need to address all three motivational systems, thereby enabling the toning down of threat sensitivities, a facilitation of reward seeking and joyful exploration and play, and the ability to feel safe in social contexts.

In addition, motives can be classified into social and non-social. Social motives have been called *social mentalities* because, unlike non-social motives, they require specific and specialized competencies to *detect* and *respond* to specific social signals from conspecifics and also to send signals relating to specific social roles and relationships (Gilbert, 1989, 2017, 2022a). Derived from evolutionary approaches (Buss, 2019; Workman *et al.*, 2020), Gilbert (1989, 1992, 2005, 2017) explored the relationship of five basic social mentalities that organize patterns of social relating: caregiving, care-seeking, cooperating and group belonging, competing and social ranking, and mating. Social mentalities have their own evolutionary trajectory and psychophysiological and contextual regulators. Social mentalities operate through dynamic, reciprocal, fluctuating interactions of communication. For example, sexual behaviour requires that participating partners can both send and receive/respond to sexual communications that impact their physiologies and enable them to engage in mating behaviour. If one participating member is not motivated or interested, cannot process sexual signals, or processes the sexual signal as a threat, or cannot send appropriate signals of interest-engagement, then the role relationship between them will fail. Cooperating requires competencies to detect potential cooperators and to coordinate actions in reciprocal, dynamic, interacting ways. Again, being motivated to cooperate (and not cheat or fear being cheated) and being competent in the skills of cooperation are important.

The evolution of a social mentality for caring (seeking and receiving) which underpins compassion, brought with it feature detectors for 'distress and need' that would trigger physiological responses that orientated an animal to act to alleviate distress and address need. One of the main (but not only) drivers for caring behaviour was parental caring and attachment formation. Although children can object to the boundaries and limits parents may put on them, for the most part care-focused and cooperative motives and behavioural interactions are prosocial, operate a strategy of *care and share* and are consensual (Gilbert, 2021).

The experience of reciprocity differs when it comes to competitive behaviour. Seeking to advance oneself over others can be voluntary, while losing and how others exert control over the self are not consensual or voluntary. Life goals and tasks are also about *competing* with others who are going after the same resources (called contest competition) and where one individual can be a resource or reward for another, as in sexual opportunity or getting others to work for one's goals. Competitive motives focus on the ability and strategy *to control and hold* resources and power, and/or defend against others' use of power against the self (Gilbert, 1992, 2021). The activation of motives for social competition and of concerns to 'control and hold power' over others can give rise to a narcissistic and egocentric orientation towards life or a fearful, defensive, submissive and appeasing one. Being in unwanted or involuntary low-rank positions, or subject to bullying is clearly not consensual and is linked to a variety of mental health problems including post-traumatic stress disorder (PTSD) (for reviews, see Gilbert, 1992, 2020b; Siddaway *et al.*, 2015; Taylor *et al.*, 2011; Troop and Hiskey, 2013).

When people are able to compete in appropriately assertive ways and promote their own views, values and interests while being fair, empathic and caring of others (i.e. not harmfully narcissistic), it gives rise to self-confidence (which is different to self-arrogance). This social (competitive and rank-focused) mentality can be highly problematic for people who have been traumatized. They may be easily triggered into aggressive defences or submissive-withdrawal ones. Such oscillations of the threat system, which has not matured an adaptive threat-regulating infrastructure, can undermine the abilities to compete (to secure resources) and appropriately defend themselves in the world with confidence. Facilitating confidence and appropriate (non-callous) ways of asserting and competing in the world, with wisdom and courage, is therefore part of a compassion process because these are qualities that prevent suffering.

Looked at this way, it is clear that many motives are coordinating and co-regulating each other, creating complex patterns of excitation and inhibition of motives. For example, we want to compete but so as not to cause harm to others we will forgo our own pursuit of resources in order to help others. We can experience guilt if our 'selfishness' is harmful and that pulls us back to concern for others. If the motivation to be caring is low, however, guilt may be hardly stimulated, in which case there is little conflict and harmful behaviour can result. For example, individuals who are highly competitive and narcissistic are less orientated to compassion, whereas those orientated to prosocial behaviour and who are empathic are less narcissistic (Basran *et al.*, 2019). The motivation to care can compete for control in decision making and therefore be a major inhibitor on potentially harmful, competitive behaviours. Further, in regard to co-regulation, motives can themselves be different. One individual seeks power because they want to use their power to help others, whereas another uses their power to self-advance (wealth) or to bully and inflict harm. Sexual motivation can be based on the desire for a close, loving or playful relationship or a harmful one, as in rape.

To add to the complexity, many conflicting processes can be unconscious (Bargh, 2017; Gilbert, 2000a; Huang and Bargh, 2014). Abbas (2015) highlights how traumatized children can have non-conscious problems in processing anger and can feel guilt at their own anger impulses, including in the transference. He notes how some individuals who struggle with unconscious anger can have difficulty with appropriate assertiveness and have somatized problems. Hence, psychotherapy needs to facilitate the working through of these unconscious conflicting motives: between wanting to care and be cared for, and wanting to hurt (with vengeance, control, retaliation and defence) (Abbas, 2015).

CFT also considers the issue of 'fear of retaliation', as in dominant subordinate power hierarchies (i.e. children can be severely threated or injured if they show anger or aggression to the parent), as causes for the non-conscious inhibition of anger impulse defences (Gilbert, 2022a). People can be worried about disobeying or offending God in case they end up in hellfire. The types of terrifying fantasies humans can create indicate a fear of vicious retaliation. Bowlby (1980) refers to the process as 'defensive exclusion', whereby children learn not to process the potential harmfulness of a parent in order to maintain some sense of connectedness. It can be better and far less frightening to see oneself as bad in a universe with a loving God than the other way around!

Compassion, therefore, will require building the courage and wisdom to acknowledge these (non-conscious) inhibiting processes, acknowledge the hurt that drives the rage, and then move to positions of appropriate assertiveness. Because the brain works as an integrated, interactive system, where motives and emotions are co-regulating each other, this is partly why CFT *seeks to change the pattern of pursued motives within people*. For example, the cultivation of compassion has important impacts on competitive behaviour (Gilbert and Simos, 2022). Indeed, one of the core dimensions that runs through all of our motivational systems, and this is crucial for CFT, is the degree to which the compassion motive seeks to be, and is mindful of being, helpful versus harmful and thereby textures social motives (Dalai Lama, 1995; Gilbert, 2000a). This is why the contemplative traditions and CFT place compassion as the core mind-organizing motivational system.

A central dimension that runs through all the social mentalities is not only how they impact threat processing but also resource-seeking drive, positive affect and reward function. Some individuals, for example, can experience what is called *social anhedonia*, where they show little interest in or gain little pleasure from social relationships, which may include friendship, play or sexual activity (Barkus and Badcock, 2019). Despite these difficulties, loneliness can still be a major issue for these individuals. Crucially, given that we are a social species – many of our psychophysiological regulating systems are stimulated and organized through social relationships (Keltner *et al.*, 2014; Mikulincer and Shaver, 2014; Slavich, 2020) – social anhedonia represents a particular problem as it involves losing the ability to access and use these psychophysiological regulators. Because CFT focuses on stimulating prosocial motives of affiliative cooperation, caregiving and receiving, it is possible it can help social anhedonia (Forster and Kanske, 2021).

With a cognitively complex species like humans, major life task goals and social mentalities give rise to many sub-goals. For example, the motive to acquire resources may lead to forms of social competition, such as studying at university to be able to pursue a good career with status and resource access. These, in turn, can be linked to self-identity goals (to become a doctor or a teacher) and to groups one wants to belong to. However, competitive goals and power-seeking control can have damaging antisocial impacts on political, social and intimate relationships (Gilbert, 1989). Human motives for caring have become extended into many forms of prosocial behaviour such as volunteering, teaching, and rescue and medical services, where the primary motivation is to help people in distress or need, or just to promote their welfare. Hence, although it can appear that humans have a huge variety of potential motives, and things they want to achieve and pursue, from an evolutionary point of view, they tend to be rooted in four or five vital domains of evolved functioning. This is key because it can enable us to identify psychophysiological mechanisms underpinning different motivational processes.

Emotions

Emotions function in the service of motives (Keltner *et al.*, 2018). Without a motive for something, emotions are unlikely to arise. The evolutionary psychiatrist Nesse (2019) puts it simply:

> Emotions are specialised states that adjust physiology, cognition, subjective experience, facial expressions, and behaviour in ways that increase the ability to meet the adaptive challenges of situations that have reoccurred over the evolutionary history of a species... (p.53)

Panksepp (1998) offered an important overview and classification of the evolutionary functions of emotion, including distinctions between threat and resource-seeking emotions. In CFT, emotion functions are linked to the adaptive challenges that gave rise to the three basic motives.

- *Harm avoidance* emotions are linked to the perception of threat and harm avoidance. There are two types. One is linked to behavioural activation, the other to inhibition and demobilization. The activation threat emotions are mostly ones for anxiety, anger and disgust. Social mentality derivatives can include those of shame, envy and vengeance. However, sometimes the threat response has to be one of deactivation or demobilization, for example freezing or 'playing dead' (Beck *et al.*, 1985; Marks, 2013). In a predator situation, movement can trigger attack and therefore not moving is the defence. Evolved defences, however, are not just for short-term use but must accommodate to dangerous and threatening environments *that are not changing*. Learned helplessness, for example, highlighted that animals can go into demobilized and 'shutdown' states when confronted by uncontrollable stress (Seligman, 1975). In some environments, where individuals are subject to bullying and harassment (under aversive control), they will adopt submissive profiles to signal to a dominant their 'non-challenging, appeasing low status' and reduce explorative and resource-seeking behaviour. There is now a large literature indicating that when people are subjected to situations where they are threatened and cannot escape (trapped), they show defeat shutdown states. These states are highly associated with depression (Gilbert, 1992; Gilbert and Allan, 1998) and anhedonia (Gilbert *et al.*, 2002). Defeat and shutdown states are associated with trauma (Siddaway *et al.*, 2015; Taylor *et al.*, 2011; Troop and Hiskey, 2013). Although there is overlap between social defeat states and loss of control (e.g. from electric shock), as in learned helplessness, threats coming from non-social versus social sources require quite different defences. In the latter case, the source of threat is constantly present and moving away or towards 'with intention'. Hence, defensive detection must involve sensitivity to the mental state of the other. In addition, an individual's defensive behaviour will be anger-aggressive or fearful-avoidant and appeasing. For the latter, the defence has downregulated the attack motives in the potential attacker/bully (Gilbert, 2000a, 2000b). Different defences are needed if the threat is abandonment.

Demobilized states can also be seen in children who have been separated from their secure attachments and go into what attachment theorists have described as protest-despair states (Bowlby, 1980; Music, 2022). If the young is separated in the wild, then protesting for a while to attract the attention of the parent may be helpful, but after a point it will only attract predators or get lost and therefore it has to hunker down and wait for rescue (Gilbert, 1992). That closing down and reducing of explorative behaviour, movement and interest in the environment has been called despair (Bowlby, 1980).

- *Acquisition and resource-seeking* emotions are associated with gaining resources and exerting control. They are regarded as 'rewards' in behavioural science. They are associated with feelings of interest, pleasure, excitement and joy. Social derivatives can include ones of pride, affection and caring. As noted above, trauma and neglect can significantly disrupt the drive-seeking motives and hence the emotions associated with reward seeking and acquisition. Individuals may find it difficult to anticipate or gain enjoyment from certain activities, and this loss of positive emotion is also regarded as a form of anhedonia. These problems are especially noted in certain types of depression, which in turn can be driven by trauma (Craske *et al.*, 2019). As noted above, trauma can lead to the pursuit of numbness.

- *Rest and digest* emotions are linked to feelings of contentment, peacefulness and safeness. These emotions arise when threat emotions and acquisition emotions are not active. Rest and digest emotions are usually experienced positively and are associated with lower sympathetic arousal, and clearly distinguished from drive and energizing emotions (Depue and Morrone-Strupinsky, 2005). These emotions are particularly associated with feelings of affiliation-linked social safeness (Armstrong *et al.*, 2021; Kelly *et al.*, 2012). This can be important for traumatized children because trying to stimulate a sense of social safeness can also stimulate a sense of aloneness or abandonment. These brain states show complex patterns in the sense that practised meditators utilize vagal and balanced autonomic processes but also have alert awareness. Hence, what is involved here is not so much 'arousal' states as what is happening in psychomotor and movement systems (Gilbert, 2022a).

There is increasing data on the psychophysiological distinctions between these systems. For example, Duarte and Pinto-Gouveia (2017) found that heart rate variability (HRV) was associated with positive emotions of feeling safe and content, but not with excitement or lack of arousal. Kirschner *et al.* (2019) looked at the effects of a short self-compassion training and found it improved HRV. They noted that changes in HRV may precede feeling safe and connected. Most emotion systems in everyday life are experienced as blends. For example, excitement involves some degree of controllable risk and threat/anxiety, whereas play involves some degree of activation-exploration as well as a sense of safeness. Hence, understanding how different psychophysiological systems are balanced and co-regulate each other is important. One of the noted problems with children who are traumatized, particularly if they go on to develop personality difficulties, is that their emotional arousal systems are unstable. They can quickly switch from trusting and openness to distrusting and anger. Part of the reason for this is because the vagal-linked emotion regulation system that evolved with the attachment system is not functioning as an emotional coordinator and regulator (see below). Hence, this system is a target in CFT.

Competencies

Motives and emotions are different from (cognitive) competencies. Competencies can be recruited by any motive or emotion because they facilitate processing and action. For example, birds need wings to fly but also a brain to navigate them in the air. Why they are flying (motive for) and the emotions while flying are independent of their competencies to fly. It is similar for cognitive competencies. CFT focuses on three major human competencies:

1. Non-social reasoning: this uses problem-solving, thinking and analysing of non-social phenomena, and is the basis of the scientific mind and insight (Byrne, 2016).
2. Social reasoning: this uses empathy and mentalizing, which are specialist processing competencies for insight into the complex of motives, desires and emotions behind people's behaviours and communications (Luyten *et al.*, 2020). One does not mentalize a thunderstorm but uses non-social reasoning to track it and determine how to avoid it; whereas one does mentalize in order to avoid or win an argument, or to impress, assert, please or appease.
3. The ability to be aware that one is conscious: in other words, a consciousness of being conscious. This provides the basis for becoming mindful, mindfully aware and a mind observer (Austin, 2009; Gilbert and Choden, 2013; Manuello *et al.*, 2016). Research has shown that some animals, particularly primates, have self-awareness in the sense of self-recognition in a mirror, and have some awareness of their impact on others, but it seems doubtful that they are 'aware that they are aware' and can deliberately choose to be mindful, and with knowing insight choose how to work with their own 'tricky' minds.

Just as motives and emotions can be significantly affected by trauma so, too, can all three types of cognitive competency. The cognitive therapies (Hofmann *et al.*, 2013) have outlined many dimensions of cognitive, mostly non-social, reasoning, such as attention, rumination, prediction and attribution, that assign meaning to distressing events. This can become a focus for therapy (Cohen and Mannarino, 2015). Dialectical behaviour therapy (DBT) addresses a number of these different cognitive competencies, and recently Bohus and colleagues have integrated CFT interventions into DBT with good results (Bohus *et al.*, 2020; Kleindienst *et al.*, 2021).

Mentalizing therapists focus more on social reasoning (empathy and mentalizing processes) that enables us to have insight into the minds of others and recognition that people do things because of their own motives, emotions and beliefs (Luyten *et al.*, 2020). People with early trauma have problems mentalizing, which makes it a focus for therapy (Oehlman Forbes *et al.*, 2021). This therapy has also been developed for people with trauma (Luyten *et al.*, 2020). Traumatized children can struggle with understanding the minds of others as they have lacked a secure base, did not have emotions validated or empathically connected with, and are focused on picking up threat (Oehlman Forbes *et al.*, 2021). The third competency, mindfulness (the ability to become an observer of the mind with knowing awareness and intentionality), has been integrated into many different therapies (Didonna, 2009; Germer *et al.*, 2005; Williams, 2008). Therapists help clients become more mindfully observant and less engaged/fused with the contents of mind as their 'experience' happens moment by moment. A client who tends to be 'in' an emotion and says, 'I am angry' may shift to 'I am experiencing anger flowing through me'. Wise observation (mind awareness) can offer an opportunity for clients to reflect and consider more helpful ways to work with an emotion.

CFT explores all three key processes and competencies. Crucially, all of these interventions are guided, contextualized and utilized via the motivation for care and compassion. For example, in helping people stand back and re-examine their thinking, CFT may first activate a compassion brain state with various breathing exercises, visualizations and awareness of intention (see Section 5). Empathy and mindfulness are competencies, *not* motives, and therefore can be used for any motive, some of which might be harmful. Helping clients connect to an inner desire for helpfulness sets the context for utilizing these competencies.

Behaviours

Behaviour therapists have highlighted the importance of 'how' we learn about the world, particularly through processes such as classical and operant conditioning, exploration, practice and guided discovery. These underpin Epstein's (1994, 2003) concept of two core processing systems: the experiential system, which is direct learning from experience, and a slower, more cognitive, reflective system (see also LeDoux, 2022). Van der Kolk's book, *The Body Keeps the Score* (2014), directs attention to body-based classical conditioning where physiological systems can be directly changed by the environment and trauma. This has some similarity to Porges' (2017, 2021) concept of neuroception, which describes a *non-conscious* capacity to pick up threat and safety signals. Defensive behaviours can be activating as in the fight and flight responses, or deactivating as in faint, submissive, numbing and shutdown responses. At times, there may be conflict between these potential defences (Dixon, 1998). LeDoux (2022) suggested distinguishing between the behavioural programmes of defence, which can be rapid and activated from low(er) brain centres, and the issues of feelings, which are linked to higher, more recently evolved cognitive processes. Importantly, the rapid activation of behavioural motor programmes for fight or flight might be inhibited due to the reasons noted above. For example, we might feel the urge to shout or hit out but choose to smile instead and walk away. Hence, it is the motor programme (impulse to hit or run) of the emotion (not just a feeling) that can be intensified or inhibited. Abbas (2015) suggests that the innovation of such motor impulses can be linked to classically conditioned brain systems and that the innovation occurs before it gets into higher cognitive processing. He draws a distinction between how these defences play out in different muscle groups such as the striatal muscle versus the smooth muscle, giving rise to different symptoms and problems.

Behaviour therapists also focus on the contextual regulators of behaviour. This is particularly noted in therapies such as acceptance commitment therapy (Hayes *et al.*, 2011). In terms of the change process, it is well known that learning takes place not only through exposure but also action. No matter how much one intellectually knows about driving or playing the piano, unless one actually drives or plays, one cannot become good at it. Many therapies therefore involve specific behavioural practices that address both exposure aspects and also skills training. That is very much the case for CFT too (Tirch *et al.*, 2014).

Taken together, this biopsychosocial approach is concerned with the complex interactions in information flow within and between different mental processes, rather than focusing on only one or a few processes. It is from the interactions and co-regulations that new and different brain states and different maturational pathways unfold. Hence CFT is trying to change the pattern of these processes, which gradually gives rise to new personal insights and motivation for compassionate identities.

Section 2: The evolution and nature of compassion

To explore how compassion as a motivation can be used as a focus in psychotherapy requires insight into its basic evolved functions and processes. There seem to be at least three evolved pathways into compassion. These are important to be familiar with because different clients seek out different aspects of compassion. One is via rescuing behaviour and caring for the sick and injured. A second is via close attachment, particularly the complex coordination that occurs between infant and mother. A third is via reciprocity and reputation that supports belonging and social integration. In regard to the first dimension of rescuing and caring for the sick and injured, Kessler (2020) reviewed how many species engage in rescuing behaviour. For example, even ants will carry injured conspecifics back to the nest where their chances of recovery are improved. Spikins (2015, 2022) highlighted that the archaeological record indicates that early humans who had been severely injured or ill survived, which could only have occurred if they had been looked after and cared for. Humans are well known for the disposition to want to rescue others and care for the ill and injured (Spikins, 2015). Consider all of the rescue services, including medicine and many others that people dedicate themselves to. Importantly, this behaviour does not require any affiliative attachment to the injured person, and commonly, medical and rescue services do not know the people they are helping. This is not so much the case in the second pathway.

A second pathway to caring and compassion, which is more bounded and gene focused, has come through the evolution of infant caring and attachment (Buss, 2019). We will explore this route in more detail below. However, briefly, we can mention that parental caring involves the motives and competencies to be sensitive and attentive to the distress and needs of the infant and also to provide the appropriate response such as to feed, rescue, keep warm or play with. As noted below, these two qualities of 'sensitivity to' and 'appropriate action' underpin compassion algorithms.

A third pathway is related to our hunter-gatherer lifestyle, which characterized one to two million years and 95 per cent of our evolution (Dunbar, 2014; Narvaez, 2017; Ryan, 2019). In hunter-gatherer groups, which rarely numbered above 150, caring and sharing were central for survival and reproduction. Developing a reputation for caring, sharing and helpfulness facilitated one being chosen as a friend, ally and potential sexual partner (Goetz et al., 2010). It supported belonging. Aggressive and selfish individuals were shunned (Boehm, 1999). Over time, compassion and altruism, and the expression of altruistic traits became adaptive (Ryan, 2019). Today, humans are well recognized as a species that likes to be seen as helpful, as evidenced by the extraordinary sharing of information on the internet and other places.

Clinically, some clients are looking for a sense of rescue and protection, and issues of trust and safety are crucial. Other clients feel more emotionally empty and are trying to work out how to get a sense of connectedness and empathic resonance from others and the therapist. Yet other clients are wanting to have a sense of social value, of mattering and feeling they have something to offer that is valued by others – the wish to be esteemed and desired. Many of these processes blend together but also conflict. For example, people who have been abused and seek protection may fear being wanted, liked or desired because that is a threat. It can be useful to be discuss these different dimensions of care and compassion, and that at times we can want different things from compassion, thus providing clients with a framework to make sense of their experiences and to tune into their own needs.

Motives and algorithms for compassion

Like all motives, care-compassion operates with a basic *if-then* stimulus-response algorithm of *if* A, *then do* B. For example, for harm avoidance, the algorithm is: *if* threat is detected, *then* stimulate threat processing (e.g. in the amygdala) and take defensive action. For a sexual motive, the algorithm is: *if* a sexual (signal) opportunity presents itself, *then* activate appropriate (pituitary) arousal and engage mating behaviour. For caring (e.g. as in parental caring), stimulus feature detection is: *if* there are signals of distress or need in another, *then* activate appropriate actions to alleviate distress and meet need. The algorithm for caring-compassion leads directly to the definition of compassionate motivation as *a sensitivity to suffering in self and others with a commitment to try alleviate and prevent it* (Gilbert, 2014). Although there are variations, this type of definition is shared by many researchers (Mascaro *et al.*, 2020; Seppälä *et al.*, 2017). Gilbert and Choden (2013) argue that *prevention* is implicit in Buddhist thinking and should be part of the definition. Clearly, this means that compassion has to be sensitive to 'needs' and future thinking, planning and creating, not just reacting.

A major implication of taking an algorithmic approach is that we can distinguish between the two processes of stimulus-response. First, are the motives, emotions and competencies that enable us to be sensitive to (stimuli indicating) suffering in ourselves and others, to approach and tolerate it (rather than avoid or deny). Second, are the processes and competencies that guide wise and courageous action (response). These are outlined in Figure 7.2.

CFT identifies six core processes that aim at helping clients to detect and turn towards rather than away from suffering:

1. Becoming motivated to come to therapy for trauma and to set on a healing path, which will involve engaging with painful experience.
2. Developing sensitivity and mindfulness to distress.
3. Expanding mind awareness and acknowledging (distressed) reactions to sensitivity and awareness (called sympathy for self).
4. Developing tolerance to distress linked to the therapeutic process, as in the emergence of memories or emotions, fantasies and impulses.
5. Increasing empathic understanding of the nature and causes of what comes into mind and the nature of their distress.
6. Taking a non-judgemental stance towards their own mind.

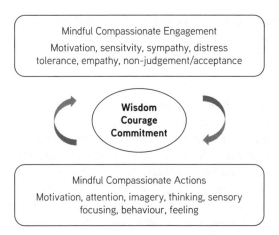

Figure 7.2: Building compassionate mind for engaging with suffering and its causes. Adapted from Gilbert and Choden (2013)

These competencies help facilitate the two crucial processes that underpin CFT: *courage* and *wisdom*. Given the way trauma affects so many psychological processes, particularly those linked to threat, courage and wisdom are essential qualities.

The second part of the algorithm is the response function. In CFT, clients engage with suffering so as to develop some degree of tolerance and non-judgemental empathic insight into the nature of the difficulty. However, this must trigger the response function; otherwise, people can get stuck in empathic distress. Gilbert *et al.* (2017) showed that sensitivity to distress without shifting to considering what would be helpful was associated with *increased* depression, anxiety and stress. Hence, people can be sensitive to their suffering but do not know what to do. CFT suggests six competencies or processes that support wise and courageous responses to suffering:

1. Switching attention to what is likely to be helpful.
2. Using various forms of imagery to stimulate bodily states and run scenarios in the mind of what is likely to be helpful.
3. Using various cognitive and other interventions to explore styles of thinking, problem solving, perspective taking – mentalizing, and reflecting.
4. Engaging in and practising behaviours that will develop compassionate courage and wisdom.
5. Utilizing the body to stimulate physiological systems which are underpinned by compassion, such as breathing exercises that stimulate the vagus nerve and facilitate grounding in the body.
6. Being able to understand and tolerate the emotions that are likely

to emerge in the pathway to taking action. For example, if actions require assertiveness, then clients develop the courageous wisdom for assertiveness. If, however, some degree of exposure and desensitization is required, then again they learn to tolerate the emotions that arise in the process.

Together, these make up the 12 therapeutic targets of CFT, and they underpin courage and wisdom, which are the centre for compassion in many contexts (Gilbert, 2009, 2022a). Courage without wisdom can be reckless or misguided, and wisdom without courage can be ineffective.

Clearly, there can be differences in how this algorithm works or fails to be activated. Callousness represents an *insensitivity* to the suffering of self or others in order to pursue self-focused goals and values. Individuals may see helping others they do not know as not worth bothering about because it is too costly. Individuals may know their behaviour is harmful, such as various forms of criminality, or individuals working in harmful industries, but self-interest prevails. Forms of self-callousness could be when we knowingly do harmful things to ourselves such as overeating and drinking but self-care loses out to other concerns or desires. For the most part, the suffering caused by callousness is simply a byproduct of the pursuit of self-interest. Harmfulness is not the intention of the behaviour.

Cruelty, in contrast, is where individuals do deliberately wish to cause suffering and to see the signals of fear and suffering in others for reasons of control, power and vengeance or even sexual pleasure. In many primate species, dominant individuals deliberately seek to intimidate subordinates and generate fear and a submissive response (Gilbert, 2000b). In forensic populations, where childhood trauma and abuse are highly represented, some individuals only feel safe if they know that others are frightened of them (Gilbert, 2022b). As we will note later, some forms of trauma can involve both callousness and cruelty. 'Hurt people hurt people', as they say, especially if hurt is linked to shame (see below). Compassion work therefore requires exploration of the nature of callousness and cruelty to understand their driving processes. The world has suffered immensely from traumatized children becoming people striving for power and, on the way to getting it and holding onto it, instigating horrific repressions, tortures and wars. Genghis Khan is a terrifying example.

Caring algorithms and physiological processes

Another crucial aspect of CFT is recognition that different motivational systems are underpinned by different physiological ones (Gilbert, 1989, 2015). Care and compassion are forms of prosociality, and there has been a rapid growth in insight into the psychophysiological processes of prosociality (Keltner *et al.*, 2014; Wu and Hong, 2022). Care and compassionate motives and behaviour are now linked to neurohormonal process such as oxytocin (Carter *et al.*, 2017; Kucerova *et al.*, 2023), circuits in the central nervous system (Kim *et al.*, 2020; Singer and Engert, 2019; Vrtička *et al.*, 2017) and the autonomic nervous system, such as the vagus nerve and HRV (Di Bello *et al.*, 2020, 2021; Petrocchi and Cheli, 2019; Petrocchi *et al.*, 2022).

Understanding the physiological underpinnings of motives like compassion offers many therapeutic benefits and is necessary for a biopsychosocial approach. First, if physiological systems are not changed in therapy, therapy may have less impact, and not a lasting impact. Steffen *et al.* (2020) found that those who did well with CFT showed changes in HRV, while those who did less well, did not. There is also increasing evidence that specific practices have specific physiological effects and therefore what people practise impacts on what physiological changes will result. For example, Singer and Engert (2019) report that empathy training, mindfulness training and compassion training have overlapping but also different impacts on neurocircuits and behaviour. As they say, 'it matters what you practise'.

Caring and the evolution of attachment

Many (but not all) of these basic psychophysiological mechanisms are believed to have evolved in the context of caring and attachment behaviour (Cassidy and Shaver, 2016; Depue and Morrone-Strupinsky, 2005; Mayseless, 2016; Mikulincer and Shaver, 2017). They are stimulated through the triggering of care-focused motivational systems (e.g. the detection of suffering or need, with the desire to do something about it) *and* the expression and the reception of affiliative and caring signals of affection and warmth (Brown and Brown, 2015; Carter *et al.*, 2017; Cozolino, 2014; De Bello *et al.*, 2020; Gilbert, 1989, 2000a, 2020ab; Keltner *et al.*, 2014; Porges, 2007, 2021; Slavich, 2020).

Attachment theorists highlighted the importance of parental input not only for physical protection and survival but also psychological development in the form of a secure base and safe haven. These create a context that facilitates important biopsychosocial maturational processes (see Bowlby, 1969, 1973, 1980; Cassidy and Shaver, 2016; Music 2017; Siegel, 2020 for reviews). Briefly, a *secure base* provides the context for protection and encouragement to explore the environment, develop skills, and (for humans) to have emotions validated and empathically understood. A secure base is activating and supports exploration and the developing of the courage to engage life, take risks and grow. A *safe haven* has soothing functions such that if a child (or adult) becomes distressed, threatened or needy, the parent (or helpful other) is able to provide the inputs to bring the child (or adult) back into regulation. These functions are ideally provided with emotional textures of warmth, positive affect and 'positive regard' (Cassidy and Shaver, 2016; Holmes and Slade, 2017; Music, 2017). In addition, there

is increasing evidence that these close interactions have a range of physiological impacts (Hofer, 1984), including forms of synchronization in visual
logical activity (Lunkenheimer *et al.*, 2018). The functions of a secure base
and safe haven are briefly outlined in Figure 7.3 and are crucial therapeutic
processes when working with traumatized children and adults (Cassidy and
Shaver, 2016; Music, 2017, 2022; Zilberstein, 2014). They are also central for
care-compassion work.

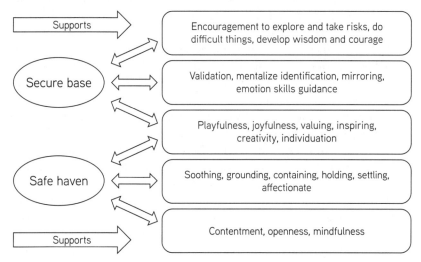

Figure 7.3: Outline of typical functions associated with a secure
base and safe haven. From Gilbert (2022a) © Paul Gilbert

The concept of a secure base and safe haven can guide the therapeutic process with children and adults (Holmes and Slade, 2017; Music, 2019, 2022).
Given that one of the roots of the evolution of compassion is parental
caring behaviour, then understanding the functions of attachment gives
insight into the psychological functions of care-compassion as a therapy
(Gilbert, 2020a, 2022d and discussed below). This means that when we
are being compassionate to ourselves, to others, or when others are being
compassionate to us, we can experience the functions of a secure base and
safe haven (Gilbert, 2022d). In other words, as depicted in Figure 7.3, for
self-compassion we can be self-encouraging, self-validating and self-reassuring. We can mentalize our own minds, and (when appropriate) can
engage the world with confidence, creativity and playfulness.

In CFT, self-compassion is not just an individual, personal task we do
for ourselves, it is also an awareness of our need for others and our ability
to turn to others for help when we need it, be able to respond to it and be
appreciative of it, taking joy from receiving rather than being begrudging or
ashamed or needing. Because compassion is a flow between self and others,

it means that we can we experience others as being encouraging and validating to us, and we can be encouraging and validating to others (Gilbert *et al.*, 2017). To achieve these outcomes, we weave together compassion motivations, emotions and competencies. Hence, the CFT therapist seeks to provide these basic therapeutic frameworks.

Emotional warmth and affection

Even in the absence of specific traumas, a lack of needed caring inputs can have a range of adverse effects on brain development (Cassidy and Shaver, 2016; Gilbert, 1989; Mayseless, 2016; Music, 2017; Siegel, 2020). Rohner (1986) developed concepts of parental acceptance-rejection that are underpinned by experiences of warmth and highlighted that the lack of warmth is significantly linked to a range of psychological adjustment difficulties and mental health problems (Gilbert, 1989; Rohner, 1986; Rohner *et al.*, 2012). Hence, in support of providing and experiencing a secure base and safe haven, the CFT therapist delivers these with warmth and affection, expressed via various sensory modalities such as touch, affectionate voice tones, facial expressions, appropriate response to distress and empathic validation, praising, encouragement and 'joyful play' to mature the highly social brain such as we humans have (Cassidy and Shaver, 2016; Music, 2017, 2022; Siegel, 2020). Indeed, play is the key domain for working with trauma in children (Goodyear-Brown, 2019).

Gilbert and colleagues (Richter *et al.*, 2009) developed a self-report measure to tap into memories of warmth and safeness in childhood and found that having positive emotional memories of feeling warm, safe and cared for in early life was associated with less vulnerability to psychological distress, with reduced self-criticism and greater ability to self-reassure and to experience positive affect. Vagos *et al.* (2017) developed a shorter version of this measure and found that girls and boys reported similar levels of early warmth and safeness, but this was much lower in youth in custodial settings. Naismith *et al.* (2019) showed that low warmth, invalidation and physical abuse had different impacts on dispositions to self-compassion and personality disorder symptoms. Low warmth is linked to dispositions towards callousness. Bisby *et al.* (2017) also showed that low maternal warmth and cold 'parenting' were more strongly associated with callousness than either emotional or physical neglect.

Matos *et al.* (2015) demonstrated that early memories of warmth and safeness were associated with reduced external and internal shame later in life and buffered against the deleterious effects of shame memories on psychological distress. Thus, having shame memories in the context of an early positive affiliative environment may provide opportunities for reconnecting with others and buffer against the negative impact of those shame experiences. In the absence of positive affiliative memories, one may feel unsafe, alone and disconnected, and more vulnerable to the negative impact of shame-related trauma. Affiliative relationships may therefore lay down positive emotional memories of the self-in-relationship-to-others that provide a source of social safeness and connectedness and enable adaptive affect regulation through access to soothing others. These connections offer opportunities to repair shame, self-soothe distress and regulate arousal caused by threat (Matos *et al.* 2020). In essence, then, childhood trauma cannot be understood only in terms of the threat system but also in terms of the problems with the psychophysiological systems for social safeness and social connectedness (Gilbert, 2020a, 2022d).

There is a long history of research on the value of social support throughout life, how it acts as a buffer to stress and is a resource for coping and affiliative relating. Ditzen and Henrichs (2014) outline multiple biopsychosocial systems that social support impacts, with a central finding that social support tones down threat processing (see also Slavich, 2020). Because compassion is rooted in the evolution of caring motives and behavioural systems (Gilbert, 2000a, 2010, 2014; Gilbert and Simos, 2022), when applied as a therapy, it seeks specifically to provide secure base and safe haven functions (Holmes and Slade, 2017; Music, 2017; Siegel, 2020). It also uses various compassionate mind-training processes (see below) to stimulate and cultivate the development of an *internalized* secure base and safe haven textured with warmth and positive affect in the client (Gilbert, 2000a, 2020a, 2022d). This not only involves addressing psychological processes such as distress tolerance and empathy but also the physiological processes that underpin caring, such as balancing the autonomic nervous system and stimulating the vagus nerve (Porges, 2007, 2017) and the neurophysiological mechanisms of compassion (Kim *et al.*, 2020; Singer and Engert, 2019). By targeting such processes, CFT attempts to realign and balance the neuropsychophysiological systems disrupted by attachment trauma. In this context, CFT is a therapeutic journey of learning to address unmet emotional and psychological (archetypal) needs that are vital inputs for the maturation and the strengthening of these systems (Lee, 2022).

Evolution, hunter-gatherer societies, attachment and childhood trauma

Before exploring the impacts of trauma in more detail, we wish to bring attention to the fact that many of our vulnerabilities to mental health problems are linked to social changes in human living and child-rearing that emerged from agricultural practices and changes to hunter-gatherer group formation. This is called mismatch theory (Chaudhary and Salali, 2022). For around 95 per cent of our evolution, we lived in small hunter-gatherer bands of around 150 members or fewer which were mutually supportive and open (Dunbar, 2014; Ryan, 2019). The importance of community and a sense of social embeddedness to creating well-being is now well established (Armstrong *et al.*, 2021; Mikulincer and Shaver 2014; Taylor, 2011). There is currently general agreement that the pattern of parenting (e.g. mother–infant) changed radically with the onset of agriculture, the growth of group size, and the movement away from mutual dependency into hierarchical, often aggressive, control (Narvaez, 2017; Narvaez and Bradshaw, 2023; Spikins, 2023).

For a variety of reasons to do with the evolutionary changes that made birthing more painful and dangerous, women needed helpers and supporters, before and post-birth (Hrdy, 2009). Importantly, infants born into hunter-gatherer communities were not just restricted to two parents, or at times one parent, as can happen often today. In hunter-gatherer societies, children were able to go to many care providers, including siblings, aunts, uncles, grandparents and known, trusted members of the community, for experiences of caring and sharing, and hence for the provision of secure base and safe haven functions from various members of the community (Narvaez, 2017). Children being traumatized would become known quickly to the community, and those who may have lost their parents would be supported by trusted community members and relatives.

Children being hidden away in homes where abuse is secret and, if taken into care, being cared for by strangers in foster homes or other establishments, is grossly abnormal. To some extent, then, childhood trauma can be seen as a result of grossly abnormal child-rearing environments, where isolated children are raised in isolated parental relationships. Parents may lack the support or watchful eye of the community, be struggling with mental health problems, be highly stressed, and be affected by the legacy of their own experience of childhood trauma. While we can seek solutions for individuals, for families or for children long term, this requires a more considered approach to parenting in general and, where possible, necessitates revisiting the concept of parenting as a community rather than just a family responsibility. This raises the very important area of how we build *communities* to support children (Tucci *et al.*, 2017).

How attachment provides a 'second' threat regulation and source of positive affect

Threat processing is critical for people who have been traumatized. However, CFT has long made an important distinction between safety and safeness in regard to threat processing (Gilbert, 1993, 2022a). Basically, safety concerns focus on the presence and absence of threat, harm and issues of prevention. Safeness is more like the secure infant who is not worried about threat because they sense they are in a supportive, caring environment. Safety tends to be regulated through the threat system of the amygdala and the sympathetic nervous system, whereas safeness is regulated through the presence of signals of helpfulness and through the parasympathetic system (Porges, 2017). Accessibility to helpful others promotes a sense of safeness that facilitates resting but with open exploration (Bailey and Wood, 1998). Figure 7.4 depicts these different processes and the value of two quite different threat-processing systems.

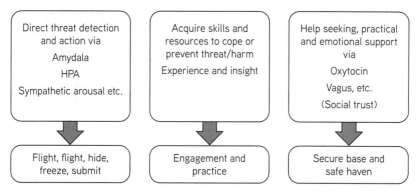

Figure 7.4: Depiction of two threat-regulation systems. © Paul Gilbert (2022a)

The left-hand side of Figure 7.4 highlights the process by which animals and humans directly engage with a threat. Threat signals stimulate the threat system via, for example, the HPA axis, the amygdala and sympathetic arousal (LeDoux, 2022; Terpou *et al.*, 2019). Unconditioned and conditioned responses (defence cascade; Schauer and Elbert, 2010) trigger safety-seeking responses (vigilance, fight, flight, submission, freeze). These can be via non-conscious processing but can also be modified by conscious cognitive processes. For example, we may feel the urge to fight or take flight but choose not to enact either. Hence, the middle column highlights that animals, and humans in more complex ways, can learn to deal with a threat that includes how to fight or escape, or how to reappraise a threat by assigning new meaning to it. These processes are relatively idiosyncratic and specific to context and to individuals. They provide the basis for a lot of contemporary psychotherapy which focuses on (say) exposure via deliberate threat activation linked to practising distress tolerance and regulating threat through helpful cognitive reframing of threat and meaning.

The third column of Figure 7.4 highlights another, very different, way to regulate threat. This occurs not by one's own individual efforts to cope but through seeking help from others. With the evolution of attachment, rather than 'the young' dealing with threats and needs directly, the child 'calls to' or seeks the input of others to regulate threat activation. First, they may need protection, need the parents to come and rescue them, or need the provision of a secure base where the parent guides the child to deal with a threat and supports them in doing so. However, the child also requires emotion regulation, which the parent may provide through the function of a safe haven and soothing. The caring, guiding, supporting, reassuring and soothing signals the parent offers the infant to regulate the threat, operate through different neuronal circuitry from that of the amygdala and the sympathetic safety-seeking systems (Kim *et al.*, 2020). The neurocircuitry for helping and being helped is linked to oxytocin, the frontal cortex and the vagus nerve (Brown and Brown, 2015; Gilbert, 1989, 1993; Kim *et al.*, 2020; Porges, 2017). This threat-regulation system means that, under threat, we might turn to others to elicit helpful, caring signals that tone down threat processing (Brown and Brown, 2015; Hostinar and Gunnar, 2015; Mayseless, 2016; Slavich, 2020). When we come to help ourselves, we may use these same processes of self-validation, self-encouragement, self-reassurance and so forth.

Safety and safeness
CFT makes a distinction between safety and safeness (Gilbert, 1993, 2022a). Safety and safety seeking involve regulating threat through the actual threat system by removing or dealing with threat-eliciting stimuli. Threat is evaluated through dimensions such as its predictability, uncertainty and controllability, its impact and the potential short- and long-term harm it could cause. Judgements of safety are to do with the presence or absence of signals that stimulate the threat system. Individuals basically feel they have safety when the threat system is not being stimulated (absence of threat), or they have confidence they can deal with it. Safeness, on the other hand, comes from the presence and availability of what is helpful. When we are using our safeness system, we are drawing on our connectedness to others, their support, grounding and encouragement to stimulate a secure base and safe haven.

Clearly, these are not independent; however, the key is that we can experience safety but not necessarily a sense of safeness in that we are embedded in a supportive environment. This is important clinically because some clients can experience safety and have confidence in their ability to deal with threats, but they may lack a sense of social connectedness, experience feelings of loneliness, and through those mechanisms be brought back into the threat of aloneness. In other words, the absence of safeness cues can itself represent a threat. For instance, you might see two doctors for an operation who are equally competent. One is highly technical, does not smile and appears cold and detached; the other is open, empathic and friendly. Which one is the more reassuring and settling? People who have been traumatized as children can struggle with social trust and be relatively wary of such signals. Hence, CFT discusses these differences with clients and works with trying to facilitate experiences that are both safety (no threat) and safeness.

Section 3: The impacts of trauma and on psychophysiological development

There is debate among clinicians and academics about what constitutes types of traumatic experience. Distinctions are made between Type I trauma, which is one-off and unexpected, such as a car accident, and Type II trauma, which involves repeated exposure to inescapable forms of trauma (Rothbaum, 2020). Traumatic experiences include physical threats, violence and injury (Kovler *et al.*, 2021), sexual abuse (Kalaf *et al.*, 2017), physical neglect (Evans and Burton, 2013), and emotional neglect (Music, 2022). Trauma can also arise in the context of ongoing mental health problems, such as that experienced during depression or psychotic episodes. This further complicates the ability to cope with, process and recover from trauma. Depressed, withdrawn, shy and socially anxious children are more vulnerable to bullying which intensifies anxiety (Lund *et al.*, 2010). Children with autism spectrum disorder are also more vulnerable to experiences of childhood trauma, including abuse and bullying (Maiano *et al.*, 2016). Hence, traumatic experiences differ in many dimensions, such as their form, nature, intensity, duration, anticipated versus non-anticipated nature, recovery trajectory, social versus non-social quality, and in terms of being inflicted by strangers versus familiars. Childhood trauma from a severe illness such as cancer, or a single incident like a car accident, will lay down different dispositional and threat sensitivities in different brain systems compared to physical or sexual abuse by those who should have cared for and loved a child.

The motives, emotions and competencies noted in Section 1 can all be impacted by trauma. A number of researchers have identified two or more parallel processing systems in relation to threat processing (Epstein, 1994, 2003; Haidt, 2001). These have been labelled rational versus experiential and are sometimes also regarded as slow reflective versus emotional-impulsive. LeDoux (2022) highlighted that we have fast-reacting behavioural systems for emotions but also slower more cognitive regulators and meaning generators for 'feelings'. Trauma can impact the fast-reacting behavioural systems for threat and reduce the capacity for the slower, reflective cognitive-regulating processes, particularly as trauma can affect the frontal cortex (Cassiers *et al.*, 2018).

Brewin *et al.* (1996) distinguished between different memory systems: one that is verbally accessible and one that is more of a felt sense that is difficult to verbalize and is located in different physiological systems. Heightened states of arousal influence cognitive systems by stimulating amygdala processing but compromising hippocampal functioning. The hippocampus, which matures later than the amygdala, processes the time and place of events as well as opportunities for verbal recall and processing. Hence, when trauma compromises the hippocampus, it affects people's abilities to process intense threat-based emotional experiences associated with trauma (Brewin *et al.*, 1996, 2010). Part of therapy can involve generating physiological shifts that can tone down the amygdala and make processing via our more complex cognitive competencies possible. Indeed, compassion training is known to impact the amygdala's sensitivity to threat (Weng *et al.*, 2018).

Trauma, then, can have very direct effects on many physiological systems, including epigenetics and the neural organization of emotions, making some easy to trigger and others difficult to trigger. Given that some of this can be non-conscious, as noted above, this means that people's emotions can be difficult for them to understand (Brewin *et al.*, 1996). Indeed, people's cognitive and verbal explanations can be post hoc efforts to make sense of what they feel rather than an accurate account of what created the emotional experience (Bargh, 2017; Haidt, 2001). In addition, when confronted by trauma, people can often have multiple emotional experiences and behavioural impulses that can be in conflict, some of which they may be aware of and some of which they may not (Abbas, 2015).

For example, a client recalling when his father lost his temper with him was able to recognize multiple experiences at the time. Being shouted at and hit in the way he was gave him the experience that 'he had done something terrible' and there was something 'very bad about him'. In addition, there was 'intense fear', including fear of 'being physically hurt and injured'. In addition, there was a sense of 'entrapment and being unable to get away', as well as a recognition that there would be 'no rescue' and that he experienced this attack 'alone' and would be 'left alone' afterwards (see Gilbert, 2022e, pp.186–187). Helping this client recognize *the multiplicity* of different emotions (not just fear) encoded in the trauma memory helped him recognize why at times he could dissociate. He was being flooded by many powerful and conflicting emotions at the same time, plus the recall of his father's feelings, judgements and accusations of him that were fused in the mix of emotions and defences. Later, what can also be encoded are reflections, where individuals look back and feel angry that they were not protected, or angry with themselves for not better defending themselves. CFT uses specific interventions and exercises that facilitate their guided discovery in the inherent multiplicity of mind. In creating a compassionate sense of self, it then becomes possible to process these individual emotions/experiences one at a time. In particular, CFT focuses on what is called the big three: anger, anxiety and sadness/grief (Gilbert, 2022c, 2022d)

PTSD can be associated with the repeated re-experiencing of fragmented and decontextualized amygdala-based sensory experiences related to the original trauma (Lee, 2022). One of the consequences of compromised information processing (compromised hippocampal processing) is an incoherent, disorganized, decontextualized sense of self and poor emotion regulation skills (Lee, 2022). In parallel with these distinctions, competencies can also be described in terms of function. Various traumas linked to abuse and neglect can impact a variety of psychophysiological systems, including epigenetics (Cowan *et al.*, 2016; O'Donnell and Meaney, 2020), the central nervous system (Cassiers *et al.*, 2018; Kavanaugh *et al.*, 2017; Terpou *et al.*, 2019), the autonomic nervous system (van der Kolk, 2014), and the immune system (Lippard and Nemeroff, 2020). In addition, there are impacts on psychological processes such as motivation, emotion balance and disposition to threat, and competencies such as empathy, self-identity, confidence, social trust and cognitive biases (van der Hart *et al.*, 2006; van der Kolk, 2014; Porges, 2011). The bottom line is that, as outlined in Figure 7.4, traumatized children can struggle because the threat-safety system has been overly sensitized to threat cues. In addition, traumatized children may find it almost impossible to access the vagal-oxytocin soothing system, because it has not been 'developed' and may even be conditioned to threat. Indeed, one of the major propositions that attachment therapists (Holmes and Slade, 2017; Music, 2017; Siegel, 2020) and CFT (Gilbert, 1993, 2022c) make is that trauma can significantly rupture the ability to use the care-seeking system for threat regulation and for building trusting, affectionate, soothing and reassuring social connections.

This is particularly problematic where parents and care providers do not offer a secure base or safe haven, and at the same time they directly stimulate the infant's threat system by being threatening and unable to regulate their own harmful desires or emotions themselves. When the infant cannot use their parental attachment figure to protect, encourage or soothe them, indeed on the contrary, when the parent or caregiver themselves is the source of threat, the infant is in an *impossible approach-avoidance conflict*. This conflict can have a major organizing effect on processing. In fact, Pavlov was one of the first to show that approach-avoidance conflict can produce serious disorganization of response systems (Lidell, 1947). Later, Mineka and Kihlstrom (1978) argued that (lack of) control and unpredictability are also central aspects of response disorganization. Many have asserted that approach-avoidance type conflicts, linked to lack of control and unpredictability, can be at the heart of the problems of traumatized children (Liotti, 2011). When threatened, the child experiences *threat without resolution* from a (non-)caring other (Liotti, 2011). In addition, the child may be trapped (e.g. in the home) and unable to use fight, flight or submissive defences. In essence, then, at such times as the infant would normally seek the secure base or safe haven functions of a parent, if they have become frightened of their parent, they will experience elevated threat when that motivational system to seek care is triggered. The motor programme for seeking care must be blocked. There are many ways this can be understood, including classical conditioning of approach-avoidance conflict that can produce significant disorganization of the behavioural repertoire (Gilbert, 1993, 2022c; Liotti, 2011)

Liotti (2000, 2011) also discussed problems that arise when unresolved loss and trauma in a parent (caregiver) lead to an ease in triggering their own trauma memories, which can interfere with nonverbal communication and their ability to provide a secure base and safe haven and can send ambivalent messages to the infant (Iyengar *et al.*, 2014). Even if parents intentionally wish to provide affectionate caring, they might struggle with their nonverbal communications. Hence, when the parent is needed to be comforting, they might be either rejecting, aggressive, or their facial expressions and manner might indicate fear and confusion, stimulating the infant's threat system that becomes coded within the infant's attachment-seeking system.

The impact of trauma on social mentalities and relating styles

Attachment researchers have highlighted that attachment ruptures and dysfunctions, including those generated by abuse and neglect, significantly disrupt the maturation of the various social relating systems and social mentalities (Cassidy and Shaver, 2016). Researchers have typically identified different types of interpersonal relating style, which have been labelled variously as anxious attachment, avoidant attachment, and ambivalent disorganized, fearful and dismissing (Cassidy and Shaver, 2016). Early life experiences orientate individuals to different strategic and social mentality ways of engaging the world. In safe and caring environments, it is advantageous for individuals to mature capacities for creating caring and sharing and safeness-giving relationships with others. However, in more neglectful or hostile environments, these strategies can be dysfunctional, and strategies for self-defence, self-promotion and safety-first orientated behaviour are advantageous – because these individuals' orientation to life is more one of limiting damage and preventing harm (Gilbert, 2021).

Figure 7.5 shows this distinction, highlighting that individuals who grow up in neglectful or threatening environments will be orientated to the competitive and social rank and power dimensions of relationships. Competitive motivation tends to downregulate caring motivation. In this approach, what is sometimes called anxious attachment would be seen as threatened low rank, where individuals tend feel inferior, lack social confidence and are shame prone, submissive and appeasing. Caring behaviour tends to be orientated to being liked rather than based on genuine empathic concern (Catarino *et al.*, 2014). In contrast are individuals who are up-rank orientated, can develop narcissistic, egocentric and manipulative traits and show elements of the dark triad (Machiavellianism and narcissism and psychopathy; Sheikhi and Aminiha, 2022).

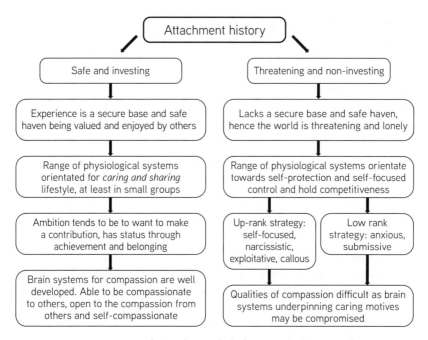

Figure 7.5: Attachment history linked to competitiveness and compassion. Adapted from Gilbert 2005. © Paul Gilbert

Hence children who are not able to develop social safeness and trust or to experience positive emotion from caring, are forced into utilizing a more ancient social motivational system which is rooted in social competition, a social ranking system and resource acquisition (Gilbert, 1989, 2005, 2022a; Liotti, 2011). When this motivation dominates the child's orientation to the world, they become highly sensitive to issues of social power and social control. Here, the strategic choices are to adopt a 'damage limitation' and 'better safe than sorry' approach to life that utilizes the down- or low-rank subordinate defences of freeze, flight, appeasement, ingratiation and submissive withdrawal. The contrasting strategy of going for control and hold and seeking up-rank and power positions over others is the more risky, but has a higher pay off. This orientates towards narcissistic defences of fight, arrogance, hubris and entitlement. Partly because competitive strategies are not rooted in care and share, concerns for others are notably absent. These strategies can be very contextual in that sometimes people will express both as a means of stabilizing their position within a rank, aptly described by Vonk (1998) as 'upward licking and downward kicking'. In therapy, too, traumatized children as adults can oscillate between these strategies, at times feeling inferior and lacking confidence and being submissive but at other times becoming arrogant and exploitative. Crucially, CFT seeks to shift people out of this (rank-focused competitive) motivational system altogether and move into a care-focused orientation to themselves and life in general. It is the shift in motivation which changes the psychophysiological underpinnings and hence many other psychological processes with it.

The role of shame

Shame proneness is a common problem linked to attachment disruption and early trauma. As such, it is a major target for therapy (Gilbert, 1998, 2022bc; Matos *et al.*, 2020 for reviews). From an evolutionary perspective, shame is a potential response to (competitive) social threat. There are three forms of shame (Gilbert, 2003, 2007, 2019; 2022bc):

- External shame is the sense of having a poor or damaged reputation in the minds of others and being judged as flawed, inferior, bad, undesirable and rejectable (Gilbert, 1998, 2007; Matos *et al.*, 2013a, 2013b; Sznycer *et al.*, 2016).
- Internal shame relates to one's own self-judgement, driven by self-criticism of being flawed, inferior, bad, undesirable and rejectable (Gilbert *et al.*, 2004, 2022c);
- Reflected shame is linked to the shame one can bring to others by association or that others bring to the self (e.g. children can feel shamed by the actions of their parents, or parents by their children; Gilbert, 2007). Parents can be aggressive towards their children if they feel their children show them up, for example in public (Kirby *et al.*, 2019). Extreme forms of shame can generate 'honour killing' (Sanghera, 2009).

People with interpersonal trauma can develop all three forms of shame; for example, a client worried how her new partner would perceive her if he knew she was abused as a child, and also if his parents found out. Children are particularly vulnerable to shame because they are clearly in the smaller, weaker position compared to the adult, with lower control over interactions, are often trapped and unable to escape from the orbit of the abusing adult, and are vulnerable to their threats and physical attacks, and to verbal descriptions from the adult: *'You are stupid; you are bad; you are pathetic; you are a nuisance; I wish I never had you.'*

Early shame experiences, particularly from attachment figures, act as traumatic memories, eliciting intrusions, hyperarousal and avoidance symptoms, and have a wide-range of effects on self-identity and emotion regulation (Matos *et al.*, 2013c, 2014; Pinto-Gouveia and Matos, 2011). Such shame traumatic memories increase proneness to external and internal shame, and symptoms of depression, anxiety and stress in adulthood (Matos and Pinto-Gouveia, 2010). Thus, these interpersonal trauma memories can engender a sense of ongoing threat to one's psychological integrity and relational safeness. Individuals can feel and believe they are seen by others as unattractive, inferior, defective, unlovable, inadequate, someone to reject, and hence others are unsafe (Matos and Pinto-Gouveia, 2010; Matos *et al.*, 2012). Early shame experiences can play a major role in overstimulating concerns with social rank which become central to one's self-identity. This shapes attentional focus: what one must display and what one must keep hidden from display; what one can allow and what one must avoid; who one can trust and who one should not trust; what one should aspire to and what failures to avoid. Hence, shame can result in a focus on concealment or compensation (trying to make up for perceived deficits; Gilbert, 1998, 2007, 2022b; Pinto-Gouveia and Matos, 2011). This partly explains why children who feel ashamed by, and blame themselves for, sexual abuse have more mental health problems than those who do not self-blame (Quas *et al.*, 2003). Shame also predicts PTSD, while self-criticism predicts depression, and poor coping predicts depression and suicidal ideation (Alix *et al.*, 2020). Self-criticism maintains trauma-related shame (Lawrence and Lee, 2014).

Self-criticism

It has been known for a long time that rather than developing supportive, compassionate and self-reassuring responses to the distress of trauma, people can become intensely and harshly self-critical (Gilbert, 2022c; Shahar, 2015; Werner *et al.*, 2019). Whelton and Greenberg (2005) showed that it was not just the content of self-criticism but the hostility (anger and contempt) that made it particularly pathogenic. Recent research supports these suggestions, and especially the link between hostile forms of self-criticism and trauma (Harman, Lee, and Barker, 2009). Consider this example from a person with an eating disorder, from Tierney and Fox's (2010) exploration of the 'anorexic voice':

> ...when I see myself in the mirror I cry because my head is screaming 'dirty fat bitch... disgusting failure, not good enough, lose weight you pathetic piece of crap, worthless, useless idiot, don't DARE eat! Where are the rest of your bones? Don't DARE eat you fat, DESPICABLE, HIDEOUS waste of space... (p.247)

Some forms of self-criticism are literally a form of raging. It is not uncommon for people to swear at themselves, calling themselves names such as 'useless, fake, pathetic, shithead' (Gilbert, 2022c). Ashfield, Chan and Lee (2021) looked at the process of change in people using group-based CFT for complex PTSD and again highlighted the harshness of their self-relationships. For example, one client noted that:

...I deserved all that happened to me, so everything that's happened I absolutely deserved it, that I'm pathetic, I'm a failure, that I'm weak ... and everything that's happened is pretty much my fault ... it was the bottom line, you know it was, I deserved it, everything... (p.292)

There is now considerable evidence that these forms of self-to-self relating are highly stimulant of the threat system, particularly the amygdala (Kim *et al.*, 2020; Longe *et al.*, 2010) and the sympathetic nervous system (Kirschner *et al.*, 2019). In effect, whether 'the attack' is coming from the outside or the inside, it stimulates the same physiological systems (see below). Whether we see something sexual or just fantasize it, it stimulates the same physiological systems. This is explained to clients in CFT. Indeed, some people develop beliefs that hostile self-criticism is actually trying to help them change, but in a misguided way. CFT highlights this is not the case and invites clients to explore their self-criticism in detail using function analysis. This approach commonly reveals quite intense hostility to the self (see Gilbert 2022c for worked examples). Over time (and it can take time), clients are then invited to explore what they are shamed or self-critical about through the eyes of their compassionate mind (brain state). CFT helps clients recognize that harsh self-criticism can be linked to an internalized judgement from others, and also emerges out of fear of being rejected. Hence, CFT works with the generators of the self-critical process, for example, helping people process their experiences and fear of 'not being good enough', of rejection and hostility from others. In other words, we switch the person out of the threat system and into the compassion system rather than trying to work with or challenge the self-critical process itself.

Hostile self-support

Hostile feelings towards the self are not just present in self-criticism. One of the observations that inspired CFT was discovering *they can also be present in efforts to be helpful* (Gilbert, 2022a, 2022c). Cognitive therapy helps people identify styles of thinking and stand back and generate more helpful alternatives. However, some people struggle with using cognition to change emotion (Stott, 2007). While working with chronically depressed people, Gilbert (2009), using cognitive therapy, began to ask clients to speak out aloud their 'alternative helpful' thoughts in the way they heard them in their minds. He was somewhat shocked to discover that, while they could generate helpful and supportive content such as 'I have been successful in the past; I have friends that care for me' and so on, their emotional tone was cold or more commonly extremely hostile and contemptuous. For example, a client could have a thought like 'I've been successful in the past' but with a hidden emotional texture of 'For goodness' sake, pay attention to what you've done successfully, you stupid person; stop dwelling on the negative!'

Clients were often embarrassed and reluctant to acknowledge the hostile tone of their efforts at 'helpful' thinking. So, it became clear that the problem of hostile feeling towards the self was not just carried in cognitive channels but also in the emotional textures and *relationship* with the self (Whelton and Greenberg, 2005), even when one was trying to be helpful and not self-critical. It became clear that one had to attend to the emotional textures of 'helpful-alternative' thinking. The obvious solution was to guide people to generate 'kind' tones, with compassion motivation underpinning cognitive reappraisal. That led to the second shock, which was that many clients did not want to do that because they saw it as unhelpful and weak and, partly because of their background, they did not know how to do it. It felt alien, odd and cold. The third shock was that, as clients did begin to try to generate genuine compassion motivation and emotion-based efforts at reappraisal, it opened up a lot of unprocessed attachment trauma as we note below.

Section 4: Compassion focused therapy (CFT)

CFT is an evolution-informed, biopsychosocial approach to therapy that seeks to use evidence-based interventions for each domain of physiology, psychology and social behaviour. It integrates interventions from different schools of psychotherapy but with a special focus on the care motive system to promote caring and prosocial behaviour to self and others. Hence, the therapeutic relationship and therapeutic interventions are contextualized within a compassion motivation orientation, with the appropriate psychophysiological impacts on processing (Gilbert, 2000a; Gilbert and Simos, 2022). There is increasing evidence for CFT's effectiveness in trauma (Ashfield *et al.*, 2021; Au *et al.*, 2017; Cowles *et al.*, 2020; Lawrence and Lee, 2014; Lee, 2022; Lucre and Corten, 2013; Willis *et al.*, 2023). In addition to outcome evidence, there is a wealth of process evidence on the biopsychosocial impacts of compassion (Gilbert and Simos, 2022; Seppälä *et al.*, 2017)

There is now considerable evidence that priming people with attachment memories and stimulating care-focused processing have major impacts on how people process threat (Gilbert, 2020a, 2020c; Gillath and Karantzas, 2019). Hence, in the present chapter we have indicated why CFT is about motivational switching and cultivating because care-focused motivations evolved with important psychophysiological processes which facilitate threat regulation and promote prosocial behaviour towards self and others. Enabling people to gain access to these processing systems is a focus of the therapy. This is set against the context that childhood trauma compromises the ability to develop the biopsychosocial functions of care as provided by secure attachment. This can mean that from early trauma people can find it difficult and challenging to use the:

- *physiological* processes of the care-support, threat-regulation system that recruits the vagus, care-based neurocircuits, oxytocin and other relevant physiological systems (see Figure 7.4)
- *psychological* processes of a secure base and safe haven such as self-validation, self-reassurance and self-encouragement for the self (see Figure 7.3). This will make it difficult to deal with issues of shame and harsh self-criticism. In addition, they may find attempts to be self-compassionate and self-reassuring threatening (Kim *et al.*, 2020; Longe *et al.*, 2010; Rockliff *et al.*, 2008)
- *social* process of the care motive systems. They can have fewer experiences of positive emotions from feeling loved and connected. They may struggle with certain competencies such as mentalizing. They may struggle with appropriate assertiveness and social trust, and find it frightening if people get close; for example, they may fear being shamed. They get caught in complex and difficult approach-avoidance conflicts.

CFT draws a distinction between the therapeutic process, which involves the therapeutic relationship, assessment, formulation, contracting and the other common therapeutic processes (Gilbert, 2022; Holmes and Slade, 2017), and compassionate mind training. Working with trauma clients requires a careful and complex interweaving of the therapeutic process with compassionate mind training (Bohus *et al.*, 2020; Gilbert and Procter, 2006). Indeed, all of the core processes known to be important in the therapeutic relationship are essential to CFT (Gilbert, 2022a; van der Kolk, 2014), including how the therapist is aware of non-conscious processing and defences such as projection and projective identification (Abbas, 2015).

Fears, blocks and resistances (FBRs) to compassion

People can be fearful and avoidant not just of frightening or painful states of mind, but also positive mental states including happiness (Gilbert *et al.*, 2014) and compassion (Gilbert *et al.*, 2011). Based on a large meta-analysis, Kirby *et al.* (2019) showed that fears of self-compassion and of being open to receiving compassion from others are highly linked to mental health difficulties. In process research studies, Gilbert *et al.* (2006) showed that low self-critical students who imagined doing less well in a course assignment than hoped for, were able to imagine being compassionate to themselves, whereas higher self-critical students found that difficult to do. In addition, they were much more able to create hostile critical images and messages for the setback. Rockliff (2008) demonstrated that compassionate imagery had a general positive effect on HRV but was associated with a worsening of HRV for people with higher self-criticism and poor attachment. Compassion and reassurance for these people were experienced as a threat.

Rockliff *et al.* (2011) found similarly with oxytocin, that many found oxytocin supported the capacity to create and experience compassion imagery but some people higher in self-criticism experienced oxytocin negatively. Neurophysiological studies have also shown that when self-critical people try to be self-compassionate, they can stimulate their threat systems (Kim *et al.*, 2020; Longe *et al.*, 2010). Pauley and McPherson (2010) found that depressed people thought compassion for themselves was almost impossible, feeling it was of little value, somewhat threatening, and that they did not deserve it. Lawrence and Lee (2014) explored the unfolding process of experiencing compassion in a CFT trauma therapy group. They found that for some, compassion felt alien, frightening and unpleasant, and that clients could not really see how it would help.

Trauma, then, does not just make access to the caring psychophysiological processes difficult, but it can also create fear and resistance to being compassionate to oneself and open to (trusting) compassion from others and to others (Kirby *et al.*, 2019). This can be because all motive systems carry their own trauma memories with conditioned emotional responses of the algorithms (Gilbert, 1992, pp.365–369). For example, if a child repeatedly experiences rejection when seeking comfort from their attachment figure, they will come to experience conditioned anxiety or anger to the triggering of that motive. This may also link to shame of 'need' for comfort. Liotti (2000) also highlighted that early trauma is coded in the care and attachment motive system. If this system is accessed in therapy, what can first appear are the emotions linked to trauma memory. In a study examining the origins of fear of compassion, Matos *et al.* (2017) found that shame experiences, encoded as traumatic memories, and central to self-identity, along with a lack of experiencing warmth and safeness as a child, were significantly linked to the development of fear of compassion for the self, for others and of receiving compassion from others. This in turn increased people's vulnerability to the effects of such early experiences on a range of psychopathological symptoms. Hence, trauma impacts the three biopsychosocial processes noted above.

Figure 7.6 depicts how, through empathic, kind and caring signals in the therapeutic relationship, and through specific exercises, clients can have their 'care and attachment' systems stimulated but also their threat defences. The unwary therapist can be surprised at the pushback, detachment or even hostility that this can trigger. However, insight into these processes enables the therapist to discuss 'wisdom protection': that if there is trauma in the care system, then that would explain the pushback and the seeking to protect oneself from the memories of trauma perhaps, or from unprocessed rage, or grief, yearning and loss (Gilbert, 2023). Given that FBRs present challenges to the therapist, in a qualitative study Steindl *et al.*

(2022) explore how therapists perceive and work with FBRs. They found four most helpful strategies to address these problems were:

- trying to get alongside the client and to see what sits behind the FBRs
- integrating a central theme of 'not your fault' that helps to soften potential shame around working with compassion
- understanding the importance of using experiential and in-the-moment interventions
- reconsidering FBRs as wisdoms of protection.

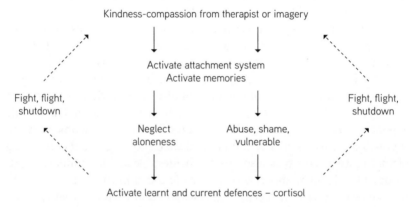

Figure 7.6: Fears, blocks and resistances. © Paul Gilbert (2009)

Fear of compassion may be directly linked to oxytocin. For example, Ebert *et al.* (2018) studied blood levels of oxytocin (OT) in relation to fears of compassion (FOC) and a measure of parenting (FEE) in people with borderline difficulties (BPD). Summarizing the results, they found:

> ...BPD patients had significantly lower OT plasma levels than healthy controls and differed significantly on all FOC and FEE scales; BPD patients had higher FOC scores (indicating more aversion of being compassionate to themselves and others and receiving compassion from others). They also differed in recalled parenting. In the BPD group, scores of the FOC scale 'fear of compassion from others' were significantly negatively correlated with OT levels. Moreover, recalled 'emotional warmth' of their parents during childhood was positively correlated with OT plasma levels of BPD subjects. No such correlations were found in the control group... (p.50)

FBRs can be linked to non-conscious processes, particularly rage and grief. Abbas (2015) suggests that anger and retaliation against hostile neglectful others generates guilt that renders these states difficult to process. Children can become terrified of retaliation should they show anger or need. The fear of guilt is an internal process, whereas the fear of retaliation can come from outside oneself. It is not uncommon for early trauma clients to experience intense, at times sadistic, rage, which makes them feel unlovable and reject-able. Hence, as some individuals engage with this rage, they fear losing the very thing they want: to be loved, lovable and protected. Clients may not be aware of their rage or intense grief, and this can take time to work through with small steps to exposure (Gilbert and Simos, 2022).

In the context of a large threatening event like the Covid-19 pandemic, a multinational study using data collected across 21 countries worldwide indicated that fears of compassion had a universal magnifying effect on the damaging impact of the pandemic on mental health and feelings of social safeness (Matos *et al.*, 2021a). Along with people feeling lonely and discon-nected from others, it increased symptoms of PTSD across all countries (Matos *et al.*, 2021b). Much of the therapy is therefore focused on anticipat-ing and working with FBRs.

Explaining compassion

Psychoeducation is a key part of creating a framework for the therapy and compassionate mind training. Sometimes, FBRs to compassion arise because clients are not aware of the scientific approach the therapist is taking (McEwan and Minou, 2023). Hence, the therapist invites the client to discuss their definitions of compassion, which can reveal such problems. Typically, they may see compassion as niceness, kindness or softness or as needing to 'love' (McEwan and Minou, 2023). These are common ideas, so the therapist introduces the scientific (motive algorithm) way to think about compassion. First, they invite the client to explore their intuitive wisdom of compassion, by using a guiding discovery. The therapist asks the client to bring to mind somebody they care about, a friend perhaps (for about 15 seconds or so), and to imagine the friend phones them up in a distressed state. They have to go to hospital for an operation but are frightened. The therapist invites the client to reflect on how they would react to their friend. From the client's responses, the therapist is usually able to point out that they are sensitive and concerned about their friend's distress. The therapist highlights that is one of the first key themes of compassion, our distress sensitivity combined with the courage and wisdom to engage with distress. Second, the therapist invites the client to think about how they would help their friend, what they would want to do. Not uncommonly, the client suggests they would go with them to hospital (although sometimes this is not so spontaneous, if the client is equally fearful of hospitals). However, because CFT is rooted in motivation, the therapist would ask, 'What would you like to do if you were not anxious?' Third, the therapist discusses why having somebody who cares about you, who will be with you when things are frightening, is helpful and that the client has intuitive wisdom for why that it would be helpful. The therapist weaves in the importance of how caring helps develop courage and wisdom because that will be necessary on the journey into trauma. Sometimes you can ask the client to think about what it would be like if the roles were reversed and it was they themselves who were frightened to go to hospital. Would they be able to ask others for help, be able to accept it and feel trust and gratitude?

De-shaming and the tricky brain

External and internal shame related to trauma memory are major sources of mental health difficulties for people with trauma (Matos *et al.*, 2020). CFT seeks to undermine shame by sharing evolution-based insights. The therapist notes that all living things, including the therapist and the client, just found themselves here with bodies and brains built for them (by DNA), not by them. No lion chose to be a lion, or antelope its prey; no human chose to be born human. We can playfully ask clients if they chose the shape of their body (arms, legs and head), their need for food, and a brain with particular dispositions. Did they choose their sex or ethnicity, or the caring or harming family or culture they were born into? We are 'a consciousness' that experiences the activation of different evolved systems in our brain. The many and varied brain states we can experience evolved for survival and reproduction reasons (gene replication), not personal happiness or well-being. Hence, our brains have built-in potentials for: needs, desires, motives for harm avoidance, food, care, reproduction, and for emotions such as anger, vengeance, anxiety, excitement and joy. Clients are guided to note that all human beings can demonstrate these potentials because we are all part of what has been built into us as humans (common humanity), *not chosen or at times even wanted by us.* This is the basis of clients beginning to understand that much of what goes on in their mind is *not their fault*; rather, they are experiencing evolved designed brain patterns.

Clients are invited to reflect on this and stand back and consider that we have a mixed portfolio of wanted and unwanted emotions; helpful and harmful. Again, that is not our fault because we did not design them and we often do not choose to feel them. For example, falling into depression, panic anxiety or paranoia is not something we choose or practise. We do not go on training workshops or retreats to get better at them. They are brain states that can be triggered *against our will*. This is important because sometimes individuals can feel that there's something wrong with them rather than experiencing their defences to what was harmful.

Clients are guided to consider that what can make our brain states par-ticularly tricky are the traumas we experienced early in life because they affect how motives, emotions and other systems get 'patterned' and turned on and off, which, again, is not the client's fault. Rather, they become automatic 'trauma patterns' that shape their social lives (Lee, 2022). The discussion of the tricky brain can have profound impacts on people's sense of decentring/defusing from their motives and emotional difficulties, and also act as a de-shaming process. Clients can become aware of how powerful and conditioned some of their emotions are and how, when they are triggered, they focus attention and generate menus of thoughts and impulses for behaviour. What can help, is to bring mindful awareness through 'knowledge of the tricky brain' to enable clients to become observant, to step back and make more helpful choices. CFT suggests that mindfulness can partly be supported by people being aware of some of the evolutionary roots of what comes into mind.

De-shaming the version we have become

The second aspect of de-shaming is to share with clients that if you (as therapist) had been kidnapped as a three-day-old baby, into a violent gang, you (as therapist) would be a totally different version of yourself. It is important that *the client* makes those observations and they can look at you and see that you would be different in many ways. CFT invites the client to recognize that you 'as a therapist today' would never have chosen to be kidnapped or to have that kind of life that would have shaped you very differently. This kind of discussion sets up a common humanity bridge with the client. They can experience it as an empathic communication that you (as therapist) understand that they did not choose their traumas or to become the way they are. Clearly, clinical sensitivity is needed here for the timing of these guided discoveries, as one is not seeking to trigger the client but to offer a framework for de-shaming and common humanity.

This second social constructionist aspect of de-shaming is to explore with clients the randomness of early attachment experiences, the lack of agency to influence those experiences which shape trauma patterns, and the versions of ourselves we find ourselves to be. This allows therapists to de-shame difficulties such as impulsivity, poor control, aggression, alcohol problems and distrust as conditioned responses to threat in the absence of signals of safeness in attachment relationships. Our experiences shape us, right down to the level of how our epigenetics and our brains get wired. Hence, we can understand 'body-rooted traumatic re-experiencing and re-enactment of trauma patterns.'

CFT helps clients consider that we experience fluctuations in brain states as we move from emotions such as anger to anxiety or calmness, and that each state is an example of the version that we are in at that moment (e.g. angry self/mind, anxious self/mind). Therapists explore that, with training and understanding of the mind, we can begin to pattern our brains differently and so experience different versions of self (e.g. compassionate self). These two elements are discussed empathically, softly (rather than scientifically). We encourage opportunities for (at times if the client is able) silent reflection to note the emotional impact of these key messages of the tricky brain and the socially shaped self and that 'much of what goes on in your mind is not your fault'.

The creation of space in therapy allows for the emergence of other key processes blocked by trauma, such as grief. When clients truly begin to connect with the insight 'it's not my fault', they can access profound states of grief and loss. This can be a vital process for honouring the pain of their experiences. Clients with early trauma can be terrified of grieving because when they were sad or yearning for comfort, they may have been abused, ignored, neglected, ridiculed or shouted at. Also, the sensation of crying, losing body muscle tone, and not being able to see or breathe properly can be experienced as threatening. These are not body states that are conducive to dealing with threats. Hence, the therapist begins to create the conditions for a secure base and safe haven such that these unprocessed emotions and motives can be worked through (Gilbert, 2023; Lee, 2022).

Responsibility implications

The focus on 'not your fault' is aimed at enabling people to stand back and undermine unhelpful shame but also to enable people to tolerate guilt if harm has been caused (Gilbert, 2019, 2022b). In fact, the undermining of shame brings people 'out of hiding and avoidance', and when they come out of hiding, they are much more able to develop the courage to address their key issues. It also facilitates genuine responsibility-taking. Helping people because one wants to avoid or compensate for shame is not the genuine motivation of compassion (Catarino *et al.*, 2014). We can note that it is not our fault if we inherit genes for lung cancer, but if we smoke, we will die. The therapist gently helps the client to recognize the difference between blaming and shaming versus taking responsibility. The key is to stimulate the motive to take responsibility, which is much more likely when people are not hiding in shame. To develop responsibility involves becoming 'mind aware' and beginning to work out what is likely to be helpful based on wisdom and courage. Later, we invite the client to reflect on what version or aspects of themselves they might have developed (and would have liked to have developed) had they not experienced trauma, and move to a discussion of what aspects and versions of themselves they might want to develop now.

Compassionate mind training

Helping the body support the mind

Many therapy approaches now outline how and why therapists can work directly on helping clients develop physiological systems that support emotion regulation and prosocial motivations to self and others (Cozolino,

2017; Petrocchi *et al.*, 2022; Porges, 2011, 2021; Rothschild 2000; Schore, 2019; van der Kolk, 2014). We call this *helping the body to support the mind*. Given the importance of the many psychophysiological adaptations from the evolution of attachment and caring, CFT's focus is on the physiological infrastructures of the care system, linked to a secure base and safe haven, which involves the vagus nerve along with other physiological and neuro-physiological processes.

Breathing

There is increasing evidence that vagal dysregulation underpins many types of mental and physical health difficulties (Petrocchi and Cheli, 2019; Pet-trochi *et al.*, 2022; Porges, 2011). A number of well-known breathing prac-tices have direct effects on the autonomic nervous system and frontal cortex (Gerritsen and Band, 2018) and cortisol (Ma *et al.*, 2017). These typically involve the slowing and deepening of the breath with a particular focus on the out-breath (Balban *et al.*, 2023; Steffen *et al.*, 2021). CFT calls this sooth-ing rhythm breathing – using the breath to help settle the body. It guides clients to lift their shoulders up and back and create an inward-bending curve-shaped spine that lifts the diaphragm. They are then guided through the *rate* of the breath (five seconds for the in-breath, five seconds for the out-breath, with two seconds at the top and the bottom of the breath, approximately four breaths per minute) and the *depth* of the breath (down into the diaphragm and imagining it going to the base of the spine). Next is the *smoothness* of the breath through the nostrils. This can take time for the client to do. Clients can begin to notice that slowing and deepening the breath can have a grounding impact and helps them feel more stable in the chair. Occasionally, it is useful to do a short hyperventilation to highlight the impact of the breath on the body and the differences between anxious breathing and soothing rhythm breathing as body grounding.

If focusing on the breath alone is difficult, trauma clients can also be guided to pay attention to their feet as 'flat on the floor' or to gently rub their hands together or to use tapping. These are offered as behavioural experi-ments and for clients to 'play with'. Clients can also be guided through the breathing practice while walking or bathing or eating, where the breathing is brought into mindfulness practices. As with other aspects of CFT, the therapist provides the information and then collaborates on how to explore the practice. There are many variations on this, such as breathing through the heart or breathing in compassion or breathing in a compassion colour.

When the basic rhythm is stabilized, the therapist can guide the client to explore different facial expressions (neutral versus friendly) and the impact they feel in the body. Crucial, too, is to explore different voice tones. Clients are invited to imagine saying 'hello' or 'how are you' to themselves on the out-breath in a neutral or disinterested tone, and then in a friendly and welcoming tone. Again, the key is to notice their effects. Clients are guided through how to make deliberate efforts to pay attention to the emotional tone of their thoughts, not just the content. Later, this can be practised in the therapy room where a client may generate two or three helpful ideas and then practise saying them to themselves using compassion breathing and voice tones.

Clients with trauma can sometimes find this approach difficult and anxiety provoking of trigger flashbacks as their breathing may have been withheld during trauma, or the sound of breathing may be associated with impending harm. It may need to be supported with a gradual desensitization and associated with movement, as in tai chi or qigong (Yeung *et al.*, 2018), or with holding something (Gilbert and Procter, 2006) to divert attention away from the physical sensations of the body while building the vagal-helpful breath patterns. Here it can be important to engage with processes that de-shame and reclaim the 'traumatized breath and body' for clients (Kozlowska *et al.*, 2015; Lee, 2022; van der Kolk, 2014). There is also increasing evidence for the value of exercise, yoga and diet impacting the vagal nerve (Breit *et al.*, 2018). Bornemann *et al.* (2016) show that biofeedback alone improves HRV, which increases altruistic behaviour.

Imagery

Imagery has been used in many therapies for guided discovery, exposure, imagery rescripting, planning, role rehearsal and motivation, and is regarded as more powerful than verbal change processes (Hackmann *et al.*, 2011). Imagery is also well known to be a powerful and precise physiological stimulator. For example, creating a sexual fantasy can be extremely powerful to support arousal. It will stimulate different physiological systems than imagining one's favourite meal, a holiday or having an argument. CFT invites clients to explore specific images and visualizations. Some clients say they are not good at imagery, and this can require clarity on how imagery works. The therapist can playfully ask: 'What is an elephant or what is a banana, and how are they different?' Helping clients recognize that imagery can often be fleeting and it is the feeling in the body that is important, can be useful guides to the process of imagery. Some individuals might struggle with imagery if they have a condition called aphantasia (Zeman *et al.*, 2016).

Safe place imagery

CFT invites clients to explore images and visualizations of safeness as a way of working with their body and mind. It is important to help clients distinguish between safety and safeness and how they interact. For example, one client imagined his safe place, but it was surrounded by barbed wire and machine guns. He was highly focused on keeping out harmful others. The therapist gently acknowledged how important this was but there had been a downside: he would be trapped behind his safety barriers. The image became a metaphor for how he lived his life: damage limitation, stopping the bad. Safeness is when we do not need to be (only) vigilant to threat and can direct our attention to other processes including openness and play.

Originally, safe place imagery in CFT was rooted in a sense of calming and grounding (Gilbert, 2009), but work with clients over the years has suggested that some prefer the idea of active play. One severely traumatized client advised Gilbert's group that her image of safeness was on her motorbike, driving with the wind in her hair, on an long, straight empty road in Colorado, heading for the mountains. Safeness for her was imagined as a combination of feeling empowered, free and exhilarated and just enjoying the activity mindfully. Subsequent discussions with group members and with subsequent groups have confirmed that playfulness is important to get a feel for safeness. Inviting clients to think about what they would like to do and how they would like to play if they felt safe can be crucial for them. Clients have mentioned flying, running up mountains or tree walking. Clients have offered fascinating insights into their unique experiences of safeness – associated with joyfulness or even exhilaration. Interestingly, too, safeness in imagery is commonly experienced with mindfulness in that the individual is 'lost' in the activity and is not actively thinking – a form of self-transcendence in a way.

Imagining the compassionate other

CFT suggests that because our minds are full of social mentalities that evolved for social interactions, imagining social interactions is the most powerful way of stimulating physiologies. For example, if we want to become sexually aroused, we imagine an interaction; if we are thinking about anger and assertiveness, we imagine an interaction; if we are thinking about how to impress the boss, we imagine an interaction. We will be physiologically impacted by the textures of those imagine interactions.

Compassion focused imagery involving *visualization of dialogues and interactions* with imaginary figures has been used for thousands of years. For example, in certain Buddhist traditions, one builds one's own compassion through imaginary interactions with images of the Buddha both receiving and giving compassion (Rinpoche and Mullen, 2005; Vessantara, 1993/2023). Imagining being loved and protected by a deity also has ancient origins in various spiritual traditions. CFT makes use of these basic ways of stimulating psychophysiological processes by inviting clients to think about two types of compassion imagery – compassionate other and compassionate self.

To fantasize an ideal compassionate other, clients are invited to consider how they might imagine an ideal friend, mentor, supporter, parent, protector or guru. The focus is on what they would *most want* the 'other' to be like; their basic emotional disposition, their voice tones, talents and feelings they emanate. Clients might want an empathic, confident, joyful, affectionate warm, playful 'other'. Lee (2005) referred to this as the 'perfect nurturer' – the client imagines another mind that is 'perfect for them' regardless of how unrealistic in real life. The process of exploring in depth what one would *really want* from a caring other and possible FBRs to it can be important for moving forward. The client is then guided to imagine relating to their fantasized other in relationship to different life issues (Gilbert, 2009; Gilbert and Choden, 2013). Rockliff *et al.* (2008) showed that visualizing a compassionate other impacted heart rate variability and reduced cortisol, although not in in people with high self-criticism and insecure attachment. The fantasized caring other can function like a secure base and safe haven. Using these ideas, Brown *et al.* (2020) explored the impact of developing and relating to a compassionate image for people with paranoid beliefs. They examined how using that fantasy would help with the anxiety of paranoia by using virtual reality to enter a lift and a tube train, while imagining being accompanied by their imagined compassionate coach. As for CFT, they indicate:

> ...the aim is to harness the experience of being nurtured and eventually internalise it, so that a new and distinctive memory is created that can be easily accessed. A compassionate coach can have any identity, but must embody all the qualities of compassion, including strength, warmth, wisdom and kindness, and should encourage the individual to be kind toward themself... (p.2).

Clients are invited to think about the qualities of courage and wisdom (for our tricky brain) their image embodies. Trauma clients will sometimes choose archetypal rather than human images, such as the lion Aslan from the *Chronicles of Narnia* novels. There is little research on this, but we suspect that it is partly to do with social trust and being let down, hurt and harmed by others.

Compassion imagery can be used for helping clients engage with trauma, although they can be frightened of experiencing flashbacks. This problem can be described as the caregiving motivation system holding trauma memories rather than compassion itself. Hence, therapists may need to work directly with these fragmented memories that act like conditioned emotional trauma responses, and replace them with compassion (i.e. vagal) responses (Lee, 2022, 2015, 2013, 2022; Lee and James, 2013). As noted above, Gilbert *et al.* (2006) found that self-critical individuals found it quite easy to imagine a critical other, but much harder to imagine a compassionate supportive other, whereas the opposite was found for people who had low levels of self-criticism. Naismith *et al.* (2018) demonstrated that people with personality disorders also struggled to develop compassionate imagery due to having few experiences of compassion, weak imagery and fear of compassion. If a person has not received much in the way of empathy or care, then it will take time for them to begin to work with it. Practising imagery, however, can gradually ease people into these experiences.

Imagery of the compassionate self

A second focus for comparison imagery is the self. Creative imagination of a version of oneself, and examining its impact on coping, has been explored in different ways. For example, Meevissen *et al.* (2010) demonstrated that imagining oneself at one's 'best possible self' and thinking about engaging in various life issues from that experience of 'that self', increased optimism. Osimo *et al.* (2015) created a virtual reality scenario where participants counselled themselves in a life difficulty as themselves or as Sigmund Freud. The Freud induction reduced depressed feelings significantly more than when they were being themselves. Similarly, practising positive-self imagery of recalling a time when one felt relaxed and positive improved self-esteem and reduced anxiety in response to anxiety-provoking vignettes (e.g. meeting your partner's parents for the first time; Stopa *et al.*, 2012). Falconer *et al.* (2014) developed a virtual reality scenario which enabled individuals to generate compassion in one virtual body and then experience themselves receiving it from their virtual body. This significantly reduced self-criticism in non-depressed (Falconer *et al.*, 2014) and depressed participants (Falconer *et al.*, 2016). Hence, imagining ourselves in certain roles, characters and states of being, and imagining how these 'self-constructions' would think and deal with various life events, can have many beneficial effects.

CFT invites clients to think about the nature of compassion, some of the key qualities they would identify as compassionate and would like to be able develop, and then how to practise them. These key qualities can be broken down such that people can focus on improving one aspect at a time, like mindful awareness, patience, grounding, friendliness, empathy and others. Inducing the compassionate self and mind state involves starting with the body, adopting the body posture, use of a facial expression and voice tones, breathing practices and grounding. The psychological focus is on the wisdom of understanding the tricky brain, and the identification of compassion as being a genuine desire to be helpful, not harmful (see the online video *Compassion for Voices*). Clients practise experimenting and experiencing these states which can be minimal to start with. When a certain degree of compassion awareness has developed, this can be utilized when engaging with trauma and trauma memory. When we switch into the compassionate mind state, bringing online important physiological processes and psychological competencies for a secure base and save haven, we bring our compassionate mind to process trauma (Lee, 2022).

Using the compassionate mind

Developing the competencies of a compassionate mind enables that mind (state) to be brought to many different therapeutic tasks. When clients have some sense of their abilities to switch mind states, through using bodywork, imagery, intention focusing and behavioural practice, the compassionate mind can be brought to different dimensions of function. For example, if one wants to help clients generate helpful coping thoughts, the therapist does a short compassionate mind induction based on breathing and motivation, intention and so on, and then asks the compassionate mind to generate helpful ways of thinking. The client is encouraged to rehearse them with compassionate emotion tones and the intention to be helpful. A variation of this can also be done with chair work where individuals first talk about a life difficulty in the emotion of the difficulty, and then spend time engaging with the compassionate mind and think about the difficulty from the compassionate mind perspective (Gilbert and Basran, 2018). Various forms of chair work enable people to take up certain emotions or positions and then explore interactions with the compassionate self (Bell *et al.*, 2020).

Compassionate letter writing and journalling can be helpful for some clients, who write letters to the traumatized self from the position of the compassionate self. Clients can be invited to do this in the therapy room (the therapist may leave the room for a few minutes to facilitate it) and then read the letter to the therapist. Then the therapist reads the letter back to the client. Sometimes letters are not so compassionate and therefore the therapist gradually guides the client to become more compassionate and more empathic. Letter writing can become a practice that improves over time. Occasionally, it is hearing their own letter, their words and ideas supporting them, through the voice of the therapist, that can be particularly powerful.

Client and therapist can create compassionate practices and dialogues that can be put on their mobile phone. All these uses of a compassionate self are tested against the client's own experience of helpfulness and the shared aims of the therapy. The therapist helps the client recognize that we have a mind that is full of multiple potentials and possibilities, some helpful, some not, through no fault of our own, *but* we can use our consciousness ability to mindfully observe what is coming in and out of our awareness and mind in non-judgemental ways and then bring our compassionate mind to these emergent experiences.

Differentiating multiplicities

One core process in CFT is to support guided discovery and working with emotions that have come out of trauma. This does not require exploring details of the trauma. The therapist explains the process of bringing compassion to our different reactions to life difficulties and that it is useful to differentiate various emotions regarding the same event. This approach supports collaboration. To help people distinguish different emotions regarding the trauma, the therapist can invite the client to explore separately: their anger about the trauma, their anxiety about the trauma, and their grief associated with the trauma. Other emotions and reactions are possible, but to begin, this is called 'the big three'. The exercise itself is called multiple selves or multiple states work (see Gilbert 2022e for a worked-through example). For each emotion, the client is guided to examine: the attentional focus and thoughts of the emotion, the motives behind the emotion, the body feelings of the emotion, the felt behavioural impulses, memories linked to the emotion, and how they cope and settle the emotion. When they have gone through all three basic emotions (anger, anxiety and sadness), they are then invited to reflect on the experience of differentiating these various emotional states. They are then asked to reflect on what each emotional state thinks of the other. So 'What does your angry self think about your anxious self? What does your anxious self think about your angry self?' and so on.

Clients can experience these different potential defences as in conflict. For example, the angry part of oneself may see the anxious part of oneself as weak and pathetic, whereas the anxious self sees the angry self as frightening and dangerous. Helping clients understand the inherent *potential conflict* between different emotions and why that is a problem can be revelatory for them. These kinds of emotional conflict can also be linked to dissociation because, as noted above, intense inner conflicts create disorganization of response systems.

The client is then invited to explore the compassionate mind approach to the trauma. First, they might be invited to stand up or walk around the room as a separation from engaging with the threat emotions. Then there is a short compassionate mind induction rooted in the breathing and grounding exercises and the compassionate focusing of intention (as above). The therapist next explores the same processes of the thoughts of the compassionate mind, the motives of the compassionate mind, the felt body sense of the compassionate mind, the behavioural impulses of the compassionate mind, and any memories of compassion and how we help compassion grow in relation to the trauma. The client is then invited to reflect on how different parts of ourselves can respond to trauma in different ways. This facilitates insight into multiple self-functioning and also helps clients begin to think about how we can have multiple emotions and reactions to the same issue. This process of differentiation can be a core theme for and ongoing discussion and reflection.

Next, the therapist invites the client to consider their compassionate mind in relation to the three defence emotions, bringing compassion to their anger, to their anxiety, to their sadness and grief. Bringing the compassionate mind to these threat emotions also enables clients to understand and tolerate them and work with them helpfully rather than impulsively or by being avoidant. The therapist may guide the compassionate mind to mentalize and empathize with these different defensive emotions. This way of working can be used in many different ways, for example by sitting in a new chair and becoming (say) the depressed self, or the numb, the shamed or the envious self, and then moving into a compassion chair and, again following a compassionate mind induction, where the compassionate mind can mentalize these brain states and seek to support them.

Compassion for others

In many of the Buddhist traditions, compassion training begins with focusing on bringing compassion to another. For example, Weng et al. (2018) offered instructions:

> For each person, they imagined a time when the person had suffered, brought non-judgmental and balanced attention to reactions to suffering, and then practiced wishing the person relief from suffering. They repeated compassion-generating phrases such as, 'May you be free from suffering. May you have joy and happiness.' They were also instructed to pay attention to bodily sensations (particularly around the heart) and to envision a golden light extending from their heart to the heart of the other person... (p.4)

The rapid movement from awareness of suffering into positive wishes to be free of suffering stimulates different physiological systems (Petrocchi et al., 2022). A number of such studies have shown that practising compassion from others can have major neurophysiological effects (Weng et al., 2013, 2018). In variations of this, clients can be invited to think of key qualities that someone else might need and imagine them getting them. What is important here is not that the person should get lost in the suffering of the other but that they feel energized for wanting to help. The approach to psychotherapy called mentalizing (Luyten et al., 2020) provides fundamental training in helping people to be more sensitive empathically aware and compassionate to others. In group therapy, one can help clients develop active listening and empathic reflection, and how to ask open questions – helping clients understand the mutuality of providing a secure base and safe haven for each other builds that sense of a compassionate self. Linking to these imagery and group tasks, the therapist can also add compassionate imagery to a sense of belonging; for example, imagining that one is part of a community of people trying to develop compassion. Indeed, the therapist may encourage clients to join mindfulness groups and practise common humanity imagery.

Compassionate behaviour

Poulin (2017) highlights that people can know a lot about compassion and even be motivated to be compassionate but do not actually translate it into action. This is not so common. Many of us know how to get fit and eat healthily, but do not always translate it into action. It helps to break down actions into achievable steps. For example, one can set up one's mobile to give friendly prompts for mindfulness and compassion or for practising one healthy behaviour each day (e.g. dietary, exercise). More specific behaviours are linked to processes of assertiveness, which involves skills training, or practising doing one enjoyable thing each day, or practising one body grounding and visualization each day (e.g. stepping into the compassionate self).

There are also many behavioural practices that are focused on being compassionate to others. These can include deliberately walking down the road with a gentle facial expression and awareness of others; taking an interest in people who help you, such as shop assistants or work colleagues; helping a charity or considering what help a friend might need; feeding the birds in winter. There are a variety of meditation practices related to sending compassion to others, which have been shown to have powerful physiological effects (Weng et al., 2018). Practices can be unique to each person, but the key is to help clients regularly prime themselves for compassion because this regularly stimulates the care-focused motivational system. Important for our trauma clients are behavioural practices and experiments that encourage engagement rather than avoidance, encourage empowerment in interpersonal interactions rather than powerlessness, and encourage interpersonal boundaries.

When clients are activated in their trauma in therapy, engaging their physiological systems with other activities can be important. One researched approach is eye movement desensitization and reprocessing (EMDR). CFT has explored ways of integrating CFT and EMDR (Kennedy, 2014; Shapiro, 2001; Whalley and Lee, 2019). In addition, sometimes while discussing trauma that may be overwhelming, clients can be invited to engage in 'pulling ropes' as in playful 'tug of war' with the therapist, or running while talking about trauma, facilitating clients being able to stay within their window of tolerance (Bohus et al., 2020; Kleindienst et al., 2021; Kozlowska et al., 2015). It is known that people with psychosis can sometimes find it easier to talk if they are walking in a park or driving or doing the washing up so they do not have to look at the therapist. After discussing issues about the ways in which trauma can easily overwhelm us, Gilbert (2009) has invited clients to suck on an orange or even a lemon as an experiment, asking clients to find their own pathways of helpfulness. All these processes involve activating sensory and action systems that utilize information-processing space, enabling them and attenuating engagement with trauma memory. The more one can help clients become an observer of the round journey, and experiment with things that can be quite creative from them, the more control they feel.

Working with trauma stories to develop an integrated compassionate narrative

The development of compassionate capacities and competencies helps clients access beneficial emotional contexts to their traumatic experiences. For instance, CFT uses compassionate imagery rescripts to fulfil unmet emotional needs in flashbacks and memories. Imagery helps provide a multisensory update to flashbacks and nightmares (Lee, 2013; Lee and James, 2013). In addition, CFT might rescript a flashback, to update a felt sense of 'being overpowered' to a felt sense of 'embodied empowerment'. CFT uses various types of imagery in trauma:

- Safe place imagery (secure base and safe haven).
- Safe base imagery (perfect nurturer or internalized caring or loving other.
- Connectedness imagery (compassionate friends and flow).

All are important and serve different functions depending on the unmet emotional need. For instance, if we are working with flashbacks where clients felt unsafe, we might use safe place imagery to promote an inner sense of safeness. If working on memories of abandonment, we might use safe base imagery such as perfect nurturer to promote caring/being cared for feelings. If we are working with trauma memories where clients felt alone, or in need of courage and support, we might use connectedness imagery, common humanity imagery, or group member imagery (if our clients attend a group). These techniques are worked out in collaboration with the client with a clear understanding about what and why they are being explored (for an extensive discussion, see Lee, 2005, 2013; Lee and James, 2013).

In general, the compassion-focused processes for healing and integrating fragmented decontextualized trauma memories help clients create a compassionate (i.e. motivated to be helpful, supportive and engaged) account of their life story. This is essentially a mapping out of trauma experiences, contextualizing by updating the meaning of trauma experiences from shame/self-blame to compassionate insight and care for well-being. This goes with developing a coherent autobiographical account of their experiences. There are different ways to approach the framework of narrative (e.g. Pennebaker, 1997; Schauer et al., 2012). It can be helpful to develop a full account of the client's trauma story, narrated through the lens of their compassionate mind, with attention paid to contextualizing flashbacks and nightmares using emotional memory techniques such as compassionate rescripts, flashback updates and EMDR interweaves (see Lee, 2022, for a fuller account of these methods).

Conclusion

Section 1 explored the basic psychological functions model that underpins compassion and how these functions are all affected by trauma. Section 2 described the evolution of compassion and its underlying psychophysiological mechanisms. In Section 3, we examined compassion in relationship to the psychological functions of a secure base and safe haven. In Section 4, we considered how trauma significantly disrupts the ability to use care-focused systems for emotional regulation and social relating. Stimulating care-based psychophysiological processes and the functions of a secure base and safe haven are a key focus in the therapy (Gilbert and Simos, 2022). This section also mapped out aspects of CFT as a therapy and mind-training process. However, we always stress that this is compassion *focused* therapy, not compassion therapy, because it integrates many other therapeutic evidence-based interventions, such as a range of cognitive interventions, behavioural and emotional practices, exposure work, visualizations (imagery) and chair work as examples.

There are a variety of different types of childhood trauma that have major impacts on the psychophysiological maturation of the child. One form of trauma focuses on direct threat from physical injury through to shaming. Another focuses on the absence of caring, including many key stimulators of positive emotion, social trust, affection, warmth, confidence and encouragement (see Figure 7.1).

These traumas also compromise the ability to develop an internalized secure base, one that supports empathic and validating understanding of the self, and the courage and wisdom to engage in addressing the challenges of life and to create this sense of joyfulness and meaning. When infants and children do not receive inputs that are soothing, and emotionally and physiologically regulating (as in a safe haven), they will be unable to access their psychophysiological processes for self-soothing, reassuring, encouraging and self-regulating. While many therapies focus on the importance of safety for working with trauma, safety has to be more than the absence of threat and instead be the provision of inputs that stimulate secure base and safe haven functions, that is, safeness. CFT has always been rooted in the evolution of caring behaviour (Gilbert, 1989) and attachment processes (Gilbert, 1993, 2013, 2022c).

Similar to attachment approaches, CFT suggests that working with trauma can be advanced when therapists create a secure base and safe haven within the therapeutic relationship, help the client internalize this, and also provide a set of compassion-focused practices that are specifically designed to stimulate the psychophysiological infrastructures of a secure basis and safe haven. CFT helps individuals reorganize threat processing and be more able to feel safe in their relationships and environments, and thereby more emotionally regulated. Overall, then, CFT seeks to address all three basic motivational tasks: dealing with threat, seeking out resources and rewards, including social ones, and having the ability to feel safe and connected to one's physical and social environment.

Clients also work through their emotional patterns, becoming more tolerant of threat ones and more capable of activating positively rewarding ones. Along the way, clients learn how to use their new brain cognitive competencies for reasoning, for mentalizing and metacognition, in ways that are helpful rather than unhelpful to them. Last but not least, clients practise helpful behaviours and skills – again all grounded in generating a compassionate orientation. CFT does not concentrate on concepts such as 'good or bad' but rather on what is helpful and what is harmful, and on understanding how and why these are the case. CFT seeks to recruit compassion-grounded motivational systems and their psychophysiological processes that enable people to find the courage and wisdom to heal trauma and move forward with compassion for self and others.

KNOWLEDGE AND PRACTICE REFLECTION

Joe Tucci, Janise Mitchell, Ed Tronick and Stephen W. Porges

The significance of compassion for the trauma field is exemplified by this richly comprehensive chapter by Gilbert, Lee and Matos. The study of compassion and the development of compassion focused therapy (CFT) expands our knowledge frame into a range of different areas. The depth of the chapter speaks for itself in relation to its relevance to trauma-transformative practice.

Like Porges and Carter, compassion delves into the evolutionary nature of caregiving to explore how relationships in our history functioned to organize positive outcomes for individuals and communities as a whole. Gilbert, Lee and Matos identify the importance of three evolutionary pathways to the development of compassionate thinking and behaviour: rescuing and caring for the sick and elderly, care of infants and children, and the collective practices of living in small groups. In each, the core of compassion lies in achieving 'social good' – benefits that support and resource the individual as well as the community.

Acts of compassion respond to the ruptures in social bonds that could have the effects of ostracizing the individual and/or leaving the community worse off. By engaging in compassionate thinking and behaviour, the effects of trauma are reduced. Violent behaviour has the potential to be modified through accountability and understanding. Compassion is transformative by its nature. It links us all to our evolutionary roots, deepening the ways in which our motives connect to our internal states and our interdependencies in relationships.

CFT recognizes that the worldviews propagated by violence and trauma leave individuals with experiences of shame and self-criticism which spiral into cycles of self-blame and self-hatred. CFT cultivates compassion, kindness and self-care as antidotes to the toxic residue of trauma and violation.

In the past 20 years, knowledge about compassion has proliferated. In the time since Harris and Fallot's first paper on trauma-informed practice, the study of compassion has offered unique perspectives on healing and recovery. Even more importantly, it has offered a framework that accompanies other forms of discursive practice, such as decolonizing and anti-oppressive approaches to responding to pain and suffering. It is arguable that if more had been available about compassion at the start of the trauma-informed paradigm, it may well have been included as a core element of the construct.

For example, scaffolding compassionate behaviour, through visualization, rehearsal and reinforcement (as described by Gilbert, Lee and Matos) provides organizations and systems with innovative ways to build the inclusion of service users who have already received support from an agency into the options that provide positive peer interactions focused on engaging in acts of compassion in small groups and over time. This strategy can also support the training of organizational staff to become more mindful of their approach with service users by guiding them through regular visualizations of interactions with a compassionate figure, such as a wise and nurturing mentor or an animal that symbolizes warmth and kindness. These daily practices are designed to evoke positive emotions and help individuals cultivate a sense of warmth, self-compassion and most critically, compassion for others.

Trauma-transformative practice offers the opportunity to revisit the nature of relationships between service users and practitioners, organizations and systems and include the construct of compassion in them. By so doing, it allows for a more complex frame of reference to be built in. The study of compassion offers different metaphors, language and practice resources that pulls it towards more complex thinking and further away from simple reductionist strategies.

It also introduces a less clinical frame of reference that acknowledges that tenderness and understanding are important qualities of organizational culture to nurture. In the context of human service organizations being asked to do more and more with less and less, compassion feeds and nourishes organizational values in ways that appreciate the communal effort that is often required to provide help and support. Staff and service users benefit when their personal goals and intentions that have a collective good are encouraged and privileged.

References
References for chapter

Abbas, A. (2015). *Reaching Through Resistance – Advanced Psychotherapy Techniques*. Sacramento, CA: Seven Leaves Press.

Alix, S., Cossette, L., Cyr, M., Frappier, J.Y., Caron, P.O. and Hébert, M. (2020). Self-blame, shame, avoidance, and suicidal ideation in sexually abused adolescent girls: A longitudinal study. *Journal of Child Sexual Abuse*, 29(4), 432–447.

Armstrong III, B.F., Nitschke, J.P., Bilash, U. and Zuroff, D.C. (2021). An affect in its own right: Investigating the relationship of social safeness with positive and negative affect. *Personality and Individual Differences*, 168, Article 109670. https://doi.org/10.1016/j.paid.2019.109670.

Ashfield, E., Chan, C. and Lee, D. (2021). Building 'a compassionate armour': The journey to develop strength and self-compassion in a group treatment for complex post-traumatic stress disorder. *Psychology and Psychotherapy: Theory, Research and Practice*, 94, 286–303.

Au, T.M., Sauer-Zavala, S., King, M.W., Petrocchi, N., Barlow, D.H. and Litz, B.T. (2017). Compassion-based therapy for trauma-related shame and posttraumatic stress: Initial evaluation using a multiple baseline design. *Behaviour Therapy*, 48(2), 207–221.

Austin, J.H. (2009). *Selfless Insight. Zen and the Meditative Transformation of Consciousness*. Boston, MA: MIT Press.

Bailey, K.G. and Wood, H.E. (1998). Evolutionary kinship therapy: Basic principles and treatment implications. *British Journal of Medical Psychology*, 71(4), 509–523.

Balban, M.Y., Neri, E., Kogon, M.M., Weed, L. *et al.* (2023). Brief structured respiration practices enhance mood and reduce physiological arousal. *Cell Reports Medicine*, 4(1), 100895.

Bargh, J. (2017). *Before You Know It: The Unconscious Reasons We Do What We Do*. New York, NY: Simon and Schuster.

Barkus, E. and Badcock, J.C. (2019). A transdiagnostic perspective on social anhedonia. *Frontiers in Psychiatry*, 10, 216.

Basran, J., Pires, C., Matos, M., McEwan, K. and Gilbert, P. (2019). Styles of leadership, fears of compassion, and competing to avoid inferiority. *Frontiers in Psychology*, 9, 2460.

Beck, A.T., Emery, G. and Greenberg, R.L. (1985). *Anxiety Disorders and Phobias: A Cognitive Approach*. New York, NY: Basic Books.

Bell, T., Montague, J., Elander, J. and Gilbert, P. (2020). 'Suddenly you are King Solomon': Multiplicity, transformation and integration in compassion focused therapy chair work. *Journal of Psychotherapy Integration*, 31(3), 223–237.

Bisby, M.A., Kimonis, E.R. and Goulter, N. (2017). Low maternal warmth mediates the relationship between emotional neglect and callous-unemotional traits among male juvenile offenders. *Journal of Child and Family Studies*, 26, 1790–1798.

Boehm, C. (1999). *Hierarchy in the Forest: The Evolution of Egalitarian Behaviour*. Boston, MA: Harvard University Press.

Bohus, M., Kleindienst, N., Hahn, C., Müller-Engelmann, M. *et al.* (2020). Dialectical behaviour therapy for posttraumatic stress disorder (DBT-PTSD) compared with cognitive processing therapy (CPT) in complex presentations of PTSD in women survivors of childhood abuse: A randomised clinical trial. *JAMA Psychiatry*, 77(12), 1235–1245.

Bornemann, B., Kok, B.E., Böckler, A. and Singer, T. (2016). Helping from the heart: Voluntary upregulation of heart rate variability predicts altruistic behaviour. *Biological Psychiatry*, 119, 54–63.

Bowlby, J. (1969). *Attachment and Loss, Vol. 1: Attachment*. New York, NY: Basic Books.

Bowlby, J. (1973). *Attachment and Loss, Vol. 2: Separation: Anxiety and Anger*. London: Hogarth Press.

Bowlby, J. (1980). *Attachment and Loss, Vol. 3: Loss: Sadness and Depression*. London: Hogarth Press.

Breit, S., Kupferberg, A., Rogler, G. and Hasler, G. (2018). Vagus nerve as modulator of the brain–gut axis in psychiatric and inflammatory disorders. *Frontiers in Psychiatry*, 9, 44.

Brewin, C.R., Dalgleish, T. and Joseph, S. (1996). A dual representation theory of posttraumatic stress disorder. *Psychological Review*, 103(4), 670–686.

Brewin, C.R., Gregory, J.D., Lipton, M. and Burgess, N. (2010) Intrusive images in psychological disorders: Characteristics, neural mechanisms, and treatment implications. *Psychological Review*, 117(1), 210–232.

Brown, P., Waite, F., Rovira, A., Nickless, A. and Freeman, D. (2020). Virtual reality clinical-experimental tests of compassion treatment techniques to reduce paranoia. *Scientific Reports*, 10(1), 1–9.

Brown, S.L. and Brown, R.M. (2015). Connecting prosocial behaviour to improved physical health: Contributions from the neurobiology of parenting. *Neuroscience and Biobehavioural Reviews*, 55, 1–17.

Buss, D.M. (2019). *Evolutionary Psychology: The New Science of the Mind* (sixth edition). New York, NY: Routledge.

Byrne, R.W. (2016). *Evolving Insight: How It Is We Can Think about Why Things Happen*. Oxford: Oxford University Press.

Carter, S., Bartal, I.B. and Porges, E. (2017). The Roots of Compassion: An Evolutionary and Neurobiological Perspective. In E.M. Seppälä, E. Simon-Thomas, S.L. Brown, M.C. Worline, C.D. Cameron and J.R. Doty (eds), *The Oxford Handbook of Compassion Science* (pp.178–188). Oxford: Oxford University Press.

Cassidy, J. and Shaver, P.R. (2016). *Handbook of Attachment: Theory, Research and Clinical Applications* (third edition). New York, NY: Guilford Press.

Cassiers, L.L., Sabbe, B.G., Schmaal, L., Veltman, D.J., Penninx, B.W. and Van Den Eede, F. (2018). Structural and functional brain abnormalities associated with exposure to different childhood trauma subtypes: a systematic review of neuroimaging findings. *Frontiers in Psychiatry*, 9, 329.

Catarino, F., Gilbert, P., McEwan., K. and Baião, R. (2014). Compassion motivations: Distinguishing submissive compassion from genuine compassion and its association with shame, submissive behaviour, depression, anxiety and stress. *Journal of Social and Clinical Psychology*, 33, 399–412.

Chaudhary, N. and Salali, G.D. (2022). Hunter Gatherers, Mismatch and Mental Disorder. In R. Abed and P. St John-Smith (eds), *Evolutionary Psychiatry: Current Perspectives on Evolution and Mental Health* (pp.64–83). Cambridge: Cambridge University Press.

Cohen, J.A. and Mannarino, A.P. (2015). Trauma-focused cognitive behaviour therapy for traumatised children and families. *Child and Adolescent Psychiatric Clinics*, 24(3), 557–570.

Cowan, C.S.M., Callaghan, B.L., Kan, J.M. and Richardson, R. (2016). The lasting impact of early-life adversity on individuals and their descendants: Potential mechanisms and hope for intervention. *Genes, Brain and Behaviour*, 15(1), 155–168.

Cowles, M., Randle-Phillips, C. and Medley, A. (2020). Compassion-focused therapy for trauma in people with intellectual disabilities: A conceptual review. *Journal of Intellectual Disabilities*, 24(2), 212–232.

Cozolino, L. (2014). *The Neuroscience of Human Relationships: Attachment and the Developing Social Brain* (second edition). (*Norton Series on Interpersonal Neurobiology*). New York, NY: W.W. Norton.

Cozolino, L. (2017). *The Neuroscience of Psychotherapy: Healing the Social Brain* (second edition). (*Norton Series on Interpersonal Neurobiology*). New York, NY: W.W. Norton.

Craske, M.G., Meuret, A.E., Ritz, T., Treanor, M., Dour, H. and Rosenfield, D. (2019). Positive affect treatment for depression and anxiety: A randomised clinical trial for a core feature of anhedonia. *Journal of Consulting and Clinical Psychology*, 87(5), 457–471.

Dalai Lama. (1995). *The Power of Compassion*. New York, NY: Harper Collins.

Davey, G.C. (2018). *Psychology*. Hoboken, NY: John Wiley and Sons.

Depue, R.A. and Morrone-Strupinsky, J.V. (2005). A neurobehavioural model of affiliative bonding. *Behavioural and Brain Sciences*, 28, 313–395.

Di Bello, M., Carnevali, L., Petrocchi, N., Thayer, J.F., Gilbert, P. and Ottaviani, C. (2020). The compassionate vagus: A meta-analysis on the connection between compassion and heart rate variability. *Neuroscience and Biobehavioural Reviews*, 116, 21–30.

Di Bello, M., Ottaviani, C. and Petrocchi, N. (2021). Compassion is not a benzo: Distinctive associations of heart rate variability with its empathic and action components. *Frontiers in Neuroscience*, 15, 223.

Didonna, F. (2009). *Clinical Handbook of Mindfulness* (Vol.18, pp.5–18). New York, NY: Springer.

Ditzen, B. and Heinrichs, M. (2014). Psychobiology of social support: The social dimension of stress buffering. *Restorative Neurology and Neuroscience*, 32(1), 149–162.

Dixon, A.K. (1998). Ethological strategies for defence in animals and humans: Their role in some psychiatric disorders. *British Journal of Medical Psychology*, 71, 417–445.

Duarte, J. and Pinto-Gouveia, J. (2017). Positive affect and parasympathetic activity: Evidence for a quadratic relationship between feeling safe and content and heart rate variability. *Psychiatry Research*, 257, 284–289.

Dunbar, R.I. (2014). *Human Evolution: A Pelican Introduction*. London: Penguin.

Dunkley, B.T., Wong, S.M., Jetly, R., Wong, J.K. and Taylor, M.J. (2018). Post-traumatic stress disorder and chronic hyperconnectivity in emotional processing. *NeuroImage: Clinical*, 20, 197–204.

Ebert, A., Edel, M.A., Gilbert, P. and Brüne, M. (2018). Endogenous oxytocin is associated with the experience of compassion and recalled upbringing in borderline personality disorder. *Depression and Anxiety*, 35(1), 50–57.

Epstein, S. (1994). Integration of the cognitive and the psychodynamic unconscious. *American Psychologist*, 49, 709–724.

Epstein, S. (2003). Cognitive-Experiential Self-Theory of Personality. In T. Million and M.J. Lerner (eds), *Comprehensive Handbook of Psychology* (Vol. 5, pp.159–184). New York, NY: Wiley.

Evans, C.B. and Burton, D.L. (2013). Five types of child maltreatment and subsequent delinquency: Physical neglect as the most significant predictor. *Journal of Child and Adolescent Trauma*, 6(4), 231–245.

Falconer, C.J., Rovira, A., King, J.A., Gilbert, P. *et al.* (2016). Embodying self-compassion within virtual reality and its effects on patients with depression. *British Journal of Psychiatry Open*, 2(1), 74–80.

Falconer, C.J., Slater, M., Rovira, A., King, J.A. *et al.* (2014). Embodying compassion: A virtual reality paradigm for overcoming excessive self-criticism. *PLoS ONE*, 9(11), e111933.

Fan, J., Liu, W., Xia, J., Li, S. *et al.* (2021). Childhood trauma is associated with elevated anhedonia and altered core reward circuitry in major depression patients and controls. *Human Brain Mapping*, 42(2), 286–297.

Forster, K. and Kanske, P. (2021). Exploiting the plasticity of compassion to improve psychotherapy. *Current Opinion in Behavioural Sciences*, 39, 64–71.

Frewen, P.A. and Lanius, R.A. (2006). Toward a psychobiology of posttraumatic self-dysregulation: Reexperiencing, hyperarousal, dissociation, and emotional numbing. *Annals of the New York Academy of Sciences*, 1071(1), 110–124.

Germer, C.K., Siegel, R.D. and Fulton, P.R. (2005). *Mindfulness and Psychotherapy*. New York, NY: Guilford Press.

Gerritsen, R.J. and Band, G.P. (2018). Breath of life: The respiratory vagal stimulation model of contemplative activity. *Frontiers in Human Neuroscience*, 397.

Gilbert, P. (1984). *Depression: From Psychology to Brain State*. Hilldale, NJ: Lawrence Erlbaum.

Gilbert, P. (1989). *Human Nature and Suffering*. Hilldale, NJ: Lawrence Erlbaum.

Gilbert, P. (1992). *Depression the Evolution of Powerlessness*. London: Psychology Press.

Gilbert, P. (1993). Defence and safety: Their function in social behaviour and psychopathology. *British Journal of Clinical Psychology*, 32, 131–153.

Gilbert, P. (2000a). Social Mentalities: Internal 'Social' Conflicts and the Role of Inner Warmth and Compassion in Cognitive Therapy. In P. Gilbert and K.G. Bailey (eds), *Genes on the Couch: Explorations in Evolutionary Psychotherapy* (pp.118–150). London: Psychology Press.

Gilbert, P. (2000b). Varieties of Submissive Behaviour: Their Evolution and Role in Depression. In L. Sloman and P. Gilbert (eds), *Subordination and Defeat. An Evolutionary Approach to Mood Disorders* (pp. 3–46). Hilldale, NJ: Lawrence Erlbaum.

Gilbert, P. (2003). Evolution, social roles and the differences in shame and guilt. *Social Research*, 70, 1205–1230.

Gilbert, P. (2005). Social Mentalities: A Biopsychosocial and Evolutionary Reflection on Social Relationships. In M. Baldwin (ed.), *Interpersonal Cognition* (pp.299–333). New York, NY: Guilford Press.

Gilbert, P. (2007). The Evolution of Shame as a Marker for Relationship Security. In J.L. Tracy, R.W. Robins, and J.P. Tangney (eds), *The Self-Conscious Emotions: Theory and Research* (pp.283–309). New York, NY: Guilford Press.

Gilbert, P. (2009). *The Compassionate Mind: A New Approach to the Challenge of Life*. Chicago, IL: Constable and Robinson.

Gilbert, P. (2010). *Compassion Focused Therapy: The CBT Distinctive Features Series*. New York, NY: Routledge.

Gilbert, P. (2013). Attachment Theory and Compassion Focused Therapy for Depression. In A.N. Danquah and K. Berry (eds), *Attachment Theory in Adult Mental Health: A Guide to Clinical Practice* (pp.35–47). New York, NY: Routledge.

Gilbert, P. (2014). The origins and nature of compassion focused therapy. *British Journal of Clinical Psychology*, 53, 6–41.

Gilbert, P. (2015). A Biopsychosocial and Evolutionary Approach to Formulation. In N. Tarrier (ed.), *Case Formulation in Cognitive Behaviour Therapy: The Treatment of Challenging Cases* (second edition) (pp.50–89). New York, NY: Wiley

Gilbert, P. (2017). Compassion as a Social Mentality: An Evolutionary Approach. In P. Gilbert (ed.), *Compassion: Concepts, Research and Applications* (pp.31–68). New York, NY: Routledge.

Gilbert, P. (2019). Distinguishing Shame, Humiliation and Guilt: An Evolutionary Functional Analysis and Compassion Focused Interventions. In C.-H. Mayer and E. Vanderheiden (eds), *The Bright Side of Shame* (pp.413–432). New York, NY: Springer.

Gilbert, P. (2020a). Compassion: From its evolution to a psychotherapy. *Frontiers in Psychology*, 11, 3123.

Gilbert, P. (2020b). Evolutionary Functional Analysis: The Study of Social Mentalities, Social Rank and Caring-Compassion. In J.N. Kirby and P. Gilbert (eds), *Making an Impact on Mental Health* (pp.4–42). New York, NY: Routledge.

Gilbert, P. (2021). Creating a compassionate world: Addressing the conflicts between sharing and caring versus controlling and holding evolved strategies. *Frontiers in Psychology*, 11, 3572.

Gilbert, P. (2022a). Compassion Focused Therapy as an Evolution Informed, Biopsychosocial Science of the Mind: History and Challenge. In P. Gilbert and G. Simos (eds), *Compassion Focused Therapy: Clinical Practice and Applications* (pp.24–89). New York, NY: Routledge.

Gilbert, P. (2022b). Shame, Social Status and the Pain of Social Disconnection. In P. Gilbert and G. Simos (eds), *Compassion Focused Therapy: Clinical Practice and Applications* (pp.122–163). New York, NY: Routledge.

Gilbert, P. (2022c). Internal Shame and Self-Disconnection: From Hostile Self-Criticism to Compassionate Self-Correction and Guidance. In P. Gilbert and G. Simos (eds), *Compassion Focused Therapy: Clinical Practice and Applications* (pp.164–206). New York, NY: Routledge.

Gilbert, P. (2022d). The Evolved Functions of Caring Connections as a Basis for Compassion. In P. Gilbert and G. Simos (eds), *Compassion Focused Therapy: Clinical Practice and Applications* (pp.90–121). New York, NY: Routledge.

Gilbert, P. (2022e). Meeting the Challenges of a Multi Mind and the Role of Grieving. In P. Gilbert and G. Simos (eds), *Compassion Focused Therapy: Clinical Practice and Applications* (pp.313–344). New York, NY: Routledge.

Gilbert, P. (2023). An Evolutionary and Compassion Approach to Yearning and Grief for What One Did Not Have. In D.L. Harris and A.H.Y. Ho (eds), *Compassion-Based Approaches to Loss and Grief* (pp.18–27). New York, NY: Routledge.

Gilbert, P. and Allan, S. (1998). The role of defeat and entrapment (arrested flight) in depression: An exploration of an evolutionary view. *Psychological Medicine*, 28, 584–597.

Gilbert, P., Baldwin, M., Irons, C., Baccus, J. and Palmer, M. (2006). Self-criticism and self-warmth: An imagery study exploring their relation to depression. *Journal of Cognitive Psychotherapy: An International Quarterly*, 20, 183–200.

Gilbert, P., Allan, S., Brough, S., Melley, S. and Miles J.N.V. (2002). Anhedonia and positive affect: Relationship to social rank, defeat and entrapment. *Journal of Affective Disorders*, 71, 141–151.

Gilbert, P. and Basran, J. (2018). Imagining one's compassionate self and coping with life difficulties. *EC Psychology and Psychiatry*, 7(12), 971–978.

Gilbert, P., Catarino, F., Duarte, C., Matos, M. *et al.* (2017). The development of compassionate engagement and action scales for self and others. *Journal of Compassionate Health Care*, 4(1), 1–24.

Gilbert, P. and Choden (2013). *Mindful Compassion*. Chicago, IL: Constable Robinson.

Gilbert, P., Clarke, M., Hempel, S., Miles, J.N.V. and Irons, C. (2004). Criticising and reassuring oneself: An exploration of forms, styles and reasons in female students. *British Journal of Clinical Psychology*, 43(1), 31–50.

Gilbert, P., McEwan, K., Catarino, F., Baião, R. and Palmeira, L. (2014). Fears of happiness and compassion in relationship with depression, alexithymia, and attachment security in a depressed sample. *British Journal of Clinical Psychology*, 53(2), 228–244.

Gilbert, P., McEwan, K., Matos, M. and Rivis, A. (2011). Fears of compassion: Development of three self-report measures. *Psychology and Psychotherapy*, 84, 239–255.

Gilbert, P. and Procter, S. (2006). Compassionate mind training for people with high shame and self-criticism: Overview and pilot study of a group therapy approach. *Clinical Psychology and Psychotherapy*, 13(6), 353–379.

Gilbert, P. and Simos, G. (eds.) (2022). *Compassion Focused Therapy: Clinical Practice and Applications*. New York, NY: Routledge.

Gillath, O. and Karantzas, G. (2019). Attachment security priming: A systematic review. *Current Opinion in Psychology*, 25, 86–95.

Goetz, J.L., Keltner, D. and Simon-Thomas, E. (2010). Compassion: An evolutionary analysis and empirical review. *Psychological Bulletin*, 136(3), 351–374.

Goodyear-Brown, P. (2019). *Trauma and Play Therapy: Helping Children Heal*. New York, NY: Routledge.

Hackmann, A., Bennett-Levy, J. and Holmes, E.A. (2011). *Oxford Guide to Imagery in Cognitive Therapy*. Oxford: Oxford University Press.

Haidt, J. (2001). The emotional dog and its rational tail: A social intuitionist approach to moral judgment. *Psychological Review*, 108, 814–834.

Harmen, R., Lee, D.A. and Barker, C. (2009). The role of self-attack and self-soothing in the maintenance of shame-based PTSD. *Clinical Psychology and Psychotherapy*, 17(1), 13–24.

Hayes, S.C., Strosahl, K.D. and Wilson, K.G. (2011). *Acceptance and Commitment Therapy: The Process and Practice of Mindful Change*. New York, NY: Guilford Press.

Hofer, M.A. (1984). Relationships as regulators: A psychobiologic perspective on bereavement. *Psychosomatic Medicine*, 46, 183–197.

Hofmann, S.G., Asmundson, G.J. and Beck, A.T. (2013). The science of cognitive therapy. *Behaviour Therapy*, 44(2), 199–212.

Holmes, J. and Slade, A. (2017). *Attachment in Therapeutic Practice*. London: Sage.

Hostinar, C.E. and Gunnar, M.R. (2015). Social support can buffer against stress and shape brain activity. *AJOB Neuroscience*, 6(3), 34–42.

Hrdy, S.B. (2009). *Mothers and Others: The Evolutionary Origins of Mutual Understanding*. Boston, MA: Harvard University Press.

Huang, J.Y. and Bargh, J.A. (2014). The selfish goal: Autonomously operating motivational structures as the proximate cause of human judgment and behaviour. *Behavioural and Brain Sciences*, 37, 121–175.

Iyengar, U., Kim, S., Martinez, S., Fonagy, P. and Strathearn, L. (2014). Unresolved trauma in mothers: Intergenerational effects and the role of reorganization. *Frontiers in Psychology*, 5, 966.

Kalaf, J., Coutinho, E.S.F., Vilete, L.M.P., Luz, M.P. *et al.* (2017). Sexual trauma is more strongly associated with tonic immobility than other types of trauma – A population based study. *Journal of Affective Disorders*, 215, 71–76.

Kavanaugh, B.C., Dupont-Frechette, J.A., Jerskey, B.A. and Holler, K.A. (2017). Neurocognitive deficits in children and adolescents following maltreatment: Neurodevelopmental consequences and neuropsychological implications of traumatic stress. *Applied Neuropsychology: Child*, 6(1), 64–78.

Kelly, A.C., Zuroff, D.C., Leybman, M.J. and Gilbert, P. (2012). Social safeness, received social support, and maladjustment: Testing a tripartite model of affect regulation. *Cognitive Therapy and Research*, 36, 815–826.

Keltner, D., Kogan, A., Piff, P.K. and Saturn, S.R. (2014). The sociocultural appraisals, values, and emotions (SAVE) framework of prosociality: Core processes from gene to meme. *The Annual Review of Psychology*, 65, 425–460.

Keltner, D., Oatley, K. and Jenkins, J.M. (2018). *Understanding Emotions*. New York, NY: Wiley Global Education.

Kennedy, A. (2014). Compassion-focused EMDR. *Journal of EMDR Practice and Research*, 8(3), 135–146.

Kessler, S.E. (2020). Why care: Complex evolutionary history of human healthcare networks. *Frontiers in Psychology*, 11, 199.

Kim, J.J., Parker, S.L., Doty, J.R., Cunnington, R., Gilbert, P. and Kirby, J.N. (2020). Neurophysiological and behavioural markers of compassion. *Scientific Reports*, 10(1), 1–9.

Kirby, J.N., Grzazek, O. and Gilbert, P. (2019). The role of compassionate and self-image goals in predicting psychological controlling and facilitative parenting styles. *Frontiers in Psychology*, 10, 1041.

Kirschner, H., Kuyken, W., Wright, K., Roberts, H., Brejcha, C. and Karl, A. (2019). Soothing your heart and feeling connected: A new experimental paradigm to study the benefits of self-compassion. *Clinical Psychological Science*, 7(3), 545–565.

Kleindienst, N., Steil, R., Priebe, K., Müller-Engelmann, M. *et al.* (2021). Treating adults with a dual diagnosis of borderline personality disorder and posttraumatic stress disorder related to childhood abuse: Results from a randomised clinical trial. *Journal of Consulting and Clinical Psychology*, 89(11), 925.

Kovler, M.L., Ziegfeld, S., Ryan, L.M., Goldstein, M.A. *et al.* (2021). Increased proportion of physical child abuse injuries at a level 1 pediatric trauma center during the Covid-19 pandemic. *Child Abuse and Neglect*, 116, 104756.

Kozlowska, K., Walker, P., McLean, L. and Carrive, P. (2015). Fear and the defense cascade: Clinical implications and management. *Harvard Review of Psychiatry*, 23(4), 263–287.

Kucerova, B., Levit-Binnun, N., Gordon, I. and Golland, Y. (2023). From oxytocin to compassion: The saliency of distress. *Biology*, 12(2), 183.

Lawrence, V. and Lee, D.A. (2014). Exploration of people's experiences of compassion-focused therapy for trauma, using interpretative phenomenological analysis. *Clinical Psychology and Psychotherapy*, 21(6), 495–507.

LeDoux, J.E. (2022). As soon as there was life, there was danger: The deep history of survival behaviours and the shallower history of consciousness. *Philosophical Transactions of the Royal Society B*, 377(1844), 20210292.

Lee, D.A. (2005). The Perfect Nurturer: A Model for the Development of Compassionate Processes Within the Context of Cognitive Therapy. In P. Gilbert (ed.), *Compassion: Nature and Use in Psychotherapy* (pp.326–351). New York, NY: Routledge.

Lee, D.A. (2013). Compassion Focused Cognitive Therapy for Shame-Based Trauma Memories and Flashbacks in PTSD. In N. Grey (ed.), *A Casebook of Cognitive Therapy for Traumatic Stress Reactions*. London: Brunner-Routledge.

Lee, D.A. (2015). Case Formulation in Complex PTSD: Integrating Theory with Practice. In N. Tarrier (ed.), *Case Formulation in Complex Cases* (second edition). New York, NY: Routledge.

Lee, D.A (2022). Using Compassion Focused Therapy to Work with Complex PTSD. In P. Gilbert and G. Simos (eds), *Compassion Focused Therapy: Clinical Practice and Applications* (pp.565–583). New York, NY: Routledge.

Lee, D.A. and James, S. (2013). *The Compassionate-Mind Guide to Recovering from Trauma and PTSD: Using Compassion-Focused Therapy to Overcome Flashbacks, Shame, Guilt, and Fear.* Oakland, CA: New Harbinger.

Liddell, H.S. (1947). The experimental neurosis. *Annual Review of Physiology*, 9, 569–580.

Liotti, G. (2000). Disorganized Attachment, Models of Borderline States and Evolutionary Psychotherapy. In P. Gilbert and B. Bailey (eds), *Genes on the Couch: Explorations in Evolutionary Psychotherapy* (pp. 232–256). New York, NY: Brunner-Routledge.

Liotti, G. (2011). Attachment disorganization and the controlling strategies: An illustration of the contributions of attachment theory to developmental psychopathology and to psychotherapy integration. *Journal of Psychotherapy Integration*, 21(3), 232–252.

Lippard, E.T. and Nemeroff, C.B. (2020). The devastating clinical consequences of child abuse and neglect: Increased disease vulnerability and poor treatment response in mood disorders. *American Journal of Psychiatry*, 177(1), 20–36.

Longe, O., Maratos, F.A., Gilbert, P., Evans, G. *et al.* (2010). Having a word with yourself: Neural correlates of self-criticism and self-reassurance. *NeuroImage*, 49, 1849–1856.

Lucre, K.M. and Corten, N. (2013). An exploration of group compassion-focused therapy for personality disorder. *Psychology and Psychotherapy: Theory, Research and Practice*, 86(4), 387–400.

Lund, I., Ertesvåg, S. and Roland, E. (2010). Listening to shy voices: Shy adolescents' experiences with being bullied at school. *Journal of Child and Adolescent Trauma*, 3(3), 205–223.

Lunkenheimer, E., Tiberio, S.S., Skoranski, A.M., Buss, K.A. and Cole, P.M. (2018). Parent–child coregulation of parasympathetic processes varies by social context and risk for psychopathology. *Psychophysiology*, 55(2), e12985.

Luyten, P., Campbell, C., Allison, E. and Fonagy, P. (2020). The mentalising approach to psychopathology: State of the art and future directions. *Annual Review of Clinical Psychology*, 16, 297–325.

Ma, X., Yue, Z.Q., Gong, Z.Q., Zhang, H. *et al.* (2017). The effect of diaphragmatic breathing on attention, negative affect and stress in healthy adults. *Frontiers in Psychology*, 874.

Maiano, C., Normand, C.L., Salvas, M.C., Moullec, G. and Aime, A. (2016). Prevalence of school bullying among youth with autism spectrum disorders: A systematic review and meta-analysis. *Autism Research*, 9(6), 601–615.

Manuello, J., Vercelli, U., Nani, A., Costa, T. and Cauda, F. (2016). Mindfulness meditation and consciousness: An integrative neuroscientific perspective. *Consciousness and Cognition*, 40, 67–78.

Maratos, F.A., Duarte, J., Barnes, C., McEwan, K., Sheffield, D. and Gilbert, P. (2017). The physiological and emotional effects of touch: Assessing a hand-massage intervention with high self-critics. *Psychiatry Research*, 250, 221–227.

Marks, I.M. (1987). *Fears, Phobias, and Rituals: Panic, Anxiety, and their Disorders.* Oxford: Oxford University Press on Demand.

Marks, I.M. (1987/2013). *Fears and Phobias.* Cambridge, MA: Academic Press.

Mascaro, J.S., Florian, M.P., Ash, M.J., Palmer, P.K. *et al.* (2020). Ways of knowing compassion: How do we come to know, understand, and measure compassion when we see it? *Frontiers in Psychology*, 11, 547241.

Matos, M., Duarte, J. and Pinto-Gouveia, J. (2017). The origins of fears of compassion: Shame and lack of safeness memories, fears of compassion and psychopathology. *The Journal of Psychology: Interdisciplinary and Applied*, 151(8), 804–819.

Matos, M., McEwan, K., Kanovský, M., Halamová, J. *et al.* (2021a). Fears of compassion magnify the harmful effects of threat of COVID-19 on mental health and social safeness across 21 countries. *Clinical Psychology and Psychotherapy*, 28(6), 1317–1333

Matos, M., McEwan, K., Kanovský, M., Halamová, J. *et al.* (2021b). The role of social connection on the experience of COVID-19 related post-traumatic growth and stress. *PLoS ONE*, 16(12), e0261384.

Matos, M. and Pinto-Gouveia, J. (2010). Shame as a traumatic memory. *Clinical Psychology and Psychotherapy*, 17(4), 299–312.

Matos, M., Pinto-Gouveia, J. and Costa, V. (2013c). Understanding the importance of attachment in shame traumatic memory relation to depression: The impact of emotion regulation processes. *Clinical Psychology and Psychotherapy*, 20, 149–165.

Matos, M., Pinto-Gouveia, J. and Duarte, C. (2012). Above and beyond emotional valence: The unique contribution of central and traumatic shame memories to psychopathology vulnerability. *Memory*, 20(5), 461–477.

Matos, M., Pinto-Gouveia, J. and Duarte, C. (2013b). Internalising early memories of shame and lack of safeness and warmth: The mediating role of shame on depression. *Behavioural and Cognitive Psychotherapy*, 41(4), 479–493.

Matos, M., Pinto-Gouveia, J. and Duarte, C. (2015). Constructing a self-protected against shame: The importance of warmth and safeness memories and feelings on the association between shame memories and depression. *International Journal of Psychology and Psychological Therapy*, 15(3), 317–335.

Matos, M., Pinto-Gouveia, J. and Gilbert, P. (2013a). The effect of shame and shame memories on paranoid ideation and social anxiety. *Clinical Psychology and Psychotherapy*, 20, 334–349.

Matos, M., Steindl, S., Gilbert, P. and Pinto-Gouveia, J. (2020). Shame Memories that Shape Who We Are. In P. Gilbert and J. Kirby (eds), *Making an Impact on Mental Health: The Applications of Psychological Research* (pp.97–126). New York, NY: Routledge.

Mayseless, O. (2016). *The Caring Motivation: An Integrated Theory*. Oxford: Oxford University Press.

McEwan, K. and Minou, L. (2023). Defining compassion: A Delphi study of compassion therapists' experiences when introducing patients to the term 'compassion'. *Psychology and Psychotherapy: Theory, Research and Practice*, 96, 16–24.

Meevissen, Y.M., Peters, M.L. and Alberts, H.J. (2011). Become more optimistic by imagining a best possible self: Effects of a two-week intervention. *Journal of Behaviour Therapy and Experimental Psychiatry*, 42(3), 371–378.

Mikulincer, M. and Shaver, P.R. (eds). (2014). *Mechanisms of Social Connection: From Brain to Group*. Washington, DC: American Psychological Association.

Mikulincer, M. and Shaver, P.R. (2017). An Attachment Perspective on Compassion Altruism. In P. Gilbert (ed.), *Compassion: Conceptualizations, Research and Use in Psychotherapy* (pp.187–202). New York, NY: Routledge.

Mineka, S. and Kihlstrom, J.F. (1978). Unpredictable and uncontrollable events: A new perspective on experimental neurosis. *Journal of Abnormal Psychology*, 87(2), 256–271.

Music, G. (2017). *Nurturing Natures: Attachment and Children's Emotional, Sociocultural and Brain Development* (second edition). New York, NY: Routledge.

Music, G. (2019). *Nurturing Children: From Trauma to Growth Using Attachment Theory, Psychoanalysis and Neurobiology*. New York, NY: Routledge.

Music, G. (2022). *RESPARK: Igniting Hope and Joy after Trauma and Depression*. London: Mind-Nurturing Books.

Naismith, I., Kerr, S., Mwale, A. and Feigenbaum, J. (2019). A thematic analysis of compassion-focused imagery for people with personality disorder: Inhibitors, facilitators and clinical recommendations. *Clinical Psychologist*, 23(3), 213–224.

Naismith, I., Zarate Guerrero, S. and Feigenbaum, J. (2018). Abuse, invalidation, and lack of early warmth show distinct relationships with self-criticism, self-compassion, and fear of self-compassion in personality disorder. *Clinical Psychology and Psychotherapy*, 26(3), 350–361.

Narvaez, D. (2017). Evolution, Child Raising and Compassionate Morality. In P. Gilbert (ed.), *Compassion: Concepts, Research and Applications* (pp.31–68). New York, NY: Routledge.

Narvaez, D. and Bradshaw, G.A. (2023). *The Evolved Nest. Nature's Way of Raising Children and Creating Connected Communities*. Berkeley, CA: North Atlantic Books.

Nesse, R.M. (2019). *Good Reasons for Bad Feelings: Insights from the Frontier of Evolutionary Psychiatry*. New York, NY: Dutton.

O'Donnell, K.J. and Meaney, M.J. (2020). Epigenetics, development, and psychopathology. *Annual Review of Clinical Psychology*, 16, 327–350.

Oehlman Forbes, D., Lee, M. and Lakeman, R. (2021). The role of mentalisation in child psychotherapy, interpersonal trauma, and recovery: A scoping review. *Psychotherapy*, 58(1), 50–67.

Osimo, S.A., Pizarro, R., Spanlang, B. and Slater, M. (2015). Conversations between self and self as Sigmund Freud – A virtual body ownership paradigm for self-counselling. *Nature Scientific Reports*, 5, 13899.

Panksepp, J. (1998). *Affective Neuroscience*. Oxford: Oxford University Press.

Pauley, G. and McPherson, S. (2010). The experience and meaning of compassion and self-compassion for individuals with depression or anxiety. *Psychology and Psychotherapy: Theory, Research and Practice*, 83(2), 129–143.

Pennebaker, J. (1997). Writing about emotional experiences as a therapeutic process. *Psychological Science*, 8(3), 162–166.

Petrocchi, N. and Cheli, S (2019). The social brain and heart rate variability: Implications for psychotherapy. *Psychology and Psychotherapy: Special edition: Building an Integrative Science for Psychotherapy for the 21st-Century*, 92, 208–223.

Petrocchi, N., Di Bello., M., Cheli, S. and Ottavianni, C. (2022). Compassion Focused Therapy and the Body: How Physiological Underpinnings of Prosociality Informed Clinical Practise. In P. Gilbert and G. Simos (eds), *Compassion Focused Therapy: Clinical Practice and Applications* (pp.345–359). New York, NY: Routledge.

Pinto-Gouveia, J. and Matos, M. (2011). Can shame memories become a key to identity? The centrality of shame memories predicts psychopathology. *Applied Cognitive Psychology*, 25(2), 281–290.

Porges, S.W. (2007). The polyvagal perspective. *Biological Psychology*, 74(2), 116–143.

Porges, S.W. (2011). *The Polyvagal Theory: Neurophysiological Foundations of Emotions, Attachment, Communication, and Self-regulation* (*Norton Series on Interpersonal Neurobiology*). New York, NY: W.W. Norton.

Porges, S.W. (2017). Vagal Pathways: Portals to Compassion. In E.M. Seppälä, E. Simon-Thomas, S.L. Brown, M.C. Worline, C.D. Cameron and J.R. Doty (eds), *The Oxford Handbook of Compassion Science* (pp.189–202). Oxford: Oxford University Press.

Porges, S.W. (2021). Polyvagal theory: A biobehavioural journey to sociality. *Comprehensive Psychoneuroendocrinology*, 7, 100069.

Poulin, M.J. (2017). To Help or Not to Help: Goal Commitment and the Goodness of Compassion. In E.M. Seppälä, E. Simon-Thomas, S.L. Brown, M.C. Worline, C.D. Cameron and J.R. Doty (eds), *The Oxford Handbook of Compassion Science* (pp.355–367). Oxford: Oxford University Press.

Quas, J.A., Goodman, G.S. and Jones, D.P. (2003). Predictors of attributions of self-blame and internalising behaviour problems in sexually abused children. *Journal of Child Psychology and Psychiatry*, 44(5), 723–736.

Richter, A., Gilbert, P. and McEwan, K. (2009). Development of an early memories of warmth and safeness scale and its relationship to psychopathology. *Psychology and Psychotherapy: Theory, Research and Practice*, 82(2), 171–184.

Rinpoche, R.T. and Mullen. K. (2005). The Buddhist Use of Compassionate Imagery in Mind Healing. In P. Gilbert (ed.), *Compassion: Conceptualizations, Research and Use in Psychotherapy* (pp.218–238). New York, NY: Routledge.

Rockliff, H., Gilbert, P., McEwan, K., Lightman S. and Glover, D. (2008). A pilot exploration of heart rate variability and salivary cortisol responses to compassion-focused imagery. *Journal of Clinical Neuropsychiatry*, 5, 132–139.

Rockliff, H., Karl, A., McEwan, K., Gilbert, J., Matos, M. and Gilbert, P. (2011). Effects of intranasal oxytocin on compassion focused imagery. *Emotion*, 11, 1388–1396.

Rohner, R.P. (1986). *The Warmth Dimension: Foundations of Parental Acceptance-rejection Theory*. New York, NY: Sage.

Rohner, R.P., Khaleque, A. and Cournoyer, D.E. (2012). Introduction to parental acceptance-rejection theory, methods, evidence, and implications. *Journal of Family Theory and Review*, 2(1), 73–87.

Rothschild, B. (2000). *Body Remembers: The Psychophysiology of Trauma and Trauma Treatment*. New York, NY: W.W. Norton.

Ryan, C. (2019). *Civilised to Death: The Price of Progress*. New York, NY: Simon and Schuster.

Sanghera, J. (2009). *Daughters of Shame*. New York, NY: Hachette.

Schauer, M. and Elbert, T. (2010). Dissociation following traumatic stress: Etiology and treatment. *Journal of Psychology*, 218(2), 109–127.

Schauer, M., Neuner, F. and Elbert, T. (2012). *Narrative Exposure Therapy (NET): A Short-term Intervention for Traumatic Stress Disorders* (second edition). Gottingen, Germany: Hogrefe and Huber.

Schore, A.N. (2019). *Right Brain Psychotherapy*. New York, NY: W.W. Norton.

Seligman, M.E.P. (1975). *Helplessness: On Depression, Development and Death*. San Francisco: CA: Freeman.

Seppälä, E.M., Simon-Thomas, E., Brown, S.L., Worline, M.C., Cameron, C.D. and Doty, J.R. (eds) (2017). *The Oxford Handbook of Compassion Science* (pp.399–420). Oxford: Oxford University Press.

Shahar, G. (2015). *Erosion: The Psychopathology of Self-criticism*. Oxford: Oxford University Press.

Shapiro, F. (2001). *Eye Movement Desensitisation and Reprocessing: Basic Principles, Protocols, and Procedures* (second edition). New York, NY: Guilford Press.

Sheikhi, M. and Aminiha, A. (2022). Mediating role of mentalisation in the relationship between childhood adversity and dark triad personality. *Mental Health: Research and Practice*, 1(2), 43–53.

Siddaway, A.P. Taylor, P.J., Wood, A.M., and Schulz, J. (2015). A meta-analysis of perceptions of defeat and entrapment in depression, anxiety problems, posttraumatic stress disorder, and suicidality. *Journal of Affective Disorders*, 184, 149–159.

Siegel, D. J. (2020). *The Developing Mind: How Relationships in the Brain Interact to Shape Who We Are* (third edition). New York, NY: W.W. Norton.

Singer, T. and Engert, V. (2019). It matters what you practice: Differential training effects on subjective experience, behaviour, brain and body in the ReSource Project. *Current Opinion in Psychology*, 28, 151–158.

Slavich, G.M. (2020). Social safety theory: A biologically based evolutionary perspective on life stress, health, and behaviour. *Annual Review of Clinical Psychology*, 16, 265–295.

Spikins, P. (2015). *How Compassion Made Us Human: The Evolutionary Origins of Tenderness, Trust and Morality*. Barnsely: Spear and Sword Books.

Spikins, P. (2022). *Hidden Depths: The Origins of Human Connection*. Yorkshire: White Rose University Press.

Steffen, P.R., Bartlett, D., Channell, R.M., Jackman, K. *et al.* (2021). Integrating breathing techniques into psychotherapy to improve HRV: Which approach is best? *Frontiers in Psychology*, 12, 191.

Steffen, P.R., Foxx, J., Cattani, K., Alldredge, C., Austin, T. and Burlingame, G.M. (2020). Impact of a 12-week group-based compassion focused therapy intervention on heart rate variability. *Applied Psychophysiology and Biofeedback*, 46, 61–68.

Steindl, S., Bell, T., Dixon, A. and Kirby, J.N. (2022). Therapist perspectives on working with fears, blocks and resistances to compassion in compassion focused therapy. *Counselling and Psychotherapy Research*. doi.org/10.1002/capr.12530.

Stevens, J.S., Kim, Y.J., Galatzer-Levy, I.R., Reddy, R. *et al.* (2017). Amygdala reactivity and anterior cingulate habituation predict posttraumatic stress disorder symptom maintenance after acute civilian trauma. *Biological Psychiatry*, 81(12), 1023–1029.

Stopa, L., Brown, M.A. and Hirsch, C.R. (2012). The effects of repeated imagery practice on self-concept, anxiety and performance in socially anxious participants. *Journal of Experimental Psychopathology*, 3(2), 223–242.

Stott, R. (2007). When the head and heart do not agree: A theoretical and clinical analysis of rational-emotional dissociation (RED) in cognitive therapy. *Journal of Cognitive Psychotherapy: An International Quarterly*, 21, 37–50.

Sznycer, D., Tooby, J., Cosmides, L., Porat, R., Shalvi, S. and Halperin, E. (2016). Shame closely tracks the threat of devaluation by others, even across cultures. *Proceedings of the National Academy of Sciences*, 113(10), 2625–2630.

Taylor, P.J., Gooding, P., Wood, A.M. and Tarrier, N. (2011). The role of defeat and entrapment in depression, anxiety, and suicide. *Psychological Bulletin*, 137(3), 391–420.

Terpou, B.A., Harricharan, S., McKinnon, M.C., Frewen, P., Jetly, R. and Lanius, R.A. (2019). The effects of trauma on brain and body: A unifying role for the midbrain periaqueductal gray. *Journal of Neuroscience Research*, 97(9), 1110–1140.

Tierney, S. and Fox, J.R. (2010). Living with the anorexic voice: A thematic analysis. *Psychology and Psychotherapy: Theory, Research and Practice*, 83(3), 243–254.

Tirch, D., Schoendorff, B. and Silberstein, L.R. (2014). *The ACT Practitioner's Guide to the Science of Compassion: Tools for Fostering Psychological Flexibility*. Oakland, CA: New Harbinger Publications.

Troop, N.A. and Hiskey, S. (2013). Social defeat and PTSD symptoms following trauma. *British Journal of Clinical Psychology*, 52(4), 365–379.

Tucci, J., Mitchell, J., Lindeman, M., Shilton, L. and Green, J. (2017). *Strengthening Community Capacity to End Violence: A Project for NPY Women's Council*. Alice Springs: NPY Women's Council and Australian Childhood Foundation.

Vagos, P., Ribeiro da Silva, D., Brazão, N., Rijo, D. and Gilbert, P. (2017). The Early Memories of Warmth and Safeness Scale for adolescents: Cross-sample validation of the complete and brief versions. *Clinical Psychology and Psychotherapy*, 24(3), 793–804.

van der Hart, O., Nijenhuis, E.R. and Steele, K. (2006). *The Haunted Self: Structural Dissociation and the Treatment of Chronic Traumatisation*. New York, NY: W.W. Norton.

van der Kolk, B. (2014). *The Body Keeps the Score: Brain, Mind, and Body in the Healing of Trauma*. New York, NY: Penguin.

Vessantara (1993). *Meeting the Buddhas: A Guide to Buddhas, Bodhisattvas and Tantric Deities*. London: Windhorse.

Vonk, R. (1998). The slime effect: Suspicion and dislike of likeable behaviour toward superiors. *Journal of Personality and Social Psychology*, 74(4), 849.

Vrtička, P., Favre, P. and Singer, T. (2017). Compassion and the Brain. In P. Gilbert (ed.), *Compassion: Concepts, Research and Applications* (pp.135–151). New York, NY: Routledge.

Weng, H.Y., Fox, A.S., Shackman, A.J., Stodola, D.E. *et al.* (2013). Compassion training alters altruism and neural responses to suffering. *Psychological Science*, 24(7), 1171–1180.

Weng, H.Y., Lapate, R.C., Stodola, D.E., Rogers, G.M. and Davidson, R.J. (2018). Visual attention to suffering after compassion training is associated with decreased amygdala responses. *Frontiers in Psychology*, 9, 771.

Werner, A.M., Tibubos, A.N., Rohrmann, S. and Reiss, N. (2019). The clinical trait self-criticism and its relation to psychopathology: A systematic review – update. *Journal of Affective Disorders*, 246, 530–547.

Whalley, M. and Lee, D.A. (2019). Using compassionate resource installation in EMDR for shame-based memories. Psychology Tools: www.psychologytools.com.

Whelton, W.J. and Greenberg, L.S. (2005). Emotion in self-criticism. *Personality and Individual Differences*, 38(7), 1583–1595.

Williams, J.M.G. (2008). Mindfulness, depression and modes of mind. *Cognitive Therapy and Research*, 32(6), 721–733.

Willis, N., Dowling, C., Deehan, T. and O'Reilly, G. (2023). Exploring the impact of trauma and the role of compassion before and after a phase-orientated intervention for complex trauma. *European Journal of Trauma and Dissociation*, 7(1), 100308.

Workman, l., Reader, W. and Barkow, J.H. (2020). *The Cambridge Handbook of Evolutionary Perspectives on Human Behaviour*. Cambridge: Cambridge University Press

Wu, Y.E. and Hong, W. (2022). Neural basis of prosocial behaviour. *Trends in Neurosciences*, 45, 749–762.

Yeung, A., Chan, J.S., Cheung, J.C. and Zou, L. (2018). Qigong and tai-chi for mood regulation. *Focus*, 16(1), 40–47.

Zeman, A., Dewar, M. and Della Sala, S. (2016). Reflections on aphantasia. *Cortex*, 74, 336–337.

Zilberstein, K. (2014). The use and limitations of attachment theory in child psychotherapy. *Psychotherapy*, 51(1), 93–103.

CHAPTER 8

Transforming Multisensory Experience into an Embodied Self: Sensorimotor Implications for Trauma Treatment

Breanne Kearney and Ruth A. Lanius

Introduction

Over the past century, trauma-related symptomology has been largely observed as a manifestation of disordered higher-order cognitive processes such as memory, thought, and emotion. However, a recent shift toward post-traumatic stress dysfunction in the central nervous system as a sensory integrative breakdown calls for greater focus on brainstem and midbrain processes and their subsequent integration with higher reaches of the cortex. Arousal dysregulation, affect over- or under-modulation, fragmented sensory experiential memories, and dissociation as symptoms of trauma-related conditions further indicate that subcortical-level processes are foundational in the manifestation of post-traumatic stress dysfunction.

Further, we consider the correlation between insecure/disorganized attachment and the later development of PTSD and other trauma-related conditions. The neurobiological mechanisms of early attachment are inextricable from sensorimotor development, where sensory feedback interdigitates with affective processes. For example, the tender touch of a mother soothes and calms an infant, whereas a mother's angry voice can startle and frighten a child. Early deficits in or disruptions to sensory-affective processing are posited to have cascading effects on the ontogenetic development of higher-order cortical circuitry involved in limbic (emotional) and neocortical (cognitive) processes. An altered brainstem foundation creates a systemic vulnerability to stress, resulting in higher incidences of psychiatric conditions and trans-diagnostic symptoms such as dissociation, hyperarousal, poor concentration, and depression. Here, we offer the perspective that trauma attacks and overwhelms the sensory integrative and affective lower reaches of the brain given their involvement in primal defensive responding, raw affect generation and processing, and subconscious social relational processing (i.e. detecting threat or safety in another). Lastly, we make a case for sensorimotor-based approaches in the treatment of trauma, given their ability to target subcortical processes such as multisensory integration, arousal modulation, and affect regulation.

Multisensory integration in health and trauma

Our experience of reality is a symphony of sensory inputs from various modalities strung together in temporal congruence. This multisensory perception orients us to the world in real time and space (Harricharan *et al.*, 2021). Our experience of the world and our bodies at any given moment also encompasses biological, affective drives which motivate instinctual behaviour, affording us the richness and depth of a range of affective experiences from joy to rage (Panksepp, 1998). These raw sensory inputs and affective activations are initially processed in the subcortical brainstem and midbrain regions before being relayed to higher-order structures in a pre-processed, filtered form.

Further, top-down influences modulate raw sensory and affective information, selectively manipulating which are relevant and brought into awareness. For example, Ellingsen and colleagues (2013) found that administering a placebo for oxytocin, a neurochemical posited to reduce pain and increase pleasantness of touch, to healthy individuals elicited reports of reduced pain and heightened pleasure in conjunction with increased coupling of the periaqueductal grey (PAG), the grey matter encompassing the cerebral aqueduct in the midbrain, with the prefrontal cortex. Here, cognitive appraisal mechanisms (the expectation of changes to sensory experience) alone had the capacity to attenuate or exaggerate sensory perception. This bidirectional information flow, which we will term vertical integration, optimally is a fluid and dynamic process capable of adaptations to instinctual, bodily, and/or environmental demands.

Vertical integration as a more ancient mechanism is prerequisite for horizontal integration of the brain, where medial and lateral aspects of the phylogenetically newer neocortex communicate efficiently. How these interactions are optimized to integrate information from all modalities and amplify relevant signals while dampening others remains to be fully elucidated, and the mechanisms are likely to be complex and multidimensional. However, what is clear is that our perceptual experience is highly contingent on motivational states and contextual information, and vice versa (Ellingsen *et al.*, 2016). For instance, a caress from a loved one has a soothing effect, while the same caress from a rapist will elicit quite the opposite perceptual and affective response. Likewise, receipt of a light caressing touch or rhythmical movements during critical developmental periods, characterized by motivational states of need for physical comfort and safe handling for survival, shapes how we ascribe emotional valence and contextual memory to sensory information.

It is hypothesized that the integration and modulation of sensory input from both interoceptive (relating to the body's internal world) and exteroceptive (relating to the external environment) sources is required for a coherent sense of the body in space and its capacity for adaptive behaviour given environmental circumstances (Ayres, 1972; Harricharan et al., 2021; Kearney and Lanius, 2022). The importance of the body's sensorial experience, first detected in peripheral sensory organs or receptors, aligns with the concept of embodied cognition (Shapiro and Spaulding, 2021), which emphasizes the role that the physical body plays in cognitive and emotional capacities. Elementally, sensory input is received through somatosensory, auditory, visual, olfactory, gustatory, vestibular, and interoceptive modalities. Vestibular information is detected within the vestibular organs of the inner ear and is first relayed to the cerebellum and the vestibular nuclei located in the pons. The vestibular nuclei also receive somatosensory feedback from ocular muscles and have both upward projections to the midbrain and cortex and downward projections to the muscles and autonomic viscera (heart, lungs).

Somatosensory information, inclusive of discriminative touch, proprioception, and affective (light stroking) touch, is relayed from the peripheral sensory organs and mechanoreceptors of the skin, muscles, and joints up to the brainstem. Discriminative and affective touch arrive at the gracile and cuneate nuclei of the medulla, whereas proprioceptive input travels upward from the muscles and joints through the cuneocerebellar and spinocerebellar tracts to inform of body position and support coordination and balance-related processes in the cerebellum. Importantly, proprioceptive input also integrates with vestibular information at the level of the vestibular nuclei, continually updating the state of our antigravity musculature and posture. Auditory input is first processed at the cochlear nuclei of the upper medulla before ascending to the superior olive, as well as to the inferior and superior colliculi. Gustatory input arrives at the nucleus of the solitary tract (solitary nucleus) in the dorsomedial medulla (Cutsforth-Gregory and Benarroch, 2017) and parabrachial nucleus of the pons (Saper and Lowell, 2014), where it is relayed to higher-order regions such as the hypothalamus and insula.

Interoception, a term representing sensation that emanates from within the body and informs of its internal physiological and visceral state (Sherrington, 1906; Craig, 2002), also first arrives at the solitary nucleus of the medulla, located lateral to the motor nucleus of the vagus nerve (AbuAlrob and Tadi, 2022). Further, animal research has shown that neurons from the vestibular nuclei have direct connections to the solitary nucleus (Gagliuso et al., 2019), which would elucidate how vestibular and proprioceptive input impact and modulate sympathetic responses and interoceptive processing at the brainstem level (for a review, see Yates *et al.*, 2014). Clearly, the brainstem is crucial in the receipt and management of incoming raw sensory information, informing processes related to homeostatic regulation.

Rostral to the brainstem sits the midbrain, inclusive of the periaqueductal grey (PAG) and the superior colliculi (SC) of the midbrain tectum ('roof' of the midbrain). These structures integrate affect with sensory input and organize orienting and defense/approach behaviours in response to an affective-sensory experience (Terpou *et al.*, 2019). This sensory-affect interchange is crucial in the brain and body's response to a traumatic event, as well as in the perseverance of arousal and affect dysregulation. As opposed to its integration into conscious awareness and storage in memory, a traumatic event activates altered threat-detection circuitry and may lead to subcortically driven hyperarousal and cortical overwhelm, or cortically mediated hypoarousal and shutdown, depending on the individual's prior experience with threat. For those who have experienced event-related or repeated instances of fight/flight reactions accompanied by hyperarousal, bottom-up sensory and affective information floods the cortex suggesting cortical under-modulation of subcortical regions. This has been substantiated through dynamic causal modelling (DCM) of resting state functional connectivity (rsFC), where individuals with PTSD exhibited bottom-up directionality of increased PAG-amygdala and PAG-ventromedial prefrontal cortex (vmPFC) rsFC (Nicholson *et al.*, 2017). This cortical chaos may lead to the experience of fragmented sensory and somatic-based memories which have not been adequately integrated into memory storage, leading to re-experiencing or flashbacks.

Alternatively, those who experienced chronic, inescapable threat such as childhood physical, sexual, or emotional abuse may have developed top-down modulatory circuitry designed to suppress and numb sensory and emotional experiences in the context of affective fear (Lanius *et al.*, 2010, 2018). Indeed, enhanced top-down modulation from the vmPFC to the amygdala and PAG was displayed by individuals with the dissociative subtype of PTSD (PTSD+DS; Nicholson *et al.*, 2017), which is characterized by frequent and intense episodes of depersonalization and/or derealization (American Psychiatric Association, 2013). These individuals may experience amnesia of traumatic events, as sensory and affective affordances are prevented from engaging the autobiographical memory representation networks of the cortex. The brainstem sensory-midbrain affective interchange is also a likely seat of 'body memories', as previous traumatic events activate brainstem regions responsible for signaling muscles and joints via descending vestibular and somatosensory tracts in preparation for defensive behaviour or imminent death outside cognitive awareness.

While the vestibular nuclei send signals to postural and extensor muscles via the vestibulospinal tract, the sensory-influenced reticular nuclei also activate postural musculature and modulate muscle tone. The tectospinal tract arises from the midbrain tectum and influences the peripheral somatosensory system. These oft-neglected brainstem-body dynamics are likely to be highly involved in peripheral, somatic manifestations of trauma, which can be activated through sensory or affective triggers (Kearney and Lanius, 2022). While embodied cognition requires efficient integration of bodily sensations with motoric actions (Shapiro and Spaulding, 2021), the multisensory integrative breakdown experienced in post-traumatic conditions may induce states of disembodiment characterized by diminished emotion regulation, cognitive flexibility, motor planning, time cognisance, agency, and self-related processing.

Attachment trauma as a multisensory integrative breakdown

Ontogenetically, brainstem and midbrain regions develop before higher-order limbic and cortical brain regions, and they are enriched through nurturing sensory and affective experiences with a primary caregiver(s) in the child's formative days, months, and years. A lack of reliable and positively valenced sensory feedback during times of distress, such as being picked up and held when physically or emotionally hurt, provided with reassuring touch when experiencing overwhelming emotion, or soothed with calming and rhythmic prosody of speech, leads to insecure or disorganized attachment with resultant deficits in arousal and emotion regulation. As such, disrupted attachment processes relate to disjointed or negatively valenced sensory-affective experiences within the context of an unsafe caregiver and/or environment. This constitutes a chronically traumatic situation for the developing child; for example, the child may experience touch and nourishment with blunted affect from a depressed mother or physical abuse from an emotionally dysregulated parent. This sensory-affective mismatch, where instinctual expectations are met with a survival-threatening response, is posited to alter the developing neural circuitry for higher-order processes including self-regulation, attention, self-referential processing, motor planning, and so on.

Traumatic stress encountered later in life is likely to have a more devastating and destabilizing effect on the already tenuous multisensory integrative basis of insecure attachment. Insecure attachment style in adulthood refers to pervasive and enduring patterns of beliefs, expectations, and anxieties related to the availability and attentiveness of intimate partners or close others during times of need or distress (Bowlby, 1973).

While insecure and disorganized attachment is observed to a significantly greater degree in those who experienced childhood abuse and/or neglect (Carlson, 1998; Egeland and Sroufe, 1981), multiple studies have linked insecure attachment with the development and severity of PTSD symptoms (Besser and Neria, 2012; Muller *et al.*, 2000; Ogle *et al.*, 2015; Sandberg, 2010; Scott and Babcock, 2010; Twaite and Rodriguez-Srednicki, 2004; Zakin *et al.*, 2003; for a review, see Mikulincer *et al.*, 2015). Individuals with greater insecurity in relationships as adults have reported stronger physical responsivity to trauma memories as well as higher frequency of intrusive memories (Ogle *et al.*, 2015). Greater physical reactivity suggests a sensorimotor and/or sensory-sympathetic (arousal) response to stressors, accentuating the interweaving of attachment, sensory processing, and trauma-related processes. Further, the earlier the occurrence of traumatic events, the more the events disrupt critical sensorimotor developmental periods. The most robust sensorimotor development occurs in the first few years of life, alongside the nurturance of primary attachment relationships. This corresponds with findings that the earlier timing of trauma in the life course correlates with increased PTSD severity (Muller *et al.*, 2000). Overall, sensory integration and attachment are intertwined developmental processes, which are vulnerable to disruption through early experiences with abuse or neglect that predispose an individual to the development of post-traumatic stress dysfunction later in life.

Treatment implications: Sensorimotor-based approaches for trauma-related conditions

From this perspective, a neurobiological basis for how trauma can be 'stored in the body' begins to emerge (van der Kolk, 2015). The 'bottom-up' approaches to trauma therapy, whether termed 'somatic' or 'sensorimotor' or 'body-based,' are all predicated on the notion that sensory input from the body can influence processes in the brain. Accessing the subcortical foundation for one's sense of comfort in and control over one's body lies at the heart of these treatment approaches (Schwartz and Maiberger, 2018). As we have outlined, subcortical brain regions responsible for the integration of raw sensory input are also implicated in processes gone awry in trauma, including arousal regulation, affective and motivational state modulation, and connection of cortical awareness to the physical bodily experience (Harricharan *et al.*, 2021). Additionally, sensory modulation challenges, or difficulties regulating one's physiological and behavioural responses to sensory information, are commonplace in traumatized individuals (Engel-Yeger *et al.*, 2013; Yochman and Pat-Horenczyk, 2020). Indeed, greater interest in the role of lower brain structures in arousal regulation and behavior in trauma-related conditions has directed more attention toward the adoption of sensory integrative theory and therapeutic approaches in traumatized populations (Fraser *et al.*, 2017; Warner *et al.*, 2013). The beneficial effects of these approaches may be particularly strong for those with a history of attachment disruptions and chronic childhood traumatization.

Although sensory-based treatment approaches have been utilized mostly by occupational therapists over the past 50 years, the incorporation of somatic sensory input into psychotherapeutic approaches for traumatized populations is becoming increasingly prevalent. As the pioneer of sensory integrative therapy, Jean Ayres (1972), presciently suggested:

> ...as the natural developmental association between sensory input and psychic experience becomes better understood, the two forms of therapy [occupational therapy and psychotherapy] may profit from joining forces. What is rocking and being cuddled other than tactile and vestibular stimulation plus an interpersonal relationship? Are not the neural traces for the sensory and the social aspects of the experience laid down as one in the brain? (p.266)

Ayres emphasized the importance of the client's active, sensory-enriched engagement in any therapeutic process, and viewed the brain as a self-organizing system. As such, active sensorimotor treatment approaches incorporating touch and movement, grounded in concepts of experience-dependent neuroplasticity and Hebbian learning (Hebb, 1949; Rao and Sejnowski, 2001), are posited to evoke an organizing response conducive to environmental and self-mastery (Ayres, 1972). Self-mastery is the consistent and satisfying ability to produce meaningful goal-directed action; in other words, the self is in control of the body and has trust in its actions on the outside world.

Similar in theoretical background, sensorimotor psychotherapy (SP) (Ogden et al., 2006) and somatic experiencing (SE™) (Levine, 2010) are informed by the notion that trauma is a somatic sensory-based phenomenon. SP incorporates active movement and attends to defensive posturing while working through trauma symptoms and memories (Fisher, 2011, 2019; Ogden et al., 2006). In SE™, special attention is paid to the body's instinctual drive to complete previously thwarted or unsuccessful actions, such as turning the wheel of a car to prevent a traumatizing car accident (Payne et al., 2015). As somatic-oriented therapy approaches, SP and SE™ focus on arousal and affective dysregulation as a subcortical issue central to trauma treatment (Ogden et al., 2006; van der Kolk, 2003). Importantly, mindful attention toward sensations, bodily postures, and movements allows for the re-connection and integration of subcortical and cortical regions. These postures and movements might include a reflexive slumping of the spine and cowering of the head in response to feelings of shame, which might then be replaced with a lengthened spine and extended neck to confidently rise the head (Fisher, 2011; Ogden et al., 2006). Here, we add the importance of vestibular and somatosensory feedback from the body in its response to trauma triggers, as well as its role in reorganizing the client's experience through felt somatic modifications. Although research behind these approaches remains limited, three small to moderately sized clinical trials of SP-informed group therapy have shown promising results in arousal regulation and reductions in PTSD symptoms (Classen *et al.*, 2021; Gene-Cos *et al.*, 2016; Langmuir *et al.*, 2012).

Relatedly, Warner and colleagues (2013) have developed a treatment model entitled Sensory Motor Arousal Regulation Therapy (SMART), informed by both Ayres' SI (sensory integration) approach (May-Benson and Schaaf, 2015) and SP (Ogden *et al.*, 2006). SMART is tailored for traumatized children and adolescents, with adaptations underway for use with adults. The SMART approach emphasizes the importance of arousal regulation and vestibular and somatosensory processing to facilitate the ability to identify and regulate sensations and emotions (Warner *et al.*, 2014). It similarly acknowledges the phenomenon that when an individual's arousal is dysregulated, they are unable to access the higher cortical functions, such as language and verbal problem solving, necessary for cognitive or talk-based therapeutic approaches (Warner *et al.*, 2013). Therefore, use of language is de-emphasized until the client reaches a stage of healing where the neocortex connects to the felt subcortical experience. Research is limited, but preliminary quasi-experimental and case studies have shown significant reductions in anxiety symptoms and somatic complaints in traumatized adolescents (Finn *et al.*, 2018; Warner *et al.*, 2014)

Deep brain re-orienting (DBR), a developmentally informed treatment approach, targets the multisensory integrative brainstem and midbrain regions involved in orientation to stimuli and affective responding. Here, DBR provides a window into the enduring somatic experiences in the aftermath of trauma, which had previously resulted in arousal and affect dysregulation at the levels of the SC and PAG. Mindful attention to muscular tension elicited in response to a traumatic memory provides information on the pre-affective components of the trauma memory, where the head, neck, and body prepare to respond in a particular sequence (orienting tension-'shock'-affect) below the level of conscious affective awareness. Orienting tension, as mediated by the superior colliculi, is identified by the individual and utilized as an anchor for grounding in the present moment, which can be returned to if the ensuing somatic and affective experiences become overwhelming. Particular attention is paid to activity in the muscles around the eyes and in the neck, innervated by the vestibular and proprioceptive systems, as this has been found to be reflective of SC activation in primates (Corneil and Camp, 2018).

This orienting tension is postulated to precede the affective and more integrative defensive responses of fight, flight, or freeze at the level of the

PAG (Corrigan and Christie-Sands, 2020). The individual is then supported in experiencing the somatic sensations related to the initial trauma or attachment wound. The first steps of the sequence are slowed down in order to be fully processed and witnessed by the guiding therapist before affective visceral sensations and emotions surface. When successful, DBR clears patterns of phylogenetically and ontogenetically primal response patterns that are no longer relevant in the present context. This physical, bodily orientation toward stimuli in the present moment, as opposed to a traumatic memory, is the antithesis to dissociative flashbacks, derealization, and depersonalization.

Several other 'bottom-up' approaches, including, but not limited to, equine-facilitated psychotherapy (EFP), trauma-sensitive yoga (TSY) (Emerson and Hopper 2011; Emerson *et al.*, 2009), and expressive arts therapy (Malchiodi, 2020), utilize somatic sensory input as a means of regulating the nervous system and building trust in and connection to the body. Here, embodiment, or the mindful inhabitation of one's body during present experience and action, can be incorporated in various ways into therapeutic approaches to trauma healing (Schwartz and Maiberger, 2018). Whereas TSY focuses on guiding clients in tolerating titrated somatic sensation and/ or the affective states somatic sensory input can arouse, EFP champions the sense of mastery one builds through client-directed touch, balance, and bodily control within a therapeutic alliance with the horse. Mindful yogic movements and postures provide vestibular and somatosensory stimulation in conjunction with guided cognitive appraisal. In EFP, the client with severe early life trauma is provided with the somatic sensory ingredients necessary for co-regulation with another, the establishment of embodied trust and selfhood, and ultimately the extension of a relational self within nurturing human relationships (Naste *et al.*, 2018).

Various forms of expressive arts, including theatre, music, art, writing, and dance, tap into individuals' sense of agency by incorporating the physical body in meaningful, goal-oriented actions. This active 'doing' is inherently a multisensory experience, where the body can experience success in its creative expressions (Malchiodi, 2020). If trauma impacts the lower reaches of the brain, first developed early in life, accessing these regions requires attention to nonverbal, sensory-motor processes inherent in a variety of expressive art forms. Active engagement in artful expression can be grounding and soothing for traumatized individuals, allowing for regulation of arousal, tolerance of sensations and emotions that arise, and integration of past traumatic experiences into a coherent self-referential story.

Overall, encouraging the individual to re-connect with their felt bodily experiences within a positively valenced therapeutic alliance contradicts the previous negatively valenced multisensory experiences and attachment disruptions (van der Kolk, 2015). Importantly, we emphasize that 'bottom-up' approaches are not unidirectional; in fact, reconstructing the bridge between sensorial affect and cortical processing requires attention to top-down processes as well. Use of mindful attention to somatic experience may activate the medial prefrontal cortex (mPFC), previously shown to be engaged in mindfulness-based approaches (Creswell *et al.*, 2007; Davidson *et al.*, 2003; Siegel, 2007). The mPFC then downregulates lower regions involved in emotionality, arousal, and affect regulation, such as the amygdala, locus coeruleus, SC, and PAG. Initially, the therapist acts as an externalized mPFC by attending to alterations in posture, arousal, and movements until the client can independently take notice. The client is then able to attend to, appreciate, and better control their affective and physiological defensive responses, and a sense of agency and trust in the body is restored (or primarily developed in the case of chronic childhood trauma).

We suggest that the utilization of somatic sensory input within a framework of mindfulness, where the individual is guided in taking notice of the presence, intensity, and quality of the stimulation, will bridge the brain-body disconnect that is often so difficult to address in cognitive therapies. Titrated and individualized trauma-sensitive, somatic sensory-enriched approaches may support the individual in regulating emotional and physiological responses, building safety within the therapeutic alliance, and tolerating and integrating traumatic memories during psychotherapy sessions.

Taken together, sensory and raw affective processing at the brainstem and midbrain levels are posited to lie at the root of our responses to traumatic events and our everyday functioning. Integrated and modulated sensations and affective responses promote organized, flexible, and regulated cognitive processes that communicate fluidly with the body. However, adverse and unsafe sensory and affective experiences from chronic traumatization and insecure attachment during neurodevelopment may predispose an individual toward psychopathology, characterized by disorganization, disembodiment, and dysregulation of the nervous system. Thus, traumagenic conditions can be seen through the lens of sensory-affective processing, where sensory-based therapeutic approaches may be a crucial adjunct to optimize cognitively focused treatments and restore the brain-body connection in the aftermath of trauma.

KNOWLEDGE AND PRACTICE REFLECTION

Janise Mitchell, Joe Tucci, Ed Tronick and Stephen W. Porges

The whole focus of this exquisitely detailed chapter by Kearney and Lanius is to remind us that the impact of violation is not painful stories held in cognitive forms of memory that distract, affect or overpower the minds of victims and survivors of interpersonal violence. Trauma finds itself into, and is stored in, the body and the connecting systems which trace and shape the physiological connections from the body to the brain and back into the body.

It is important to understand the neuroscience that has made it possible for us to come to this realization and be able to pair it with the rich descriptions of those with lived and living experiences of trauma. It leads to an appreciation of how victims and survivors present to and engage with practitioners and organizations.

Sometimes, if the environment is activating earlier memories of the mistrust that accompanied the abuse, they feel out of place. They have an unfamiliar feeling in the pit of their stomach or the back of their head which tells them to move with trepidation. They know that their body is not feeling right, but they cannot explain why. They find it hard to concentrate on questions that are being asked of them. They can struggle to sit in a room on their own, waiting for a healthcare professional. They may not like to sit too close or too far away from another.

Sounds and smells can orient them to taking action. They may leave quickly. They may become immovable. They may seem confused and unable to talk about anything with much detail.

They can sometimes move uncontrollably. They can scratch and pick at scars or bites on their body – at times making them bleed and requiring assistance. They can refuse to eat because the sensation of food in their mouth or a particular texture of food in their mouth is off-putting. They find it hard to move away from something that they are engrossed with, like watching TV or interacting with their mobile phone. They can feel out of breath, find it difficult to breath, and may hyperventilate. They may not sleep. They may sleep all the time and be difficult to wake up when it is scheduled to do so. They may not want to go into a car or public transport. They may want to avoid public places and crowds.

These are all examples of the ways that the body accesses precursors to traumatic states that activate defensive mechanisms learnt over time to protect the individual from more pain. Sometimes, these states are full-blown recreations of the violation, looking as if the person has left their body and is reacting to an unknown or invisible assailant whispering the messages of fear, control and manipulation that accompanied their violation.

It is self-evident that practitioners, organizations and systems with a commitment to serving the interests of victims and survivors need to consider how environmental stimuli, relational stimuli and sensory stimuli are managed in ways that offer care, understanding and acceptance.

Including opportunities for individuals to sit away from others in a waiting room if they choose is a simple but powerful reconfiguration of supporting the nervous system of victims and survivors to settle in unfamiliar environments. Having access to natural environments is another example.

Trauma-transformative practice considers these issues deeply and commits resources and attention to integrating an understanding of the inherent capture of the body in the experience of trauma, and respect for its rhythms and reactions.

References
References for chapter

AbuAlrob, M.A. and Tadi, P. (2022). Neuroanatomy, Nucleus Solitarius. In StatPearls [Internet]. Treasure Island, FL: StatPearls Publishing.

American Psychiatric Association (2013). *Diagnostic and Statistical Manual of Mental Disorders 5th Edition*. Arlington, VA: American Psychiatric Press.

Ayres, A.J. (1972). *Sensory Integration and Learning Disorders*. Los Angeles, CA: Western Psychological Services.

Besser, A. and Neria, Y. (2012). When home isn't a safe haven: Insecure attachment orientations, perceived social support, and PTSD symptoms among Israeli evacuees under missile threat. *Psychological Trauma: Theory, Research, Practice, and Policy*, 4(1), 34–46.

Carlson, E.A. (1998). A prospective longitudinal study of attachment disorganization/disorientation. *Child Development*, 69(4), 1107–1128.

Bowlby, J. (1973). *Attachment and Loss: Volume II: Separation, Anxiety and Anger*. New York, NY: Penguin Books.

Classen, C.C., Hughes, L., Clark, C., Hill Mohammed, B., Woods, P. and Beckett, B. (2021). A pilot RCT of a body-oriented group therapy for complex trauma survivors: An adaptation of sensorimotor psychotherapy. *Journal of Trauma and Dissociation*, 22(1), 52–68.

Corneil, B.D. and Camp, A.J. (2018). Animal models of vestibular evoked myogenic potentials: The past, present, and future. *Frontiers in Neurology*, 9(489).

Corrigan, F.M. and Christie-Sands, J. (2020). An innate brainstem self-other system involving orienting, affective responding, and polyvalent relational seeking: Some clinical implications for a 'Deep Brain Reorienting' trauma psychotherapy approach. *Medical Hypotheses*, 136(109502).

Craig A.D. (2002). How do you feel? Interoception: The sense of the physiological condition of the body. *Nature Reviews Neuroscience*, 3, 655–666.

Creswell, J.D., Way, B.M., Eisenberger, N.I. and Lieberman, M.D. (2007). Neural correlates of dispositional mindfulness during affect labeling. *Psychosomatic Medicine*, 69(6), 560–565.

Cutsforth-Gregory, J.K. and Benarroch, E.E. (2017). Nucleus of the solitary tract, medullary reflexes, and clinical implications. *Neurology*, 88(12), 1187–1196.

Davidson, R.J., Kabat-Zinn, J., Schumacer, J., Rosenkranz, M. *et al.* (2003). Alterations in brain and immune function produced by mindfulness meditation. *Psychosomatic Medicine*, 65(4), 564–570.

Egeland, B. and Sroufe, L.A. (1981). Attachment and early maltreatment. *Child Development*, 52(1), 44–52.

Ellingsen, D., Leknes, S., Loseth, G., Wessberg, J, and Olausson, H. (2016). The neurobiology shaping affective touch: Expectation, motivation, and meaning in the multisensory context. *Frontiers in Psychology*, 6, 1986.

Ellingsen, D., Wessberg, J., Eikemo, M., Liljencrantz, J. *et al.* (2013). Placebo improves pleasure and pain through opposite modulation of sensory processing. *Proceedings of the National Academy of Sciences of the United States of America*, 110(44), 17993–17998.

Emerson, D. and Hopper, E. (2011). *Overcoming Trauma Through Yoga: Reclaiming Your Body*. Berkeley, CA: North Atlantic Books.

Emerson, D., Sharma, R., Chaudhry, S. and Turner, J. (2009). Trauma-sensitive yoga: Principles, practice and research. *International Journal of Yoga Therapy*, 19(1), 123–125.

Engel-Yeger, B., Palgy-Levin, D. and Lev-Wiesel, R. (2013). The sensory profile of people with post-traumatic stress symptoms. *Occupational Therapy in Mental Health*, 29, 266–278.

Finn, H., Warner, E., Price, M. and Spinazzola, J. (2018). The boy who was hit in the face: Somatic regulation and processing of preverbal complex trauma. *Journal of Child and Adolescent Trauma*, 11(3), 277–288.

Fisher, J. (2011). Sensorimotor approaches to trauma treatment. *Advances in Psychiatric Treatment*, 17(3), 171–177.

Fisher, J. (2019). Sensorimotor psychotherapy in the treatment of trauma. *Practice Innovations*, 4(3), 156–165.

Fraser, K., MacKenzie, D. and Versnel, J. (2017). Complex trauma in children and youth: A scoping review of sensory-based interventions. *Occupational Therapy in Mental Health*, 33(3), 199–216.

Gagliuso, A.H., Chapman, E.K., Martinelli, G.P. and Holstein, G.R. (2019). Vestibular neurons with direct projections to the solitary nucleus in the rat. *Journal of Neurophysiology*, 122(2), 512–524.

Gene-Cos, N., Fisher, J., Ogden, P. and Cantrel, A. (2016). Sensorimotor Psychotherapy Group Therapy in the Treatment of Complex PTSD. *Annals of Psychiatry and Mental Health*, 4(6), 1080.

Harricharan, S., McKinnon, M.C. and Lanius, R.A. (2021). How processing of sensory information from the internal and external worlds shape the perception and engagement with the world in the aftermath of trauma: Implications for PTSD. *Frontiers in Neuroscience*, 15(625490).

Hebb, D.O. (1949). *The Organization of Behaviour: A Neuropsychological Theory*. New York, NY: Wiley.

Kearney, B.E. and Lanius, R.A. (2022). The brain-body disconnect: A somatic sensory basis for trauma-related disorders. *Frontiers in Neuroscience*, 16, 1–36.

Langmuir, J.I., Kirsch, S.G. and Classen, C.C. (2012). A pilot study of body-oriented group psychotherapy: Adapting sensorimotor psychotherapy for the group treatment of trauma. *Psychological Trauma: Theory, Research, Practice, and Policy*, 4(2), 214–220.

Lanius, R.A., Boyd, J.E., McKinnon, M.C., Nicholson, A.A. *et al.* (2018). A review of the neurobiological basis of trauma-related dissociation and its relation to cannabinoid- and opiod-mediated stress response: A transdiagnostic, translational approach. *Current Psychiatry Reports*, 20(118), 1–14.

Lanius, R.A., Vermetten, E., Loewenstein, R.J., Brand, B. *et al.* (2010). Emotion modulation in PTSD: Clinical and neurobiological evidence for a dissociative subtype. *American Journal of Psychiatry*, 167(6), 640–647.

Levine, P.A. (2010). *In an Unspoken Voice: How the Body Releases Trauma and Restores Goodness*. Berkeley, CA: North Atlantic Books.

Malchiodi, C.A. (2020). *Trauma and Expressive Arts Therapy: Brain, Body, and Imagination in the Healing Process*. New York, NY: Guilford Publications.

May-Benson, T.A. and Schaaf, R. (2015). Ayres Sensory Integration® Intervention. In I. Söderback (ed.), *International Handbook of Occupational Therapy Interventions* (second edition). 633–646 Switzerland: Springer Cham.

Mikulincer, M., Shaver, P.R. and Solomon, Z. (2015). An Attachment Perspective on Traumatic and Posttraumatic Reactions. In M. Safir, H. Wallach and A. Rizzo (eds), *Future Directions in Post-Traumatic Stress Disorder: Prevention, Diagnosis, and Treatment*. New York, NY: Springer.

Muller, R.T., Sicoli, L.A. and Lemieux, K.E. (2000). Relationship between attachment style and posttraumatic stress symptomology among adults who report the experience of childhood abuse. *Journal of Traumatic Stress*, 13(2), 321–332.

Naste, T.M., Price, M., Karol, J., Martin, L. *et al.* (2018). Equine facilitated therapy for complex trauma (EFT-CT). *Journal of Child and Adolescent Trauma*, 11(3), 289–303.

Nicholson, A.A., Friston, K.J., Zeidman, P., Harricharan, S. *et al.* (2017). Dynamic causal modeling in PTSD and its dissociative subtype: Bottom-up versus top-down processing within fear and emotion regulation circuitry. *Human Brain Mapping*, 38(11), 5551–5561.

Ogden, P., Pain, C. and Fisher, J. (2006). A sensorimotor approach to the treatment of trauma and dissociation. *Psychiatric Clinics of North America*, 29(1), 265–279.

Ogle, C.M., Rubin, D.C. and Siegler, I.C. (2015). The relation between insecure attachment and posttraumatic stress: Early life versus adulthood traumas. *Psychological Trauma: Theory, Research, Practice, and Policy*, 7(4), 324–323.

Panksepp, J., (1998). *Affective Neuroscience: The Foundations of Human and Animal Emotions*. Oxford: Oxford University Press.

Payne, P., Levine, P.A., and Crane-Godreau, M.A. (2015). Somatic experiencing: Using interoception and proprioception as core elements of trauma therapy. *Frontiers in Psychology*, 6(93), 1–18. doi: 10.3389/fpsyg.2015.00093

Rao, R.P.N. and Sejnowski, T.J. (2001). Spike-timing-dependent Hebbian plasticity as temporal difference learning. *Neural Computation*, 13(10), 2221–2237.

Sandberg, D.A. (2010). Adult attachment as a predictor of posttraumatic stress and dissociation. *Journal of Trauma and Dissociation*, 11(3), 293–307.

Saper, C.B. and Lowell, B.B. (2014). The hypothalamus. *Current Biology*, 24 (23), R1111–R1116.

Schwartz, A. and Maiberger, B. (2018). *EMDR Therapy and Somatic Psychology*. New York, NY: W.W. Norton and Company.

Scott, S. and Babcock, J.C. (2010). Attachment as a moderator between intimate partner violence and PTSD symptoms. *Journal of Family Violence*, 25(1), 1–9.

Shapiro, L. and Spaulding, S. (2021). Embodied Cognition. In E.N. Zalta (ed.), *The Stanford Encyclopedia of Philosophy* (Winter 2021 Edition). Stanford, CA: Stanford University.

Sherrington, C.S. (1906). *The Integrative Action of the Nervous System*. New Haven, CT: Yale University Press.

Siegel, D.J. (2007). Mindfulness training and neural integration: Differentiation of distinct streams of awareness and the cultivation of wellbeing. *Social Cognitive and Affective Neuroscience*, 2(4), 259–263.

Terpou, B.A., Harricharan, S., McKinnon, M.C., Frewen, P., Jetly, R. and Lanius, R.A. (2019). The effects of trauma on brain and body: A unifying role for the midbrain periaqueductal gray. *Journal of Neuroscience Research*, 97(9), 1110–1140.

Twaite, J.A. and Rodriguez-Srednicki, O. (2004). Childhood sexual and physical abuse and adult vulnerability to PTSD: The mediating effects of attachment and dissociation. *Journal of Child Sexual Abuse*, 13(1), 17–38.

van der Kolk, B.A. (2003). The neurobiology of childhood trauma and abuse. *Child and Adolescent Psychiatric Clinics of North America*, 12(2), 293–317.

van der Kolk, B.A. (2015). *The Body Keeps the Score: Brain, Mind, and Body in the Healing of Trauma*. New York, NY: Viking.

Warner, E., Koomar, J., Lary, B. and Cook, A. (2013). Can the body change the score? Application of sensory modulation principles in the treatment of traumatised adolescents in residential settings. *Journal of Family Violence*, 28(7), 729–738.

Warner, E., Spinazzola, J., Westcott, A., Gunn, C. and Hodgdon, H. (2014). The body can change the score: Empirical support for somatic regulation in the treatment of traumatised adolescents. *Journal of Child and Adolescent Trauma*, 7(4), 237–246.

Yates, B.J., Catanzaro, M.F., Miller, D.J. and McCall, A.A. (2014). Integration of vestibular and emetic gastrointestinal signals that produce nausea and vomiting: Potential contributions to motion sickness. *Experimental Brain Research*, 232, 2455–2469.

Yochman, A. and Pat-Horenczyk, R. (2020). Sensory modulation in children exposed to continuous traumatic stress. *Journal of Child and Adolescent Trauma*, 13(1), 93–102.

Zakin, G., Solomon, Z. and Neria, Y. (2003). Hardiness, attachment style, and long term psychological distress among Israeli POWs and combat veterans. *Personality and Individual Differences*, 34(5), 819–829.

CHAPTER 9

Trauma-Transformative Principles in the Treatment of Complex Traumatic Stress Disorders

Christine A. Courtois and Julian D. Ford

Introduction

Complex trauma encompasses events or experiences that are:

> *Intentional interpersonal* acts that are *inescapable* and cause *injury* that is potentially *irreparable* … highly *intimate, intrusive,* and *invasive* of the body and the self of the individual, often involving *imminent threat,* the totality of which results in deformations of *identity* (including the capacity to *integrate one's identity and experience and maintain one's integrity*) and disrupting *interpersonal capacity for intimate and other* relationships. (Ford and Courtois, 2020, p.5)

Herman (1992b) originally conceptualized complex trauma as a descriptor for various forms of intrafamilial abuse (especially incest/sexual abuse and other forms of ongoing child maltreatment and domestic violence) and extreme conditions of captivity and disempowerment (as found in domestic violence and other situations of forced imprisonment). Based on her review of the then-available literature on the most common consequences of intrafamilial trauma in childhood (involving mostly female victims), she identified major developmental disruptions and maturational challenges that were in addition to those that made up the triad of criteria (re-experiencing, numbing, physiological hyperarousal) for the diagnosis of post-traumatic stress disorder (PTSD) as included in the *DSM-III* (American Psychiatric Association, 1980). These criteria were mostly derived from the study of war trauma and its impact on late adolescent or adult combatants (mostly male), a different population altogether. Herman (1992a) placed these additional symptoms into seven categories, as alterations in: 1) ability to regulate affective impulses; 2) attention and consciousness; 3) self-perception; 4) perception of the perpetrator; 5) relationships with others; 6) somatization and/or medical conditions; and 7) systems of meaning. She proposed the inclusion of a free-standing diagnosis of complex post-traumatic stress disorder (CPTSD) in the *DSM-IV* (American Psychiatric Association, 1994). Her proposal, despite being accepted by members of the anxiety disorders review committee, was overturned at a higher level of review. Instead, complex forms of PTSD were included listed as an associated feature of PTSD in the *DSM-IV* where they have remained through the current edition, *DSM-5* (American Psychiatric Association, 2013) despite subsequent proposals for inclusion.

However, the criteria for the diagnosis of PTSD in the *DSM-5* expanded from the original three categories to four (an avoidance and cognitive changes category was added) to address more complex presentations, making it more inclusive of complex trauma criteria. Also included was a dissociative sub-type of PTSD that may represent a form of complex trauma response.

As research on complex forms of trauma developed, a data base has emerged that demonstrates that complex forms of psychological trauma result in additional symptoms besides those included in PTSD (even in the newly expanded *DSM-5* criteria) (Brewin *et al.*, 2017; D'Andrea *et al.*, 2012). Based on these data, the most recent edition of the *International Classification of Disorders-11* (*ICD-11*) (World Health Organization, 2018) included a new and free-standing diagnosis of CPTSD applicable to adults, adolescents, and children with experiences of repeated, prolonged/continuous, or multiple forms of traumatic exposure and experience. This diagnosis is referred to as a 'sibling' diagnosis of 'classic or traditional' PTSD as defined in the *ICD*. It includes additional symptom criteria defined as Disturbances of Self-Organization (DSO), consisting of emotional dysregulation, negative self-concept, and interpersonal difficulties. Additionally, functional impairment was indicated as a requirement for the diagnosis, and dissociation and somatization/medical problems were noted as common in those with a history of complex trauma. A CPTSD diagnosis requires that one symptom from each of the three *ICD* PTSD diagnostic criteria are met in addition to at least one symptom from each of the DSO categories. Only one diagnosis (PTSD or CPTSD) can be made, and CPTSD supersedes PTSD.

The conceptual framework of CPTSD incorporates (neuro)developmental/maturational impact that is based on a personal and interpersonal resource loss model, a different theoretical model from the traditional conditioned fear-response model represented in the core symptom criteria of 'classic' PTSD. The inclusion of CPTSD in the *ICD* responds to the concerns of many practitioners that chronic/continuous/cumulative interpersonal violations (especially those that occur during childhood) have more broad-based impact beyond the core criteria and symptoms that make up PTSD. In turn, the impact of DSOs can extend across the entire lifespan as they undergird a wide range of mental health and somatic/medical problems, both at the time of the trauma and later. The findings of studies into adverse childhood experiences (ACEs) (Breuer *et al.*, 2020; Putnam *et al.*, 2020) and of recently conducted cross-cultural studies (Levin *et al.*, 2021; Redican *et al.*, 2021) have provided additional support for the diagnosis of CPTSD. Significant findings substantiate that those individuals with more ACEs who present for mental health treatment differ from those without such a history (Herzog and Schmahl, 2018), in ways that are consistent with the *ICD-11* formulation. Kira and colleagues recently reported that continuous traumatic stressors are the strongest predictor of CPTSD, followed by early childhood adversities, which themselves are often repetitive to the point of being continuous (Kira *et al.*, 2022).

Despite a developing body of research on complex trauma and its consequences, debate among traumatic stress professionals regarding both the reality and the utility of the CPTSD diagnosis has been continuous. On the one hand, there are those who argue that CPTSD is a redundant form of PTSD as it is now formulated and therefore is not needed. They identify PTSD symptoms as those that are most in need of treatment and amelioration and encourage a course of treatment that routinely focuses on the trauma and its processing as soon as possible. This position is buttressed by the evidence-based findings and recommendations contained within clinical practice guidelines produced by several professional organizations. For a synopsis of four of the most recent guideline documents, the reader can consult Hamblen *et al.* (2019). Proponents of this perspective posit that any additional symptoms are encompassed within the co-occurring diagnoses that accompany PTSD and can be treated separately if they do not remit with the PTSD symptom diminution.

On the other hand, CPTSD supporters counter that the current symptom description of PTSD is overly narrow in that it does not include the additional developmental and adaptive responses and symptoms that are common in those with a complex trauma history (especially from childhood adversities but also from other complex stressors at other points along the life course) and that are not entirely fear-based. Their view is that an encompassing diagnosis that takes the additional symptoms and difficulties into consideration is needed as it is more parsimonious and serves to direct a treatment process that is more broadly focused than on the trauma symptoms exclusively.

Evolving understanding and emerging types of complex trauma

In recent decades, an increase in professional and social attention to all forms of trauma and its relative ubiquity in the lives of many across the globe, including contemporary stressors (e.g. Covid-19 pandemic; the renewed reckoning of the impact of systemic racial and ethno-cultural discrimination and marginalization; political unrest and terrorism; mass shootings; and increases in the scope and severity of climate-related disasters, among others), has directed attention to its consequences. At present, several main typologies have been proposed by different groups of researchers and theoreticians. These may change going forward, but here we present one, including six different types that are generally recognized.

A major distinction can be drawn between types of trauma that are *impersonal* in their occurrence and causation (i.e. not deliberate or due to human design or action) – usually referred to as Type 1 – and those that are *interpersonal* in intent and perpetration – referred to as Type 11 (Terr, 1991). Type 1 *impersonal* trauma is usually of a sudden, unexpected, *accidental, and unintentional* (or not personally targeted) onset (e.g. accidents or catastrophes, weather- or climate-related disasters). Its occurrence is often attributed to an 'act of God or nature' or a strictly random occurrence that is due to being in the 'wrong place at the wrong time' and not due to other causation, planning, or intention on anyone's part. It is generally of short-term duration but may have a long trail of associated events and stresses (some of which may be additionally traumatic and traumatizing), as seen in the aftermath of a weather-related disaster such as a flood, fire, or hurricane that destroys homes and entire communities. It may also be long-lasting for some victims in terms of severe physical or emotional injury, including PTSD, associated anxiety and depression, and significant losses and psychosocial consequences (e.g. separation from or loss of family members, loss of home and community, struggles with bureaucratic agencies and difficulties being made whole again). The post-traumatic response may extend to the traumatized individual's loved ones and others in their community and can cause additional distress (relational stress, misunderstanding, conflict that can result in additional losses such as divorce or suicide). Less tangible losses might involve spiritual beliefs and changes in worldview. Impersonal forms of trauma can additionally include such circumstances as chronic illnesses, injuries, physical (including neurological) deformities and disabilities that occur on a random and unpredictable basis (and that sometimes involve intensive and repeated treatments used in an attempt to heal them that can additionally be traumatizing, such as burn injuries and treatment). Such illnesses and incapacities up to and including death can emerge at any time across the lifespan, causing significant life disruption and distress.

Type 11, *interpersonal* trauma, differs substantially from Type 1, primarily due to the nature of its causation, that is, the *intentional* actions of another person, alone or in a group or organization. It is sometimes referred to as 'human-induced' or 'human-produced' trauma that involves acts of interpersonal aggression and intrusion on the one hand or neglect or detachment on the other, often under the heading of 'interpersonal violence'

(IPV), directed primarily at children (child abuse) or adults (domestic or community violence). This type has two main categories:

1. Traumatic events caused or perpetrated by *strangers*.
2. Those caused or perpetrated by a *related or otherwise known* individual or group with whom the victimized person has some sort of relationship.

On average, since violations by strangers are more sudden and random/situational and those involved are unlikely to have a prior relationship or ongoing contact or access, violations of this sort are usually of a one-time or shorter duration. This scenario may be changing (creating a crossover between the two types) with the advent of the internet and social media, where those who initially made contact as strangers go on to develop a relationship over time in which grooming, provocations, violations, and victimizations are premeditated and intentional. In this case, the developing of established relationship becomes the context of the victimization, making it more like the second category where interpersonal violence perpetrated by related/known others is more likely premeditated and planned.

Victimizations perpetrated by known others are not usually sudden or committed violently or forcefully except in some cases when the intent is clearly to stun, frighten, or terrorize the victim into compliance. Instead, this form of victimization usually involves a pre-existing relationship of some sort as the context for access and then a progression of misrepresentations to rationalizations to engage/ensnare the victim into the activity. Once the violation occurs, the perpetrator continues to rationalize it or transfers responsibility for its occurrence by blaming or shaming the victim for having caused or wanted it. Thus, the relational context and the process or misrepresentation and projected blame can profoundly confuse and entrap the victim, while it allows for the repetition, continuance, and escalation of the victimization over time. The process continues when the perpetrator adds injunctions or threats to keep the behaviour hidden and secret from others, introducing the concept of wrongdoing and furthering the entrapment. Such forced silence can itself be traumatic as it interferes with disclosure and keeps the victim isolated and self-dependent in terms of coping.

The identity and role of the perpetrator, the relationship between victim and perpetrator, and the power differentials between them are particularly significant elements. The closer the relationship, the greater the degree of betrayal involved, resulting in more severe consequences for the victim, on average (Freyd, 1996). Whether interpersonal violence or other abuse/victimization occurs within a family or other context such as a fiduciary relationship or an organization, the victim's accessibility, dependence, marginalized status, and lack of power or status create additional conditions of entrapment that make recurrence likely. Moreover, when a relationship is used both to entrap a victim and to misrepresent the exploitive or abusive behaviour as a legitimate part of the relationship (referred to as grooming), as noted in the previous paragraph, the victim is often left confused and compliant, only to be devastated when the betrayal becomes apparent, whether at the time of its occurrence or years and even decades later. Research findings have determined that ambivalent attachment between abuser and victim (referred to as a trauma bond or 'Stockholm syndrome') is a quite common consequence of abuse that is relational. Nevertheless, it is frequently misunderstood and used to implicate or blame the victim and impugn their credibility.

In some cases, there is overlap between Types I and II, as is the case when what was originally understood to be a random accident, disaster, or injury is later found to be due to human impairment, malfeasance, or negligence (e.g. airline pilot or train conductor who was drunk or texting at the time of an accident; doctor who was impaired while performing medical procedures). This has been described by Terr (1991) as a *crossover* type that generally results in more distress for the victim due to the interpersonal involvement. Were it not for the individual's actions or inactions, the resultant disaster or accident would not have occurred.

The four remaining types are all variations of interpersonal trauma but place more emphasis on the victim in terms of identity, group memberships and ascribed lower social or power status and marginalization. Type III *identity-based* trauma refers to victimization that is based on major characteristics of the victim's personal identity, that are mostly permanent and unchangeable. These form the basis of or provide the rationale for discrimination and oppression that then become the gateway for additional and often insidious and continuous forms of victimization. These identity factors include the individual's gender (especially female), race (skin color, hair, facial and other body features), age, ethnicity, and sexual orientation and sexual identity, among the most prominent. Children and females have been found to be the most victimized groups in both domestic settings and in the broader community, based on their lesser size, maturation, and status (children), and gender stereotypes resulting in fewer rights, less power and status vis a vis men (girls and women) (McGinty *et al.*, 2021; Smith *et al.*, 2019), although other traumagenic or protective factors may exacerbate or mitigate gender-related vulnerability (Wilker *et al.*, 2021).

Type IV trauma is a counterpart of Type III in that it is based on another aspect of identity, this one having to do with the individual's *group membership* (Kira *et al.*, 2022). Members of the non-dominant group are identified as 'different from, the other, the infidel, the adversary, or the enemy' based on differences in nationality, ethnicity, cultural background and traditions, gender, religious beliefs and practices, political beliefs and affiliation, and innumerable other factors. These social contexts result in intergroup conflict that ranges from the occasional skirmish up to and including warfare and domination, colonization, oppression, discrimination, and, in some cases, ethnic cleansing and genocide. Combatants, prisoners of war, civilians exposed to warfare and those treated as the 'spoils of war,' captives and hostages held for ransom, political prisoners, asylum-seekers, refugees and other displaced populations living in camps or having no fixed status, address, or country all fit within this category.

Type V trauma is yet another variation of the previous two types. It involves trauma that is *intergenerational*, with discrimination and oppression as the basis of the colonization or enslavement of one group by another (Kira *et al.*, 2022). This is now identified as *ancestral* or *historical* trauma and involves the wholesale loss of property and family, tribal, or other personal and group rights and freedoms and the eradication of traditions in indigenous First Nation or other populations that are viewed as primitive or less-than in some way by those who consider themselves superior. The conquering of subjugated people by enslavers/colonizers (i.e. those with more power or status) is often accompanied by the sale/trafficking of family members and re-education/indoctrination in the ways of the dominant culture through family separations and enrollment in special camps and schools. Unfortunately, individuals in such contexts are very vulnerable to additional forms of mistreatment by those who administer those settings.

Type VI includes *cumulative, continuous*, and *insidious* trauma that encompasses multiple forms across all the different types (Kira *et al.*, 2022). Tragically, the most disenfranchised individuals and groups are at continuous and disproportionate risk for all forms of victimization, and some are re-victimized on an ongoing and continuous basis with no escape throughout their lives. Some researchers and theoreticians have recently emphasized ongoing and multiple (or intersectional) forms of trauma on some individuals, groups and populations, especially those who are marginalized, poverty-stricken, discriminated against, enslaved/trafficked or otherwise entrapped, and who have minimal resources and little power. For example, Ford and Courtois (2020) have discussed layered and continuous forms of trauma based on early life attachment trauma, abuse and poly-victimization, multiple childhood adversities, and re-victimization and the additional risks for marginalized community members. These individuals and groups bear the greatest trauma burden. Kira and colleagues (2022) have recently described these and other forms as *intersectional trauma* and referred to the past several years as the 'Covid-19 and the continuous traumatic stressors era'.

It has become apparent that most of these interpersonal traumas (and some of the impersonal ones as well) meet the defining criteria for complex trauma. That is, they are primarily interpersonal and intentional in causation (whether by an individual, group, or within an organization); occur within a relationship of some sort (familial, fiduciary, organizational, or societal) that is used to access the victim who is dependent in some way and has less power or resources (and size and maturity, in the case of children); are repeated to the point of becoming chronic and continuous, thereby creating risk for additional victimization in other contexts; are often synergistic and progressive in severity of intrusion or assault; and they entrap and disempower. As these forms of trauma are complex, as are their effects, which are discussed in the next section.

The compounded effects of complex trauma

As the diagnosis of CPTSD specifies, the symptoms of complex trauma encompass and are in addition to those that make up the diagnosis of PTSD. In the case of childhood abuse and adversities, these are developmental/maturational and, when unacknowledged or unaddressed at the time, transform into what Gelinas (1983, p.316) referred to as the 'secondary elaborations of the untreated effects.' This description can be applied to all forms of repeated and layered interpersonal trauma and their impact. These include the child's (or adult's) attempts to cope with the trauma at the time and later (referred to as survivor skills), which were adaptive in their original context of fear and danger but then become maladaptive secondary elaborations when utilized in different (often neutral or non-dangerous) contexts. Prominent examples are dissociation that becomes generalized and automatic in response to even minor stressors or out-of-context situations, the use of substances, relationships, risk-taking, violence towards self or others, or suicidality as a means of suppressing, reducing, coping with, or manifesting emotional pain. Deformations of identity and negative sense of self and self-worth create their own problems for the individual. Their relational history impacts their ability to trust others and to have healthy, mutual, and intimate relationships.

The relational setting of complex trauma, whether personal, group, organizational, or societal, creates betrayal trauma, a form initially introduced by Freyd (1996) and for which there is now considerable research support. As noted above, the closer the degree of the relationship between the participants and the greater the power differential between them, the greater the emotional damage. The victim must contend with the victimization itself in addition to its commission by someone who was in a position of responsibility to protect and safeguard rather than exploit. The betrayal-trauma concept has extended beyond its original focus on the primary perpetrator. It now applies to others who betray when they fail to provide help and protection and to bystanders who notice but do not intervene. This has previously been described as the 'second injury.' It also applies to organizations and their agents involved in not responding to reports and disclosures, instead covering up and protecting the accused (especially if they are prominent and powerful in some way) and disbelieving and blaming the complainant. This occurs so commonly that Freyd coined the term DARVO that stands for Deny, Attack, Reverse Victim and Offender, to describe this practice (Harsey and Freyd, 2020).

As discussed above, the original formulation of complex trauma was based on research findings regarding the effects of childhood abuse. In fact, our previous writing was originally focused on the complex developmental adversities and trauma in childhood and their consequences (Courtois *et al.*, 2009; Ford and Courtois, 2013, 2020). As the types of identified trauma have grown appreciably over the past decades, so has the recognition that other forms of complex trauma can occur throughout the entire life course whether *de novo* in adulthood and without a prior history or, more commonly, in layered form on top of previous traumatization. It is these many presentations and intersectionalities of complex trauma exposures and their myriad and often synergistic after-effects and secondary elaborations that we address in this contribution.

For example, research studies of veterans with a history of both war trauma and childhood traumatization have suggested that such a history (especially when unacknowledged and unresolved) impedes recovery from war-related PTSD while maintaining other life difficulties (Ford,1999; Ford and Kidd, 1998). Violations that are based on individual characteristics and group membership can form an ongoing underlay in the individual's life that involves both continuous and cumulative victimization. These can involve incessant microaggressions and unremitting forms of other types of intrusions and violations that take place on an ongoing or more ambient basis.

All of this leads to the conclusion that, although the treatment of adult-onset PTSD symptoms through evidence-based trauma-focused treatments such as prolonged exposure (PE), cognitive processing therapy (CPT), eye movement desensitization and reprocessing (EMDR), narrative exposure therapy (NET), and others has been found to be efficacious for the symptoms of PTSD, additional treatment for the supplemental symptoms of more complex variants is needed, as are different treatment models and applications. As we lead into the discussion of treatment, we wish to be explicit that there are many cases where exposure to potentially traumatic events or experiences does not result in PTSD or CPTSD (or any other mental health disturbance for that matter), nor do we wish to downplay individual resilience and the significance of supportive others and institutions (Karatzias *et al.*, 2020; Vallieres *et al.*, 2021). According to multiple research findings (Able and Benedek, 2019; Lauterbach and Armour, 2016; McGuire *et al.*, 2021), *naturalistic recovery*, where the victim experiences acute traumatic responses in the immediate aftermath that remit with time (generally within a supportive context), is a trajectory that can occur for children and adults. However, such naturalistic recovery is the exception among those victimized as children or at any developmental epoch for victims living in other more complex closed-system traumatic circumstances, especially where there is lack of effective intervention and treatment. Some individuals can naturalistically recover, especially if they receive strong emotional support and intervention that resolves trauma symptoms and interferes with the typical course of shame, self-blame, and other personal and relational distress. But we also want to express concern that many traumatized individuals do not realize they have been traumatized, have at most partial or fragmented memories of traumatic experiences, or disconnect the traumatic experiences from their symptoms (whether these were ongoing or appeared in delayed fashion).

Thus, we believe there are many 'hidden' or unacknowledged trauma survivors who would benefit both by making the association and receiving support to help them to do so. In our previous writing, we have also discussed the limitations of the current diagnostic systems for the mental health and life sequelae of complex trauma, labeled these as *complex traumatic stress disorders* and called for additional research and the ongoing evolution of definitions and formulations (Courtois and Ford, 2013; Ford and Courtois, 2020). In fact, many victims and their supporters argue to substitute the word 'disorder' with 'injury' as a means of de-stigmatizing and normalizing post-traumatic responses.

The sequenced relationship-based model of complex trauma treatment

When Herman (1992a) first introduced CPTSD, she also presented a sequenced three-phase treatment model based on the one developed by French neurologist Pierre Janet at the end of the 19th century (Herman, 1992b). His patients resembled the typical dissociative complex trauma (or dissociative sub-type of PTSD) patient in many ways, so the application of his model was seen as fitting. The sequenced model consists of three distinct but often overlapping phases, each containing treatment tasks, preceded by a period of pre-treatment and assessment. It is largely based on clinical consensus (and available and emerging treatment outcome findings) developed by those working with the complex trauma patient population. As noted above, it has generated controversy in the research and treatment community (van Vliet *et al.*, 2018) because it does not call for the immediate application of trauma-focused treatments and instead recommends an initial period devoted to safety, psychoeducation, skill-building, and the development of a treatment alliance.

Although presented in linear form that suggests a direct chronology, the approach we will describe is not intended to be rigid or lockstep in application (Ford and Courtois, 2020). Rather, it is expected that clients will move forward and back between the phases based on their individual circumstances, including their resources, deficits, motivations, and context, among many others. This will also occur based on expectable stressors in life and in the therapeutic alliance over the course of the treatment. Moreover, as some complex trauma survivors are highly dissociative (Jowett et al., 2021) and additionally at high risk for re-victimization (and might be still caught within the past or current abuse), as well as for self-harm, addictions, suicidality, and other violence to or from others, these risks and their presentation as crises in treatment deserve an urgent response (Ford, 2021). Recent integrative approaches to treatment for complex traumatic stress disorders based on new research findings (Briere and Lanktree, 2011; Briere and Scott, 2014; Ford and Courtois, 2020; Greenberg, 2021; Karatzias et al., 2021) has suggested other modes and chronologies of treatment strategies, including those that are multi-modal and are discussed in more detail below. We (Ford, 2021; Ford and Courtois, 2020) have also discussed picking and choosing strategies and treatment tasks in accordance with the client's specific needs and preferences as part of a collaborative therapeutic effort.

The relationship component of treatment

Although Herman discussed relationship aspects of treatment, including the need for connection and community, we expanded on this aspect of treatment based on recently available information from the neurosciences about attachment/relational trauma in early life and its neurobiological and psychosocial impact (Ford, 2020), including attachment style (Ford and Courtois, 2020). We further incorporated research findings about what are now known as evidence-based relational variables and their significance in the success of treatment (Norcross and Lambert, 2018), factors largely ignored in the available treatment guidelines for PTSD (Courtois and Brown, 2019). A systematic review of evidence-based relational variables and their efficaciousness in the treatment of trauma indicated that alliance was of particular important (Ellis et al., 2018). We also attended to the recent writings in relational psychoanalysis and other treatment models that emphasize the role of the relationship as a foundation of treatment (Howell, 2020). Finally, we integrated our model with the trauma-informed care and trauma-referenced philosophy and treatment orientations that emphasize the importance of an informed, supportive, and non-judgmental relationship and, in reference to interpersonal trauma, posit 'relational healing for relational injury.' Kinsler et al. (2009) and Pearlman and Courtois (2005) articulated how the relationship is both the context and catalyst for relational healing to occur and that both relationship and therapeutic techniques are called for. Kinsler (2017) expanded on this chapter in his recently published book on the same topic.

Because betrayal trauma is so common, its relational effects are brought into the treatment relationship as they are into other relationships. It is advisable for therapists to have specialized knowledge and awareness of the relatively unique challenges and treatment traps, including common transference and countertransference responses and roles in working with the traumatized, so they can anticipate them and have some idea about how to respond to and manage them (Chu, 1988). Both the challenges and the relational demands – as well as learning about the client's traumatic experiences, including humans' capacity for cruelty – can be disconcerting for the therapist. This is especially likely if their professional training has not included education or training about trauma and its treatment – unfortunately often the case (Courtois and Gold, 2009). Where a therapist has had their own history of trauma, it is advisable that they have worked to resolve it and have developed an 'earned security' attachment status that will allow them to stay emotionally regulated in response to these common challenges. These strategies are in the interest of avoiding usual pitfalls, of not inadvertently re-traumatizing the client, and of sustaining the therapist's health and career. The reader is referred to our text (Ford and Courtois, 2020) and others (Davies and Frawley, 1994; Howell, 2020; Kinsler, 2017; Muller, 2018; Pearlman and Saakvitne, 1995) for additional information about relational issues, including dissociation that occurs within and outside the treatment setting. We will return to the topic of relationship when we present our PRISM model below, after we outline the sequenced model.

The pre-treatment period – introduction, assessment, and preliminary treatment planning

This period has been presented separately from the three treatment phases, but it is an integral component of treatment that should not be omitted, nor should it be treated casually (in our individual clinical consultations, we have both had numerous experiences of therapists who have not considered nor completed anything more than a cursory assessment, something we consider a grave clinical error). It calls for an introduction and assessment as part of the intake, followed by collaborative discussion and treatment planning prior to the advent of treatment. The major exception to this would be if the client arrives in a condition of crisis or danger when immediate action might be in order, as discussed by Ford (2021). But even when that is the case, Ford recommends assessing the situation and the client as much as is possible before proceeding.

A broad and comprehensive biopsychosocial evaluation is called for that includes questions about trauma and adverse childhood and other life events, along with the more standard areas of inquiry. The therapist must be mindful that traumatized clients might have difficulty with answering questions, so explaining the purpose of the assessment and how it is conducted can be important. So is being mindful of the client throughout, with appreciation that they might not be able to answer some questions and pay attention to their responses. In the event that the client becomes overwhelmed in some way, helping them to re-orient to the situation and to slow down and have some control is necessary. Furthermore, some clients choose not to disclose some of their experiences and reactions, even if asked directly. The therapist should not assume they are being uncooperative or dishonest, merely that they are not ready. Many clients have described a need to get to know the therapist and to develop some initial trust before they can divulge secrets and other closely held information.

In addition to interview-based assessment, screening and assessment questionnaires that assess trauma history and PTSD/CPTSD (and related) symptoms can provide helpful information for both the client and the therapist (Briere and Spinazzola, 2009; Spinazzola and Briere, 2020). Briere and Lanktree (2011) have developed a comprehensive treatment model based on planned repeat assessments used to direct (or re-direct) the course of the treatment and the strategies employed. This is in keeping with the model of customizing the treatment to the client. The therapist might also want to introduce the process of in-session feedback, whether done verbally or by a short check sheet in each session. Inviting feedback in this way supports collaboration and transparency in the process. This further supports the goal of empowerment by inviting the client's participation – something that initially be very discomforting, especially for those who have had ongoing experiences of 'being done to' or 'unseen' and whose needs or point of view have gone unrecognized.

This period (usually two to four sessions, sometimes more) is a time for the potential client and therapist to get a preliminary 'read' on one another and to determine whether they can work together. They review the assessment information and the client's presenting treatment concerns and goals to arrive at collaborative goal setting and treatment planning (again in the interest of transparency). In this early phase it essential to provide the client with a general introduction to the structure and process of the treatment, along with the 'rules of the road' in a treatment contract/document that fully explains rights and responsibilities of both parties and important issues such as confidentiality/mandated reporting and other extra-treatment actions (i.e. Tarasoff warning, voluntary and involuntary hospitalization, legal actions or family cut-offs), billing and payment, boundaries and limitations, and means and times of the therapist's accessibility. These form the foundation of treatment that can be referred to when and if issues or challenges arise.

Phase 1: Safety, education, skill building, stabilization, relationship building

Phase 1 includes and builds on the education provided in the assessment period, something that continues over the entire course of the treatment. The initial focus is present-day safety and how to achieve and maintain it – a process that might take a great deal of time and attention, particularly when the client is in an ongoing circumstance of danger. This might involve learning to be as safe as possible through preventive and self-defensive strategies when lack of safety cannot be easily changed. Moreover, when the client is a direct danger to self or to or from others (still in the original abuse, domestic violence, prostitution, trafficking, etc.), strategies need to be developed through a process of repeated risk and violence assessment, development of an ongoing safety plan in collaboration with the client, and distress tolerance and impulse management training. This also involves the teaching of a variety of skills, beginning with self-calming strategies (breathing and somatic awareness) and emotion identification and modulation, followed by other life skills:

- Identifying addictions and beginning the process of achieving sobriety.
- Encouraging preliminary and mostly cognitively-based narration of the trauma, interspersed with the other tasks.
- Identifying primary modes of coping and cognitions and beliefs about the trauma and about the self and others.
- Identifying prominent symptoms of PTSD and CPTSD, such as flashbacks, emotion dysregulation, and dissociation.
- Identifying evocative or activating cues – commonly referred to as triggers – and teaching skills for grounding and managing (dis)stress reactions in the moment, and learning to deliberately avoid, distract or distance from, or otherwise handle them in order to have more control.
- Developing life stabilization, as a chaotic lifestyle is not uncommon.
- Working collaboratively to encourage assertiveness and personal empowerment as well as behavioural activation to counter disempowerment, helplessness, and depression.
- Identifying relational patterns with others and teaching new modes of interacting where indicated (at times, adjunctive couple or family counseling is indicated).
- Developing a working alliance with the therapist – not always an

easy task as authority figures are often mistrusted and relationships avoided.

As can be discerned, many of the interventions of this phase are directed at the disturbances of self-organization as well as the classic PTSD symptoms. The therapist is charged with providing a relational context that is safe and contained through reliability, consistency, and being emotionally regulated, in the process providing a new relational template for the client. Furthermore, the therapist works within the parameters of the treatment frame, introduced during the pre-treatment segment, described above. In all things, they attempt to follow Linehan's dictum (Linehan, 1993), 'reinforce the right thing', but do so in ways that attend to the client's ongoing shame and relational sensitivities.

Finally, where there are other co-morbid mental health conditions and diagnoses, such as depression, anxiety, substance abuse disorder or other addictions, or pronounced medical conditions, these may require separate assessment and concurrent treatment according to their acuity and the degree of impairment involved. Interventions might include psychopharmacology and other forms of adjunctive treatment. It is sometimes the case that addressing one issue may cause another to be remitted (e.g. identifying and changing erroneous or problematic beliefs may allow for the remission of depression) or allow another to be uncovered (e.g. developing trust in the therapeutic relationship may allow for the disclosure of previously hidden issues such as self-injury or dissociation, that then can be addressed).

There are admittedly many treatment tasks here, and the necessity of addressing them varies dramatically by client and circumstance. Some clients enter treatment with established skills and attributes and are quite resilient, while others are lacking these foundations and need more remediation and intensive treatment. In fact, Kluft (1994) identified characteristics and descriptors for clients with high, medium, and low trajectories that can be helpful in initial and repeat assessment. The low trajectory group – those with the least environmental and personal resources – might benefit greatly from the support they derive in this stage and never move beyond it. This should not be considered a failure but rather a tailoring of the treatment to the client, discussed in more detail below. Additionally, the client's attachment style is of considerable importance (Alexander and Anderson, 1994; Wallin, 2007). Those with a secure attachment background and style (an inner working model of self and others), despite their history of complex trauma, bring more personal and interpersonal resources to the treatment than do those with insecure dismissive or pre-occupied or disorganized styles. They typically have a stronger sense of self and self-worth, have skills in emotional identification and modulation, are more trusting of others and have fewer relational difficulties and a support system as a result. They are therefore likely to move through this phase more quickly and efficiently than clients with more deficits. This is especially the case for those with high internal fragmentation, and personal incoherence about their history, a disorganized style, and fewer resources, typically those who are highly dissociated, up to and including dissociative identity disorder (DID). These conditions may require the therapist to devote much more time and attention to the development of a secure attachment that, in turn, allows for the patient's self-exploration and the elaboration of more self-integration and a growing sense of positive self-worth.

Thus far, we have not directed attention to memories of past traumas or the use of trauma-focused treatments. While these might be selectively and productively applied in Phase 1, the general consensus among clinicians most experienced in treating complex trauma is that trauma-focused treatments should not be deployed until Phase 2. This is after the client has gained a foundation of greater emotional and life stability and resultant ability to manage the painful emotions that accompany trauma processing, defined as facing rather than avoiding the trauma, and experiencing the associated feelings. This issue is a major point of contention with advocates of trauma-focused treatments who make a case for the immediate use of these techniques with most traumatized clients to process their trauma symptoms in the interest of diminishing or ending them (van Vilet *et al.*, 2018). They cite the available and growing body of research findings regarding the efficacy of these techniques, even when applied almost immediately. Complex trauma proponents, by and large, do not dispute the efficacy findings but do question their wholesale applicability to complex trauma patients as an initial strategy.

Many clinicians who have extensive experience in treating individuals with complex trauma histories advocate for careful assessment and preparation prior to initiating trauma memory processing (Cloitre *et al.*, 2011). Depending on the client's preference and internal and external resources and supports, this may be accomplished quite rapidly, providing the client with a sense of security and confidence that is likely to lead to a positive therapeutic outcome in a comparable or even faster time period than if Phase 1 is skipped or greatly compressed. When Phase 1 takes longer, it is important that this is based on a careful ongoing assessment of the client's readiness, and not on an *a priori* perception by the therapist that a client with a complex trauma history is deficient in self-regulation capacities and resources.

Thus, the sequenced meta-model is not inconsistent with maximizing the efficiency and timeliness of engaging clients with complex trauma histories in trauma memory processing. It provides a personalized approach that underscores the importance of preparation of the client for memory processing based on an assessment – not an *a priori* assumption – of the client's readiness and ensuring truly informed consent by the client for engaging in this aspect of therapy. This also is consistent with evidence that client preference for the treatment approach has been shown to be an important contributor to positive outcomes in PTSD treatment (Zoellner *et al.*, 2009). Precisely how best to prepare and support clients beginning in Phase 1 remains an open question, and for that reason we will describe an adaptation of the sequential approach that we describe as PRISM principles in the next section.

Phase 2: Trauma memory processing

Phase 2 is devoted to remembrance, memory processing, and mourning, as articulated by Herman (1992b). In this phase, the client is encouraged to go beyond the cognitive recounting of the trauma (the story line) and to begin or continue to experience and express feelings associated with its occurrence and consequences. This is the phase where trauma-focused treatments, with their emphasis on directly accessing and processing traumatic memories, are most applicable. Since there are several trauma-focused treatments to choose from, they should be presented to and discussed with clients as to their method and relative benefits and risks and then selected according to the client's preference. For example, some clients clearly prefer PE due to its relative brevity and direct exposure, while others prefer EMDR since the trauma does not need to be verbalized and instead is focused on by the client. Others are not inclined towards any model, preferring instead a more chronological or even freeform recounting, that involves gradual rather than prolonged exposure. Briere and Scott (2014), Ford and Courtois (2020) and Ford (2018) have articulated methods for accessing and processing memories in this way and Courtois (1999) has provided guidance for the therapist to maintain a stance of supportive neutrality when memories are discontinuous and fragmented.

Whatever the method, all strategies involve a deconditioning of the fear response and other associated emotions. There are certainly many others, some utilizing different sense modalities. For example, some might involve directed life review writing or the development of a life chronology as used in narrative exposure therapy. The focus of such exercises might be on positive and negative experiences over the lifespan, the traumatic events, resilience and new understandings about coping and survival, or all three. Other methods might involve freeform or directed artwork and journaling/poetry writing, and somatic explorations and discussion. Where there has been moral injury, those issues might need to be addressed with a separate protocol, as described by Griffin *et al.* (2019).

Once traumatic memories have been identified and processed, the client feels able to recall them without avoidance and with psychophysiological self-regulation. They can then separate past events from the present. In the language of attachment and dissociation, the client integrates experience that has previously been cut-off, in the process becoming more cognisant or more coherent in their understanding of their experiences. This process is immediate in some cases or can take much longer, as in those with fragmented or shattered identities (including dissociative identity disorder) who must break through amnesia, depersonalization, and derealization barriers and associated internal conflict to develop a more cohesive sense of self and a more coherent life story.

Whatever its duration or intensity, processing is often accompanied by increased recognition of the toll taken and the losses accrued. This may usher in a period of deep introspection and mourning and (delayed and present-day) bereavement involving lost childhood, lost good parenting, lost lifetime, lost abilities – including the ability to be personally integrated – undeveloped aspects of self and identity apart from the trauma, unrealized relationships, lost opportunities, and so on. Often the most significant recognition occurs when the 'scales fall from the eyes' of the client in terms of primary and secondary betrayals and how significant relationships were corrupted through their objectification, exploitation, and projected blame and shame (i.e. how they were left 'holding the bag' of responsibility and distress). However, this is also a time when, as they get more in touch with themselves and their story, clients develop a nascent pride to replace the shame and become more empowered in their life and their relationships. This work continues into the next phase.

Phase 3: Life re-integration

Phase 3 involves further self-integration along with a re-integration into life apart from the trauma. It is oriented toward assessing and possibly changing or rebalancing relationships with others and is organized around safety and mutuality. Survivor clients now have more clarity about themselves and their experiences and this knowledge and their newly developed skills to negotiate and navigate relations help as they focus on the present and the future. In the case of abusive family members or others who have been enablers or bystanders, discussion and or confrontation may start the process. In some cases, it will lead to separation from those who were and remain unsafe, whether physically, sexually, or emotionally, and who refuse to make changes. In others, it will result in newly established boundaries and limits while remaining in the relationship. This process resembles the stage of addiction recovery when, in order to maintain sobriety, recovering addicts must determine who will and will not be supportive and who will put their new sobriety at risk. It is also in this phase where other unaddressed or unresolved issues come to the fore. These might include the ability to develop and maintain friendships and a support system, to develop and maintain intimate relationships, to address issues involving intimacy and sexual functioning, to improve or rebalance parenting as needed, and occupational choice, training, and functioning, among many others. Many of these are conducted in adjunctive settings such as Alcoholics Anonymous (AA) or Adult Children of Alcoholics (ACOA) meetings, and group, couple, and family therapy, to name but a few.

Although this phase might seem the easiest of the three, the transition to 'normal' can be fraught with all kinds of unanticipated challenges. The primary therapist will need to provide ongoing support, perspective, and encouragement while therapeutic gains are applied in a different context. It is helpful for the therapist to assist the client to anticipate and plan for them. For example, it is not uncommon for family members and others to resist changes in the client, deny the need for them, or maintain a stance of abuse and dismissal. They may pressure the client to 'change back' to maintain their own comfort level (which often involves denial and other minimization) rather than what is in the client's best interest. In turn, this might result in the client losing ground or relapsing in some way and they may need to return to Phase 1 to rebuild or strengthen skills. As throughout the course of therapy, this should be identified as a chance for problem solving and not as a complete failure on the client's part, although they might be tempted to see it that way.

Another challenge arises if the client chooses to take action such as making a report to criminal justice or a licensing board or mounting a civil suit or engaging in criminal proceedings. Any of these actions are best undertaken after the client has completed the bulk of their processing and is in a relatively stable status because, even today, the complainant victim's credibility is often challenged. The client should be aware of these possible consequences before making the decision to pursue action. The therapist's ongoing support is especially significant in such actions that might extend the duration of treatment.

Finally, bringing therapy to an end must be addressed, as it is a substantial relational event, involving change and loss. Kinsler (2017) has compellingly written of different ways that these treatments might end. Whenever possible, it should be undertaken mindfully and with attention to the client's history of traumatic separations and loss. Adequate time to plan for a way to say goodbye and to end the treatment is recommended to provide for a different form, or as Salzberg (2010) poignantly puts it, 'a good enough ending.'

Augmenting the sequenced meta-model with PRISM

Since the publication of our revised book on treatment approaches (Ford and Courtois, 2020), we have devised a set of recommended principles, approaches, and strategies for complex trauma treatment, fitting the acronym PRISM. This refers to treatment that is **Personalized**, **Relational**, **Integrative**, **Sequenced/Strategic**, and **Multi-Modal/Multi-Dimensional**. It is very much in line with trauma-informed care and, in fact, uses this as a foundation; it is also designed to be highly responsive to traumatized individuals, whatever their trauma types, and is trauma transformative.

Personalized treatment

Personalization of the treatment is necessitated to counter the objectification that individuals with histories of complex trauma have experienced and endured. The therapist seeks to directly counter this non-recognition and invalidation, whether it occurred by commission or omission (or both), by exhibiting a deep interest in and resonance with the client. These, along with other factors such as personal reliability and consistency, ongoing emotional regulation, and boundary management, serve to create a secure treatment relationship. It is advisable for therapists to generally determine the client's attachment style early in the treatment as it will assist them in adjusting their own interventions. Since these clients tend to be emotionally dysregulated and skittish regarding relationships (covering the spectrum from overly attached/compliant/preoccupied/protective to overly detached/defiant/contemptuous and anything in between, often exhibited in an unexpected and paradoxical way), the therapist must tailor their responses to point it out and notice with the client and to build trust incrementally. They must also expect setbacks, relapses, and ruptures, which they seek to identify and resolve with the client in the interest of relational trust and growth. Such relational repair is an essential component of developing new relational templates.

Psychophysiological approaches are incorporated into the treatment as post-traumatic responses are physiological as well as psychological. As noted by van der Kolk (2014), 'the body keeps the score,' and attention to the client's physical responses is used as a means of accessing and identifying emotions and to counter dissociation/fragmentation. Many clinicians have found that close attention to the hyperactivation and hypoactivation of the traumatic stress response as well as attention to dissociative responses can yield benefits in self-awareness and personal integration for these clients who may be highly depersonalized (Ogden, 2020).

Philosophy and principles of treatment are recognized and adhered to. These include but are not limited to many of the issues discussed above, especially respect for the individual and their right to self-determination; belief in natural healing potential and resilience; a mindset of strengths-based empowerment, including client preference about treatment strategies and their responsibility for their own motivation and healing; incorporation of principles of trauma-informed care; the use of evidence-based and supported treatments wherever possible in the treatment; specialized knowledge and training of the therapist; professional self-presentation and demeanor on the part of the therapist; and recognition of the impact of trauma on the treating therapist and others.

Professional standards and ethics are also treatment foundations. Therapists must practice within the strictures of their profession and be especially mindful of the ethics dictum, 'First, do no harm.' As pertains to traumatized clients, this can be re-phrased as 'First, do no *more* harm' (Courtois, 2015). Therapists are not expected to conduct treatments that are free of errors, but they are expected to practice personal mindfulness and self-management and to engage in ethical behavior and practice.

Relational treatment

As previously discussed, the *relationship* is a core element of successful treatment for complex interpersonal trauma. A *responsive* and *responsible* therapist extends *respect* to the client, a position that counters previous disregard and disrespect. The treatment goal is the *resolution of the trauma* and its most egregious effects wherever possible, and the client's *recovery*, including the development of a life worth living that is self-determined and largely devoid of ongoing trauma symptoms. The therapist takes a stance of *resonance with and reflection of the client* to engage them in self-exploration, leading to *restoration of self* and increased capacity for *relational engagement and intimacy*. Therapists work according to a learning and change model and expect *relapses, setbacks, and ruptures*, not perfection, in the healing process, something they teach their clients. *Relational ruptures* should be expected, and when they occur, the therapist identifies them and seeks to engage in their *repair*. as these are often very significant events in a client's relational development. Boundary management is especially important, as these clients' boundaries have been violated, often repeatedly, and many have been conditioned into dual and transactional relationships, something they might project into the therapy and onto the therapist. Awareness of *risk* and knowledge about *risk-management* in this population are also important issues for which therapists must carefully prepared (Courtois *et al.*, 2020).

Integrated treatment

The unique *identity* of the client, including issues of *intersectionality and personal contextual factors*, is ascertained to deepen understanding of the client and their exposure/experience and subjective response. This assists in providing an *individualized and integrated* treatment. As noted, this customization may include the use of many different strategies, paces, and chronologies, all adapted to the client. The *intensity of the treatment* is titrated throughout to keep the client in a window of tolerance and not in ongoing conditions of hyper- or hypoarousal. The client's *identity development* (and *integration* in cases where it is highly fragmented and dissociated) is a major goal.

The *impact of this work on the therapist* is specifically discussed in the professional and trauma-informed care literature and approach. When unacknowledged and unaddressed, vicarious trauma and secondary traumatic stress can put both therapist and client at risk. To both tolerate the strain that accompanies this work and to sustain themselves, therapists (along with their program administrators, supervisors, and colleagues) need to monitor their own emotional and physical health, their life quality and satisfaction, and receive ongoing support through consultation, supervision, continuing education, and other methods. Sustainability can also be facilitated by all working from the same overarching trauma-informed and responsive framework and philosophy.

Safety and security

This treatment begins with a focus on personal *safety*, a focus that extends throughout. Recovery is difficult if not impossible without personal, relational, and environmental safety. At times, absolute safety is impossible to achieve. When that is the case, *skills and strategies for safety* are taught and reinforced using a collaboratively devised *safety plan*. Not uncommonly, complex trauma clients lead chaotic and drama-filled lives. Where these come to light, the therapist must seek to teach life *skills for stabilization and self-regulation*. Education occurs across the entire course of treatment.

Relationally, the therapist strives to provide a '*secure base*' and a '*safe haven*' to *support* the client in self-exploration and trauma processing. As noted above, the relational context can be highly activating for the interpersonally traumatized client, who may initially respond using the 'tried and true' methods associated with their primary attachment style – that is, their coping responses and adaptations developed as defense and self-protection. The therapist must be prepared to bring these *styles of attachment and their associated strategies to the client's attention* as they introduce them to other methods. The therapist also teaches *skills for emotional and other self-regulation*, starting by co-regulating with the client as a model for an increased capacity for self-regulation. The treatment and especially the impact of a secure relationship assists the client in developing a more *secure style*, usually labeled as 'earned secure.'

The treatment is holistic in its orientation and scope. Therefore, attention to *somatic issues*, presentations, and distress are warranted. *Somatic approaches* may be used in conjunction with other strategies to assist with affective identification and self-regulation. Personal mindfulness and strategies such as breathing, yoga, directed artwork or writing, or personal journaling might be used to help the client calm their bodies and clear their minds.

The therapist places emphasis on *self-care* and components of a healthy lifestyle, something that might be quite new to the client, since illness (some of it psychosomatic) and self-neglect and inattention to personal well-being (as conclusively identified in the ACEs studies), personal risk-taking, disengagement from self, and self-neglect are so prominent in this population.

For the therapist, ongoing *sources of support including supervision and consultation* (whether individual or in a group) are highly recommended. Such activities offer outside support and a perspective that help therapists in managing their own reactions/countertransference/vicarious trauma responses, and in directing the treatment. They can be invaluable when the therapist is having a personal life crisis or when crises develop in the context of the treatment.

Multi-modal treatment

This treatment can incorporate and integrate strategies and modalities from across all therapeutic orientations. This treatment is increasingly considered *multi-modal and multi-dimensional* in application and as encompassing *multi-component models*, all selected and applied according to the therapist's training and experience and the client's needs. The intensity of the treatment is deliberately *modulated* throughout to accommodate the client's status, capacities, and resources, and to remain in the window of tolerance. Moreover, throughout the treatment, the client's *motivation* is assessed and enhanced as needed. Clients are encouraged to own and lean into their recovery efforts and are reinforced for their motivation, hard work, and treatment gains. The therapist is free to *modify* the treatment as it progresses according to client feedback, repeat assessments, and clinical observations and judgment.

Memory processing through exposure rather than avoidance is the recommended treatment for the deconditioning and resolution of the trauma response. It is not a process that can be applied to all clients, as some are unable to tolerate it and some choose not to address the trauma directly.

Conclusion

This chapter has reviewed information about complex trauma, its various types and permutations, its common after-effects, the inclusion of CPTSD as a diagnosis in the *ICD-11*, and models and strategies for psychotherapy with complex trauma survivors. Although additional empirical support is needed and is underway for both the diagnosis and its treatment, preliminary findings support the utility of a sequence of hierarchical phases and treatment tasks. We have supplemented this with principles of practice that have received empirical as well as consensus endorsement. Many complex trauma clients enter treatment in crisis and in conditions of personal and relational brokenness. While these and other factors frequently make work with this population quite challenging and even vexing, success in reversing these factors can provide powerful satisfaction for both therapist and client alike. Therapists who have treated clients with complex trauma histories in accordance with the format described here have expressed how it helped them in organizing and applying treatment. Therapists have remarked on developing vicarious resilience in parallel with their clients, whose perseverance and tenaciousness they admire.

KNOWLEDGE AND PRACTICE REFLECTION

Joe Tucci, Janise Mitchell, Ed Tronick and Stephen W. Porges

There are multiple themes inspired by the expansive territory reviewed by Courtois and Ford in this chapter. All of them are significant to the way in which practitioners, organizations and systems can better support victims and survivors of interpersonal violence.

The expanded and detailed taxonomy about the types of complex trauma is critical knowledge for trauma-transformative organizations. It establishes a richer way of understanding how different forms of violation intersect with each other, leading to more complex and amplified experiences of trauma. A summary of their analysis is presented in below. We have made a slight amendment to Type 3 so that it is clear that the identity basis of the violation is inclusive of individual and group characteristics.

Category	Form	Example
Type 1	Impersonal trauma	Sudden, unexpected, accidental, and unintentional events, such as a weather disaster or car accident.
Type 2	Trauma experienced as a result of interpersonal violation and abuse	Child physical abuse, child sexual abuse, family and domestic violence, kidnapping.
Type 2A	Trauma from interpersonal violence perpetrated by strangers	Child sexual abuse perpetrated by an adult who physically traps a child at a public place, such as a shopping centre toilet.

Type 2B	Trauma from interpersonal violence perpetrated by related or familiar individuals	Grooming of a child by someone in a position of authority, such as teacher, sporting coach or religious leader. Bullying by a peer online. Child sexual, physical and emotional abuse perpetrated by a parent. Physical and sexual assault by an intimate partner.
Type 3	Individual and group identity-based trauma experienced as a result of discrimination and oppression	Based on major characteristics of the individual or group identity (e.g. gender – especially female, race, skin color, hair, facial and other body features, age, socio-economic status, ethnicity, sexual orientation and sexual identity, geography and educational attainment.) These characteristics form the basis of or provide the rationale for prejudiced-based violation. Abuse and violence towards people with disabilities. Physical and financial abuse of the elderly.
Type 4	Group identity-based trauma experienced as a result of persecution, war, genocide	Ethnic cleansing and genocide. Combatants, prisoners of war, civilians exposed to warfare, captives and hostages held for ransom, political prisoners, asylum-seekers, refugees and other displaced populations living in detention camps.
Type 5	Group identity-based trauma experienced as a result of colonization and enslavement	Sale/trafficking of family members. Forced separation of First Nations children from families as a result of assimilationist government policies. Failure to recognize traditional ownership of land. Ongoing impact of historical massacres of First Nations people.
Type 6	Cumulative, continuous and insidious trauma that encompasses multiple forms across all the different types	Exploitation of children and young people who are living in foster and residential care. Poly-victimization of children due to concurrent and ongoing experiences of physical, sexual and psychological abuse within the family.

In this taxonomy, Courtois and Ford offer an insight into the very nature of the damaging and ongoing impact of trauma when it arises from violation by another person or group of people. There are dynamics associated with interpersonal violence which in and of themselves cause hurt and pain. The betrayal of trust and care, the use of power, the historical reverberations of colonizing violence are all elements which compel the use of trauma, not in reductionist and simplified ways, but as experiences which intensely affect the very integrity of victims and survivors.

There is power in calling out the tactics of violation. It reduces the risk of sanitized language diluting the experience itself. It also lifts the awareness about the reality of how such violence is perpetrated in ways that exploit historical and structural vulnerabilities created by discourses of power and oppression. It is why current language in trauma-informed literature that emphasizes the importance of diversity may serve to rinse out the barbarity of interpersonal violence which is always purposeful, deliberate and intentional in its ambition to inflict pain for the gratification and justification of another person or group of people with power.

Importantly, this chapter is a salient reminder of how naming and clearly demarcating the effects of such violation can bring the needs of victims and survivors into much sharper focus for practitioners and organizations.

Courtois and Ford also highlight the importance of sequencing intervention when individuals with lived and living experience of trauma seek out support. The nature of the sequence they propose parallels and integrates with the preceding chapters where safety and stability form the basis on which relational and somatic resources are offered in moments of praxis that engage the underlying neurobiology that has been altered as a direct result of complex trauma. Identifying, configuring and implementing a uniquely tailored approach that is driven by the specific needs is the ultimate goal of healing processes. In that, being driven by a comprehensive and holistic understanding of the needs of individual victims and survivors, and their networks of relationships, is a key feature of the trauma-transformative approach.

References
References for chapter

Able, M.L. and Benedek, D.M. (2019). Severity and symptom trajectory in combat-related PTSD: A review of the literature. *Current Psychiatry Reports*, 21(7), 58.

Alexander, P.C. and Anderson, C.L. (1994). An attachment approach to psychotherapy with the incest survivor. *Psychotherapy: Theory, Research, Practice, Training*, 31(4), 665.

American Psychiatric Association (1980). *Diagnostic and Statistical Manual of Mental Disorders, 3rd Revision*. Washington, DC: American Psychiatric Press.

American Psychiatric Association (1994). *Diagnostic and Statistical Manual of Mental Disorders, 4th Revision*. Washington, DC: American Psychiatric Press.

American Psychiatric Association (2013). *Diagnostic and Statistical Manual of Mental Disorders 5th edition*. Washington, DC: American Psychiatric Press.

Briere, J.N. and Lanktree, C.B. (2011). *Treating Complex Trauma in Adolescents and Young Adults*. New York, NY: Sage.

Briere, J.N. and Scott, C. (2014). *Principles of Trauma Therapy: A Guide to Symptoms, Evaluation, and Treatment* (second edition, DSM-5 update). New York, NY: Sage.

Briere, J. and Spinazzola, J. (2009). Assessment of Complex Posttraumatic Reactions. In C.A. Courtois and J.D. Ford (eds), *Treating Complex Traumatic Stress Disorders: An Evidence-Based Guide* (pp.104–121). New York, NY: Guilford Press.

Brewin, C.R., Cloitre, M., Hyland, P., Shevlin, M. *et al.* (2017). A review of current evidence regarding the ICD-11 proposals for diagnosing PTSD and complex PTSD. *Clinical Psychology Review*, 58, 1–15.

Breuer, F., Greggersen, W., Kahl, K.G., Schweiger, U. and Westermair, A.L. (2020). Caught in a web of trauma: Network analysis of childhood adversity and adult mental ill-health. *Child Abuse and Neglect*, 107, 104534.

Chu, J.A. (1988). Ten traps for therapists in the treatment of trauma survivors. *Dissociation*, 1(4), 24–32.

Cloitre, M., Courtois, C.A., Charuvastra, A., Carapezza, R., Stolbach, B.C. and Green, B.L. (2011). Treatment of complex PTSD: Results of the ISTSS expert clinician survey on best practices. *Journal of Traumatic Stress*, 24(6), 615–627.

Courtois, C.A. (1999). *Recollections of Sexual Abuse: Treatment Principles and Guidelines*. New York, NY: W.W. Norton.

Courtois, C.A. (2015). First, Do No *More* Harm. In D. Walker, C.A. Courtois and J. Aten (eds), *Spiritually Oriented Psychotherapy for Trauma* (pp.55–76). Washington, DC: American Psychological Association.

Courtois, C.A. and Brown, L.S. (2019). Guideline orthodoxy and resulting limitations of the American Psychological Association's Clinical Practice Guideline for the Treatment of PTSD in Adults. *Psychotherapy*, 56(3), 329.

Courtois, C.A. and Ford, D. (2013). *Treating Complex Trauma: A Sequenced Relationship Based Approach*. New York, NY: Guilford.

Courtois, C.A., Ford, J.D. and Cloitre, M. (2009). Best Practices in Psychotherapy for Adults. In C.A. Courtois and J.D. Ford (eds), *Treating Complex Traumatic Stress Disorders: An Evidence-Based Guide*. (pp.82–103). New York, NY: Guilford Press.

Courtois, C.A., Ford, J.D., Cloitre, M. and Schnyder, U. (2020). Best Practices in Psychotherapy for Adults. In J.D. Ford and C.A. Courtois (eds), *Treatment of Complex Traumatic Stress Disorders in Adults* (second edition) (pp.62–98). New York, NY: Guilford Press.

Courtois, C.A. and Gold, S. (2009). The need for inclusion of psychological trauma in the professional curriculum. *Psychological Trauma*, 1(1), 3–23.

Davies, J.M. and Frawley, M.G. (1994). *Treating the Adult Survivor of Childhood Sexual Abuse: A Psychoanalytic Perspective*. New York, NY: Basic Books.

D'Andrea, W., Ford, J.D., Stolbach, B., Spinazzola, J. and van der Kolk, B.A. (2012). Understanding interpersonal trauma in children: Why we need a developmentally appropriate trauma diagnosis. *American Journal of Orthopsychiatry*, 82(2), 187–200.

Ellis, A.E., Simiola, V., Brown, L., Courtois, C. and Cook, J.M. (2018). The role of evidence-based therapy relationships on treatment outcomes for adults with trauma: A systematic review. *Journal of Trauma and Dissociation*, 19(2), 185–213.

Ford, J.D. (1999). Disorders of extreme stress following war-zone military trauma: Associated features of posttraumatic stress disorder or comorbid but distinct syndromes? *Journal of Consulting and Clinical Psychology*, 67(1), 3–12.

Ford, J.D. (2018). Trauma memory processing in PTSD psychotherapy: A unifying framework. *Journal of Traumatic Stress*, 31, 933–942.

Ford, J.D. (2021). *Crises in the Psychotherapy Session: Transforming Critical Moments into Turning Points*. Washington, DC: American Psychological Association.

Ford, J.D. and Courtois C.A. (eds). (2020). *Treatment of Complex Traumatic Stress Disorders in Adults* (second edition). New York, NY: Guilford Press.

Ford, J.D. and Courtois, C.A. (eds). (2013). *Treating Complex Traumatic Stress Disorders in Children and Adolescents: Scientific Foundations and Therapeutic Models*. New York, NY: Guilford Press.

Ford, J.D. and Kidd, P. (1998). Early childhood trauma and disorders of extreme stress as predictors of treatment outcome with chronic posttraumatic stress disorder. *Journal of Traumatic Stress*, 11(4), 743–761.

Freyd, J.J. (1996). *Betrayal Trauma: The Logic of Forgetting Childhood Abuse*. Harvard, MA: Harvard University Press.

Gelinas, D.J. (1983). The persisting negative effects of incest. *Psychiatry*, 46, 313–332.

Greenberg, T.M. (2020). *Treating Complex Trauma: Combined Theories and Methods*. New York, NY: Springer.

Griffin, B.J., Purcell, N., Burkman, K., Litz, B.T. *et al.* (2019). Moral injury: An integrative review. *Journal of Traumatic Stress*, 32(3), 350–362.

Hamblen, J.L., Norman, S.B., Sonis, J. Phelps, A. *et al.* (2019). A guide to PTSD guidelines. *Psychotherapy*, 56(3), 359–373.

Harsey, S. and Freyd, J.J. (2020). Deny, attack, and reverse victim and offender (DARVO): What is the influence on perceived perpetrator and victim credibility? *Journal of Aggression, Maltreatment and Trauma*, 29(8), 897–916.

Herman, J.L. (1992a). Complex PTSD: A syndrome in survivors of prolonged and repeated trauma. *Journal of Traumatic Stress*, 5(3), 377–391.

Herman, J.L. (1992b). *Trauma and Recovery*. New York, NY: Basic Books.

Herzog, J.I. and Schmahl, C. (2018). Adverse childhood experiences and the consequences on neurobiological, psychosocial, and somatic conditions across the lifespan. *Frontiers in Psychiatry*, 9(420).

Howell, E.F. (2020). *Trauma and Dissociation Informed Psychotherapy: Relational Healing and the Therapeutic Connection*. New York, NY: W.W. Norton.

Jowett, S., Karatzias, T., Shevlin, M. and Hyland, P. (2021). Psychological trauma at different developmental stages and ICD-11 CPTSD: The role of dissociation. *Journal of Trauma and Dissociation*, 1–16.

Karatzias, T., Shevlin, M., Fyvie, C., Grandison, G. *et al.* (2020). Adverse and benevolent childhood experiences in Posttraumatic Stress Disorder (PTSD) and Complex PTSD (CPTSD): Implications for trauma-focused therapies. *European Journal of Psychotraumatology*, 11(1), 1793599.

Karatzias, T., Shevlin, M., Ford, J.D., Fyvie, C. *et al.* (2021). Childhood trauma, attachment orientation, and complex PTSD (CPTSD) symptoms in a clinical sample: Implications for treatment. *Developmental Psychopathology*, 1–6.

Kinsler, P.J., Courtois, C.A. and Frankel, A.S. (2009). Therapeutic Alliance and Risk Management. In C.A. Courtois and J.D. Ford (eds), *Treating Complex Traumatic Stress Disorders: An Evidence-Based Guide* (pp.183–201). New York, NY: Guilford Press.

Kinsler, P.J. (2017) *Complex Psychological Trauma: The Centrality of Relationship*. London: Routledge.

Kira, I.A., Aljakoub, J., Al Ibraheem, B., Shuwiekh, H.A. and Ashby, J.S. (2022). The etiology of complex PTSD in the COVID-19 and continuous traumatic stressors era: A test of competing and allied models. *Journal of Loss and Trauma*, 27, 608–628.

Kluft, R.P. (1994). Treatment trajectories in multiple personality disorder. *Dissociation*, 7, 63–76.

Lauterbach, D. and Armour, C. (2016). Symptom trajectories among child survivors of maltreatment: Findings from the Longitudinal Studies of Child Abuse and Neglect (LONGSCAN). *Journal of Abnormal Child Psychology*, 44(2), 369–379.

Levin, Y., Hyland, P., Karatzias, T., Shevlin, M. *et al.* (2021). Comparing the network structure of ICD-11 PTSD and complex PTSD in three African countries. *Journal of Psychiatric Research*, 136, 80–86.

Linehan, M. (1993). *Cognitive-Behavioural Therapy Treatment of Borderline Personality Disorder*. New York, NY: Guilford Press.

McGinty, G., Fox, R., Ben-Ezra, M., Cloitre, M. *et al.* (2021). Sex and age differences in ICD-11 PTSD and complex PTSD: An analysis of four general population samples. *European Psychiatry*, 64(1), e66.

McGuire, A., Huffhines, L. and Jackson, Y. (2021). The trajectory of PTSD among youth in foster care: A survival analysis examining maltreatment experiences prior to entry into care. *Child Abuse and Neglect*, 115, 105026.

Muller, R.T. (2018). *Trauma and the Struggle to Open Up: From Avoidance to Recovery and Growth*. New York, NY: W.W. Norton and Company.

Norcross, J.C. and Lambert, M.J. (2018). Psychotherapy relationships that work III. *Psychotherapy*, 55(4), 303.

Ogden, P. (2020). Sensorimotor Psychotherapy. In J.D. Ford and C.A. Courtois (eds), *Treating Complex Traumatic Stress Disorders in Adults* (second edition) (pp.509–532). New York, NY: Guilford Press.

Pearlman, L.A. and Courtois, C.A. (2005). Clinical applications of the attachment framework: Relational treatment of complex trauma. *Journal of Traumatic Stress*, 18(5), 449–459.

Pearlman, L.A. and Saakvitne, K.W. (1995). *Trauma and the Therapist: Countertransference and Vicarious Traumatisation in Psychotherapy with Incest Survivors.* New York, NY: W.W. Norton.

Putnam, F.W., Amaya-Jackson, L., Putnam, K.T. and Briggs, E.C. (2020). Synergistic adversities and behavioural problems in traumatised children and adolescents. *Child Abuse and Neglect,* 106, 104492.

Redican, E., Nolan, E., Hyland, P., Cloitre, M. *et al.* (2021). A systematic literature review of factor analytic and mixture models of ICD-11 PTSD and CPTSD using the International Trauma Questionnaire. *Journal of Anxiety Disorder,* 79, 102381.

Salzberg, J. (2010). *Good Enough Endings: Breaks, Interruptions, and Terminations from Contemporary Relational Perspectives.* London: Routledge.

Smith, P., Dalgleish, T. and Meiser-Stedman, R. (2019). Practitioner review: Posttraumatic stress disorder and its treatment in children and adolescents. *Journal of Child Psychology and Psychiatry,* 60(5), 500–515.

Spinazzola, J. and Briere, J. (2020). Evidence-Based Psychological Assessment for the Sequelae of Complex Trauma. In J.D. Ford and C.A. Courtois (eds), *Treatment of Complex Traumatic Stress Disorders in Adults* (second edition). (pp.125–148). New York, NY: Guilford Press.

Terr, L.C. (1991). Childhood traumas: An outline and overview. *American Journal of Psychiatry,* 148(1), 10–20.

Vallieres, F., Hyland, P. and Murphy, J. (2021). Navigating the who, where, what, when, how, and why of trauma exposure and response. *European Journal of Psychotraumatology,* 12(1), 1855903.

van der Kolk, B.A., Stone, L., West, J., Rhodes, A. *et al.* (2014). Yoga as an adjunctive treatment for posttraumatic stress disorder: A randomised controlled trial. *Journal of Clinical Psychiatry,* 75(6), e559–565.

van Vliet, N.I., Huntjens, R.J.C., van Dijk, M.K. and de Jongh, A. (2018). Phase-based treatment versus immediate trauma-focused treatment in patients with childhood trauma-related posttraumatic stress disorder: Study protocol for a randomised controlled trial. *Trials,* 19(1), 138.

Wallin, D.J. (2007). *Attachment in Psychotherapy.* New York, NY: Guilford Press.

Wilker, S., Kolassa, S., Ibrahim, H., Rajan, V. *et al.* (2021). Sex differences in PTSD risk: Evidence from post-conflict populations challenges the general assumption of increased vulnerability in females. *European Journal of Psychotraumatology,* 12(1), 1930702.

World Health Organization (2018). *International Statistical Classification of Diseases and Related Health Problems* (11th edition). Geneva: World Health Organization.

Zoellner, L.A., Feeny, N.C. and Bittinger, J.N. (2009). What you believe is what you want: Modeling PTSD-related treatment preferences for sertraline or prolonged exposure. *Journal of Behavior Therapy and Experimental Psychiatry,* 40, (3)2, 455–467.

CHAPTER 10

Self Defense and Learned Hopelessness: Adapting to Poor Care by Staying Hypervigilant for Threats and Suppressing Positive Expectations

Jonathan Baylin and Daniel Hughes

Introduction

Starting life in an environment of poor care forces the young child to develop a complex neurobiological survival strategy. Instead of Plan A, trusting and depending on caregivers, the child has to go with Plan B, mistrusting while still having to depend on caregivers (Baylin and Hughes, 2016). Incorporating recent advances in developmental neuroscience, including the science of early life stress, can help to strengthen therapeutic interventions with maltreated children and their caregivers (Shonkoff *et al.*, 2009; Teicher *et al.*, 2003; Tottenham, 2014). In our ongoing collaboration, we continue to update our approach to treatment by drawing on relevant advances in neuroscience to deepen our understanding of how children adapt initially to poor care and how we can help them to shift from Plan B toward Plan A when they find themselves in a safer, more nurturing environment of care.

Developmental neuroscience shows that two separate brain systems are centrally involved in Plan B, the adaptation to poor care that we call blocked trust: 1) the self-defense system and 2) the anti-reward system. The adaptive processes that lead to hyperactivation of these two systems in turn affect the development of a third brain system dedicated to the child's sense of self and capacity for self-awareness and self-reflection, the Default Mode Network or DMN (Raichle *et al.*, 2001; Sonuga-Barke, 2014). In what follows, we discuss the effects of early life adversity on the development of the self-defense and anti-reward systems and then relate these developmental processes to the development of the DMN. The interplay of these brain systems gets at the heart of what happens when children have to adapt to poor care. Having a model of the interplay among these three systems helps to guide interventions aimed at helping maltreated children recover the capacity to trust trustworthy adults and to develop positive self-esteem (Lanius *et al.*, 2020; Akiki *et al.*, 2018).

The self-defense system: Neuroception and chronic hypervigilance for social threats

The social self-defense system is most likely to be activated when something in another person's actions or demeanor signals potentially imminent harm. For the young child, this could be either the threat of abuse or the threat of abandonment. The self-defense system privileges speed over accuracy, categorical or global reactivity over more differentiated, nuanced, context-sensitive responses (Terpou *et al.*, 2019). This is also the brain system that supports the chronic hypervigilance that extends fear/pain-driven learning from early childhood into the future as maltreated children age (Lanius *et al.*, 2017; Liddell *et al.*, 2005).

In an environment of poor care, the child's self-defense system is prematurely activated to enable the child to detect potential threats related to abusive and neglectful behaviour by caregivers. The self-defense system relies heavily on the functioning of the midbrain threat detection system, the brain circuitry dedicated to the ultra-rapid process that neuroscientist Stephen Porges calls 'neuroception' to distinguish it from the slower process of perception (Porges, 2011). Neuroception occurs in the fast and furious time frame of less than a tenth of a second, enabling the implicit, preconscious detection of potential threats from other people.

Within the time frame of neuroception, the amygdala can detect changes in facial expressions, eye movements, tones of voice and gestures in other people which can become conditioned stimuli that predict impending harm. Early life stress sensitizes this rapid threat-detection system, lowering the threshold for the amygdala to activate sympathetic (fight or flight) and parasympathetic (immobilization) defensive reactions from brainstem regions without involving higher regions of the brain that process more detailed and context-sensitive information (Liddell, 2005).

The internal structure and functioning of different sub-regions of the amygdala reflect experience-dependent 'programming' (Ball *et al.*, 2007; Brown *et al.*, 2014). Nurturing care promotes the development of a different pattern of brain connections within the amygdala and between the amygdala and other regions of the brain than poor care develops. Good care appears to raise the threshold in the amygdala for triggering the stress system and self-defensive behaviours. Meanwhile, good care promotes development between regions of the amygdala and regions of the prefrontal cortex, hippocampal complex, and anterior cingulate that create the circuitry for regulating affect in a top-down, context-sensitive way. This 'fronto-limbic' system is under initial construction in humans during the first 18–24 months of life. Children who are fortunate enough to have reliable, trustworthy care during this period of development are more likely than maltreated children to move forward in life with the capability both to regulate strong emotions and to stay openly engaged with their environment. A well-developed fronto-limbic system supports greater emotional resilience in the face of life's challenges by enabling faster, more efficient recovery from stress reactions and from defensive reactions (Banks *et al.*, 2007).

In contrast, exposure to high levels of relational stress early in life tends to strengthen connections within the amygdala between the regions that take in sensory information and the regions that control output to the stress system and to subcortical regions that release defensive behaviours. While good care tends to raise the threshold within the amygdala for triggering stress/defensive reactions, poor care tends to lower this threshold, literally increasing the excitability within the amygdala. In a highly stressful early care scenario, the part of the amygdala (basolateral region) that can form associations between what is seen and heard and input from the pain system traveling up from the brainstem becomes more excitable, promoting stronger associations. These strong associations are then more likely to release the brakes from the output regions of the amygdala (the central and medial regions), triggering the release of defensive actions, stress hormones, and norepinephrine. This process also automatically shifts attention in an obligatory way to create a hypervigilant state of readiness to detect potential threats. Meanwhile, norepinephrine feeds back to the associative regions of the amygdala, strengthening these fear- and pain-driven connections and helping to mark them as important to remember to help avoid painful things in the future (Yu *et al.*, 2017).

Additionally, as part of this complex scenario, back projections from the amygdala to the sensory regions of the brain amplify sensations, making the multisensory memories of alarming experiences highly salient (Vuilleumier, 2009). This salience-enhancing process is the reason why fear-conditioned memories retain their vividness when triggered in the future, creating the subjective experience of reliving the original experiences, not just recalling them (Brewin, 2015; Maren, 2014).

The hyperactivation of the amygdala also suppresses the development of connections with the hippocampal system, as well as the prefrontal cortex (PFC), the brain regions that help contextualize emotionally salient experiences, regulate affect, and make better sense of what is actually going on during interactions with other people. Suppression of hippocampal functioning and of the PFC by a chronically hyperactive amygdala makes it harder for the child later in life to differentiate between present and past, to regulate strong emotions, and to learn from new relational experiences.

In effect, early life stress sensitizes the amygdala in a manner that strengthens its inherent 'negativity bias,' making it quicker to detect potential threats, to form associations, to trigger defensive reactions, all as part of nature's way of helping the young mammal survive life in a harsh environment and store this fear-driven learning for future retrieval, as needed. In a very real sense, early life adversity biases brain development toward a wilder way of living, staying vigilant for signs of danger and putting a premium on self-reliance rather than depending more fully on the care of others.

The anti-reward system: Chronic pessimism and dysphoria

In addition to understanding how early life experiences affect the midbrain self-defense system, it is helpful to understand what neuroscientists have been learning about the effects of chronic inescapable stress on the development of the brain system that typically supports active engagement with life in a safe enough environment: the dopamine-driven system supporting the motivation to seek rewards, including the comfort and pleasure of intimate relationships (Geisler and Trimble, 2008). In an environment where it could be harmful to be too ready to engage with other people, it is important that we have a demobilizing 'no go' system to help us avoid harm and disappointment from seeking reward when and where reward is unlikely to be found. So in addition to the reward system, we have an 'anti-reward system,' a brain system that helps us learn from unrewarding, disappointing, painful experiences to avoid these kinds of experiences in the future.

The anti-reward system is a brain circuitry dedicated to the process of learning from disappointing, unrewarding experiences to avoid repeating the same experiences in the future (Matsumoto and Hikosaka, 2007). This system depends heavily on a brain region called the habenula and a brain chemical called dynorphin, one of the three major types of opioids. The combined actions of the habenula and dynorphin effectively suppress the functioning of key brain systems involved in reward, pleasure, and satisfaction: dopamine, endorphins, and serotonin.

Dopamine suppression: No go

Dopamine supports mobility, active engagement with our environment and other people, being in a 'doing' mode, and learning from this doing. This includes active coping when faced with situations we want to escape, as in fight and flight reactions. This is our mobilization system or what one neuroscientist called our 'seeking' system (Panksepp, 1998). This is the 'go' system, the doing system we use to explore our world, find things we need and like, and learn ways to prevent harm or pain by taking action that is rewarded when we achieve relief, when we successfully escape. We use the dopamine system for actively engaging with life and coping with challenges, for getting the goods we need and avoiding the things that can hurt us or cause us pain.

The process of seeking rewarding experiences relies heavily on the phasic release of dopamine from the midbrain region called the ventral tegmental area or VTA. In contrast, the anti-reward system suppresses the release of dopamine from the VTA, effectively blocking the reward-seeking process. In relation to the social realm of experience, the anti-reward system helps to suppress potentially disappointing attempts to connect with other people for comfort or pleasure.

The habenula: Small but powerful

Recently, neuroscientists have been learning more about the inner workings of the anti-reward system. A key brain region that has emerged in these studies is the habenula or specifically, the lateral habenula. This is a small brain region that has been hard to study but that is now more accessible to study with newer imaging technology (Matsumoto and Hikosaka, 2007). It turns out that the lateral habenula plays a key role in the anti-reward system, essentially by suppressing the release of dopamine to avoid moving toward a potentially unrewarding thing or person (Ji and Shephard, 2007). In effect, habenula neurons 'learn to expect disappointment and thereby signal it more readily' (Kaye and Ross, 2017, p.2).

In an environment of care which is mostly safe but presents transient experiences that would be good to avoid in the future, the anti-reward and reward systems are both working to provide a balanced approach to rewarding and unrewarding things, situations, and people. In contrast, under conditions of chronically poor care, the lateral habenula apparently becomes overactive to support the process of learning to avoid engaging with caregivers except when necessary for survival. The lateral habenula has been shown to be essential to the process of making the shift from active coping with stress to the passive, immobilizing, enduring strategy required when young children have to stay and endure whatever the caregivers have to offer (Fadok et al., 2017). Over time, the habenula can become hyperactive, essentially stuck in a firing pattern that suppresses the dopamine system chronically rather than transiently. Apparently, the habenula becomes overactive as a result of a complex inflammatory process in the brain resulting from the interplay of glutamate, GABA, and the immune system.

Dynorphin: Suppressing pain while engendering dysphoria

While the lateral habenula plays a key role in suppressing the release of dopamine, another part of this anti-reward system involves the release of an opioid called dynorphin. Like endorphin, dynorphin is somewhat analgesic, helping to reduce the subjective experience of pain. However, rather than engendering a euthymic mood, dynorphin tends to promote dysphoria, a chronic state of anhedonia or difficulty experiencing pleasure from naturally rewarding things in life (Cleck and Blendy, 2008; Koob, 2009; Land *et al.*, 2008). Dynorphin is released as part of the stress reaction to chronic, inescapable conditions, probably as an evolved mechanism for helping us to endure life in a harsh, uncaring environment without experiencing overwhelming chronic pain (Land *et al.*, 2008). Also, dynorphin suppresses sensations of all kinds, and in so doing is thought to contribute to the process of dissociation, enabling a person confronted with inescapable stress to feel less 'present' – to go away affectively. Together, then, the habenula and dynorphin are part of a powerful brain system for shutting down active engagement with life in order to survive without much comfort, reward, or pleasure.

In humans, suppression of the dopamine system in combination with release of dynorphin contributes to sustained depression, to symptoms of low motivation to move, to be 'on the go,' to engage with life. While simpler mammals exhibit what neuroscientists call 'learned helplessness' in response to chronic, inescapable stress, humans exhibit what might be termed 'learned hopelessness.' Research suggests that chronic activation of the habenula affects mood, perhaps underlying the chronic negativity and pessimism seen in people who have experienced repeated disappointments. Intriguingly, researchers have found that lifting the habenula brake on dopamine neurons relieves symptoms of learned helplessness, restoring active coping behaviours in animals and reawakening reward-seeking behaviour. More importantly, there is growing evidence that targeting the habenula is helpful in treating chronic depression in people (Schlaepfer *et al.*, 2008).

The dual system strategy for surviving poor care

By combining hyperactivation of both the self-defense system and the anti-reward system, the young child's brain adapts in a way that enhances chances for surviving poor care. These twin operations help the child 1) to see bad things coming in time to deploy defensive behaviours, including fight, flight, and freeze reactions, and 2) to stay habitually pessimistic rather than hopeful about getting good things from other people. While these processes are adaptive in the short term, over time, they engender a chronic mix of hypervigilance and dysphoria that suppresses activation of higher brain regions and makes it hard for the child to awaken their brain to the news of being in a different, safer, more trustworthy environment.

This adaptation to poor care combines processes of hyper- and hypoarousal: hyperarousal for active self-defense, and hypoarousal for sustaining a chronic state of low expectations for comfort and joy. This combination of upregulating (sympathetic) and downregulating (parasympathetic) coping strategies makes children with blocked trust both hard to understand and hard to engage. Combining the ability to shift from a moody state into an active state of unmodulated self-defense in milliseconds and then rapidly back into a moody state, these children keep caregivers and themselves off balance.

No wonder adults who become caregivers for these children are at high risk of developing blocked care (Hughes and Baylin, 2012) as they try repeatedly to get close to and care for these children. Without knowledge of the effects of early life stress on children's development, caregivers cannot understand why their children are reacting to their well-intentioned approaches as something more akin to an impending attack from a predator or why their children are chronically in a negative mood, expecting to have negative experiences. When not in attack mode, these children often exhibit the core symptoms of chronic depression: anhedonia, low motivation, hopelessness, and chronic negativity.

Treatment: Calming the self-defense system and reawakening hope in children with blocked trust

Attachment focused therapy such as dyadic development psychotherapy (DDP) (Hughes and Baylin, 2012, Hughes, 2017; Hughes *et al.*, 2019, Baylin and Hughes, 2016) helps the child shift the way they are relating to the adults who are trying to care for them. Treatment has to target both the chronic activation of the self-defense system and the chronic suppression of the reward system to help the child decrease self-defensiveness and reawaken their capacity to seek engagement. Otherwise, the child is unlikely to begin to change their behaviour and, more fundamentally, their state of mind, their beliefs about themselves, other people, and the world.

Specifically, a therapy meant to reduce the impact of childhood relational trauma while building the child's sense of trust in a new caregiver has to both calm the child's hypersensitive amygdala and reawaken the child's dopamine system from chronic suppression. Treatment needs to help the child with blocked trust recover from the state of learned hopelessness, engage with caregivers, and start to process the 'news of a difference': this is not the same old harsh, untrustworthy environment experienced earlier in life.

How, then, can adults help children who have adapted to chronic stress by becoming hypersensitive pessimists make the all-important shifts in the two core brain systems that have been coopted by early life stress? How can we interrupt the child's habitual self-defense and learned hopelessness to revive the child's potential for experiencing comfort and joy in relationships?

Positive prediction errors: Creating good surprises and becoming a social bufferer

What relational processes can trigger this social buffering of the child's defense system and reawakening of the social reward system? Good surprises, relational experiences that generate what neuroscientists call 'positive prediction errors,' the brain signals triggered when something we experience with another person is unexpectedly positive. The error signal is a brain electrical pattern that can interrupt a habitual firing pattern and shift attention to something unexpected that is happening or that just happened, something that demands exploration, that triggers curiosity. The power of these positive prediction errors is strongest when we are least expecting something good – when we are mindlessly expecting something negative from another person. Adults need to know how to trigger positive prediction errors by interacting with mistrusting children in ways that are radically different from the negativity they expect from other people, especially when they are misbehaving, being mistrustful, and resisting efforts to engage them.

Social buffering and creation of mysteries: Planting the seeds of a new story of self

By surprising the child with unexpected acceptance and compassion, the adult creates a mystery, an experience that something 'wondrous strange' is happening, something that compels a second, slower look, helping the child's brain get above the neuroceptive system. As the child shifts upward toward social engagement, a new story is potentially emerging, a story that conflicts with everything the child has believed about the world and themself. It is the experience of this attention-grabbing incongruity, this big 'mismatch,' that can trigger 'interstate travel' (Baylin and Hughes, 2016), that shift up the polyvagal ladder (Porges, 2011; Dana, 2019) from habitual reactions favouring speed over accuracy to a slower approach to information processing that can foster new learning.

Here are two examples of this social buffering and interstate travel – one from history and one from the present day.

A famous case of wildness: The Wild Boy of Aveyron

Consider the case of the boy in France who in 1800 at around the age of 12 emerged from the woods where he had apparently been living in the wild for many years. After being declared a hopeless savage by several experts at the time, he was taken into the home of Dr. Itard, who took a compassionate, gradual approach to 'taming' the boy he named Victor. Here is Dr. Itard writing about spending time with Victor at bedtime. He is explaining that Victor's strongest connection is with the woman who becomes in the most meaningful sense the boy's foster mother.

> 'Yet at times', Itard writes, 'I too am welcome. They are the times I have never used for any kind of instruction. If, for example, I go to his room at nightfall when he has just gone to bed, his first movement is to sit up so that I can hug him, and then to draw me to him by taking my arms and making me sit on the bed.' (Lane, 1976, p.118)

From the case of Victor, we learn that a wild boy can come in from nature and bond with a caring adult who learns how to whisper to the young child's defense system in a way that is disarming, a way that sends strong enough safety messages into the wild one's brain to help that brain shift from mindless self-defense to social engagement and even comfort seeking and ability to receive kind care. When people poked at Victor, invading his personal space with abrupt actions, they got what they expected: aggression and 'wildness.' When Dr. Itard and his helper treated Victor kindly, they awakened his potential for connection and his underdeveloped capacity for bonding with another person.

A modern-day Wild One

Jimmy, age seven, is wanting breakfast and is expecting a pancake. His adoptive mom, Kate, tells him that she has not had time to make pancakes but he can have cereal. Jimmy has been in Kate's care for several months and he has been having frequent full-blown rage episodes in which he tries to hit and kick Kate while yelling that he will kill her. Once Kate had to lock herself in the bathroom while Jimmy raged at the door, threatening to get an axe from the basement and break through the door.

Now, as if a switch got flipped in his brain (which it did), Jimmy starts to descend into another full-blown rage attack, a brain state in which he is rapidly losing touch with his surroundings as well as losing knowledge of who is trying to provide him with breakfast. This time, though, Kate is armed with new understanding of Jimmy's reactions and how to respond in a helpful way (Hughes, 2009). She is prepared to keep her lid on and even maintain a caring state of mind towards Jimmy. In this new found compassionate state of mind, Kate has the presence to say, with intensity but not anger: 'Wow, you look like you could use a hug!!' Jimmy, verging on attack, stops in his tracks, and then responds gruffly while reaching toward Kate, 'Yes, I could!' And then amazingly Jimmy allows Kate to hug him as he softens and sinks into the warmth of her comforting, 'socially buffering' embrace. Pretty soon, Jimmy and Kate are sitting at the table eating bowls of cereal.

Like Dr. Itard with the wild boy, Viktor, Kate is becoming a compassionate 'amygdala whisperer' with new power to disarm Jimmy's chronically hyperactive self-defense system. She is giving him a chance to reawaken his blocked social engagement system and feel safe enough to seek comfort and pleasure by getting very close to another human being, letting Kate into his 'peripersonal' space within slugging and hugging distance. This is the precious territory we tend to guard against intrusions by unwanted or strange people, the space in which attachment and caregiving are enacted between trustworthy caregivers and their trusting children (offspring).

Kate provided the all-important unexpectedly positive response to Jimmy's mindless mistrust, the 'good surprise' that triggered an error signal in Jimmy's brain. This signal, triggered by the release of dopamine from Jimmy's midbrain up to his cingulate and orbitol PFC, enables him to shift his attention and modulate his affect enough to apply the brakes to his rapid downshift into self-defense. This is the 'hold your horses' mechanism that kids with blocked trust need to use in order to upshift from automatic self-defence into a more open state conducive to social engagement and connection with a trustworthy adult. Kate's ability to provide Jimmy with surprisingly positive relational experiences helps promote this interstate travel from the lower regions of Jimmy's tripartite nervous system upward to the social engagement system.

As Kate helps Jimmy shift upward toward the state of social engagement, he starts to pay attention to his immediate environment, and to Kate. Now he becomes aware that Kate is not his birth mother who hurt him; that, instead, she is his new mom who cares about him, the one with good intentions toward him who wants to comfort him and help him and teach him things about life. Jimmy is 'getting above' his mindless, categorical way of experiencing Kate to use higher brain processes that enable him to differentiate between Kate and other 'mothers.'

Re-storying: Helping Jimmy change his beliefs about himself and his world

Kate is learning to interrupt Jimmy's automatic, mindless mistrust to open a window of heightened awareness of her and of his new environment, a window of awareness in which Jimmy is open-minded enough to learn new things about his new caregivers and how they are different from the old ones. Kate is learning to engage Jimmy and help him shift from self-defense into social engagement.

But this is just the beginning of the process of helping Jimmy change his mind about himself, his own worth and the trustworthiness of his new caregivers. What could help Jimmy develop self-compassion? What would help him revise his old original story which, like most children who are mistreated early in life, is a story of low self-worth, of being 'nobody,' not worthy of being cared for, as one child said, of being 'dirt.' How can the therapist and Kate go beyond awakening Jimmy to his current environment and help him to believe that he is loveable?

Story power and the Default Mode Network

Repeated experiences of being safely seen and heard by Kate, especially at moments when Jimmy is most unlikely to expect kindness, can help to provide Jimmy with new experiences of being valued instead of devalued. Many 'reps' of this process of providing good surprises can start to embed a new version of self in the Default Mode Network (DMN). This is the brain system that activates automatically when we are awake and not busying our minds with something outside ourselves (Raichle *et al.*, 2001). Jimmy is likely to have an underdeveloped DMN, even for his age, for at least two reasons: because he has had to pay so much attention to his external environment to avoid impending harm and also because the thoughts and memories that would be activated when he does use his DMN would be negative and stressful to bring into awareness (Lanius *et al.*, 2020).

PACE and compassionate care

Let us briefly describe how DDP functions in a way to assist Jimmy to both reduce his need for vigilance regarding threats to himself and begin to approach his adoptive mom, Kate, as a source of pleasure while at the same time helping Kate to provide the comfort and joy that he so desperately needs. The DDP therapist, Sarah, first spends at least a few sessions with Kate to increase her ability to remain open and engaged with her son when he is in his defensive and often aggressive state of mind. During a part of this time, Kate focuses on understanding her own attachment history so that she is better able to inhibit her own defensive reactions. Through Sarah helping her to understand how her son's strong mistrust of her relates to his past experiences of relational distress and possibly trauma, Kate will be able to respond in a more compassionate manner to him. Finally, Kate will learn about how PACE (an acronym for an attitude of playfulness, acceptance, curiosity, and empathy) will assist her in being aware of and responsive to her son's vulnerability that lies under his angry, self-protective stance toward her.

When Jimmy joins the sessions with his adoptive mother and Sarah, he is first engaged with PACE about routine or interesting events of his daily life. Sarah focuses on establishing a conversation with him that will create a reciprocal, shared state of mind that will remain in place when she then introduces a more stressful or a shameful event in his relationship with Kate. The meaning of that event will be explored until both Jimmy and Kate are able to experience the vulnerability that underlies what occurred. In developing a story about the above event involving pancakes and cereal, Sarah is able to help them both to discover that when Jimmy heard that he would not be getting the pancakes that he wanted, he experienced that as indicating that what he wanted was not important to Kate, and even that he had become less important to her than he might have been previously. She might even regret having adopted him! As the story evolved, Kate spoke to Jimmy with acceptance and empathy for his underlying experience and he was able to accept her comfort. In the next session, with Sarah's help, Jimmy is able to begin to see how his mistrust of Kate's continuing commitment to him related to how his biological parents would often ignore him or even hit him if he asked for something from them.

Similar events that occurred in Jimmy's relationship with Kate continue to be explored, often leading to Jimmy briefly entering vulnerable states and being supported by Kate. The stories that develop about those events represent the 'reps' of soothing and positive surprises that Jimmy needs to begin the process of bringing new meanings to his life story (within the Default Mode Network). But Jimmy cannot hold on to the forward movements, and he often reverts to the prior emotional, cognitive, and behavioural patterns involving threat and mistrust. During this time, Sarah provides ongoing support for Kate so that she does not become discouraged and lose hope. Her ability to 'trust the process' and remain persistently positive is crucial if Jimmy is to integrate these fragile new relational experiences with her. Sarah also provides continuous support for Jimmy during these stressful sessions. She repeatedly co-regulates his affective state and slows the exploration process whenever he shows signs of difficulty integrating the events being explored.

During one session in the fourth month of therapy Jimmy is again able to make sense of his fragile sense of trusting Kate when he engages in challenging behaviour. While expressing empathy for Jimmy, Kate expresses intensely how much she loves him. He reacts by screaming, 'I don't want you to love me!' Kate then goes to cuddle him and he pushes her away. Sarah accepts and expresses empathy for both of them. Jimmy's intense emotional reaction decreases and he slowly moves closer to his mother. In the next few sessions Jimmy is able to explore how terrified he is of Kate's love for him. It does not fit his sense of self and he also believes that it will be taken away from him at some point in the future. Kate agrees that she understands and accepts Jimmy's hesitation, while being patient. Jimmy agrees that he will see if he might first accept Kate taking care of him, and then gradually accept Kate caring for him, and – when he wis ready – allowing Kate to love him.

The course of DDP therapy for Jimmy and Kate demonstrates well the often slow and winding course of psychological development for a traumatized child now in a new relationship with a safe caregiver. In the early stages of their relationship, the child's harm avoidance system is gradually activated less often and the child repeatedly learns to notice and respond to the safety occurring within the relationship. As safety becomes anticipated, the child also gradually begins to seek and experience pleasure within the relationship. Safety leads the way to the possibility of comfort and then to the experience of reciprocal joy.

KNOWLEDGE AND PRACTICE REFLECTION

Joe Tucci, Janise Mitchell, Ed Tronick and Stephen W. Porges

Baylin and Hughes highlight how the ever-evolving nature of neuroscience continues to shed light on what are believed to be the underlying processes of trauma arising from interpersonal violation, including the orienting reactions that are reinforced by repetitive experience of patterns of activation.

As anyone who has ever listened to Baylin and Hughes will know, they are master-class level therapists with children and their carers. They come to know each child with a depth of understanding that positions them to genuinely engage with and acknowledge their pain at neurosomatic levels (as defined by Tronick earlier in Chapter 5). They search for the meaning that the child gives to their experience, even without language. They appreciate the strengths of the child and their relationship to their carers that enable defensive patterns of responding to be accepted and gradually reconfigured. They re-story children's meanings through supporting carers to find compassionate ways to accept the needs that the child has been left unattended with. They amplify small moments of repair offered by carers to children in their moment-by-moment interactions, witnessing and supporting the joyfulness of change and hope.

> From the case of Victor, we learn that a wild boy can come in from nature and bond with a caring adult who learns how to whisper to the young child's defense system in a way that is disarming, a way that sends strong enough safety messages into the wild one's brain to help that brain shift

from mindless self-defense to social engagement and even comfort seeking and ability to receive kind care… they awakened his potential for connection and his underdeveloped capacity for bonding with another person…

In this chapter, the potential for change is celebrated. Its narrative is oriented towards the very nature of humanity to struggle to adapt to the most abject forms of violence and function in ways that find protection from the harshest of attacks. Baylin and Hughes turn to the open stance of compassionate care to find the resources that children who have been abused or neglected need to be exposed to in order for the defense systems to not be activated with their typical intensity, and allowing for newer patterns to emerge and be experienced.

Compassion is a critical quality of interactions that serves to switch off old patterns of self-protection and gently encourage victims and survivors to engage in relational dynamics that shift the ways that neurophysiological pathways become activated. It is through compassionate responses that trust is negotiated. Compassion moves into spaces that threat leaves behind when it is no longer needed. First, it is compassion for the other, followed closely by compassion for self.

Trauma-transformative practitioners and organizations appreciate the value of compassion, holding it as an invaluable resource for victims and survivors of interpersonal forms of violence. They also deeply appreciate the relational nature of healing.

References
References for chapter

Akiki, T.J., Averill, C.L., Wrocklage, K.M., Scott, J.C. et al. (2018). Default mode network abnormalities in posttraumatic stress disorder: A novel network-restricted topology approach. NeuroImage, 176, 489–498.

Ball, T., Rahm, B., Eickhoff, S.B., Schulze-Bonhage, A., Speck, O. and Mutschler, I. (2007). Response properties of human amygdala subregions: Evidence based on functional MRI combined with probabilistic anatomical maps. PloS One, 2(3), e307.

Banks, S.J., Eddy, K.T., Angstadt, M., Nathan, P.J. and Phan, K.L. (2007). Amygdala–frontal connectivity during emotion regulation. Social Cognitive and Affective Neuroscience, 2(4), 303–312.

Baylin, J. and Hughes, D. (2016). The Neurobiology of Attachment-Focused Therapy. New York, NY: W.W. Norton and Company.

Brewin, C.R. (2015). Re-experiencing traumatic events in PTSD: New avenues in research on intrusive memories and flashbacks. European Journal of Psychotraumatology, 6. doi:10.3402/ejpt.v6.27180.

Brown, V.M., Labar, K.S., Haswell, C.C., Gold, A.L. et al. (2014). Altered resting-state functional connectivity of basolateral and centromedial amygdala complexes in posttraumatic stress disorder. Neuropsychopharmacology, 39(2), 351–359.

Cleck, J.N. and Blendy, J.A. (2008). Making a bad thing worse: Adverse effects of stress on drug addiction. Journal of Clinical Investigation, 118, 454–461.

Dana, D. (2019). The Polyvagal Theory in Therapy: Engaging the Rhythm of Regulation. New York, NY: Norton.

Fadok, J.P, Krabbe, S., Markovic, M., Courtin, J. et al. (2017). A competitive inhibitory circuit for selection of active and passive fear responses. Nature, 542, 96–100. doi: 10.1038/nature21047.

Geisler, S. and Trimble, M. (2008). The lateral habenula: No longer neglected. CNS Spectrums, 13, 484–489.

Hughes, D. (2009). Attachment-focused Parenting. New York, NY: W.W. Norton and Company.

Hughes, D. (2017). Building the Bonds of Attachment (third edition). Lanham, MD: Jason Aronson.

Hughes, D. and Baylin, J. (2012). Brain Based Parenting. New York, NY: W.W. Norton and Company.

Hughes, D., Golding, K.S. and Hudson, J. (2019). Healing Relational Trauma with Attachment-Focused Interventions: Dyadic Developmental Psychotherapy with Children and Families. New York, NY: W.W. Norton and Company.

Ji, H. and Shepard, P.D. (2007). Lateral habenula stimulation inhibits rat midbrain dopamine neurons through a GABA(A) receptor-mediated mechanism. Journal of Neuroscience, 27, 6923–6930.

Kaye, A. and Ross, D.A. (2017). The habenula: Darkness, disappointment, and depression. Biological Psychiatry, 81(4), e27–e28. doi: 10.1016/j.biopsych.2016.12.004.

Koob, G.F. (2009). Neurobiological substrates for the dark side of compulsivity in addiction. Neuropharmacology, 56,18–31.

Land, B.B., Bruchas, M.R., Lemos, J.C., Xu, M., Melief, E.J. and Chavkin C. (2008). The dysphoric component of stress is encoded by activation of the dynorphin kappa-opioid system. Journal of Neuroscience, 28, 407–414.

Lane, H. (1976). The Wild Boy of Aveyron. Cambridge, MA: Harvard University Press.

Lanius, R.A., Terpou, B.A. and McKinnon, M.C. (2020). The sense of self in the aftermath of trauma: Lessons from the default mode network in posttraumatic stress disorder. European Journal of Psychotraumatology, 11(1), 1807703, doi:10.1080/2000198.2020.180773.

Lanius, R.A., Rabellino, D., Boyd, J.E., Harricharan, S., Frewen, P.A. and McKinnon, M.C. (2017). The innate alarm system in PTSD: Conscious and subconscious processing of threat. Current Opinion in Psychology, 14, 109–115.

Liddell, B.J., Brown, K.J., Kemp, A.H., Barton, M.J. et al. (2005). A direct brainstem-amygdala-cortical 'alarm' system for subliminal signals of fear. NeuroImage, 24(1), 235–243.

Maren S. (2014). Nature and causes of the immediate extinction deficit: A brief review. Neurobiology of Learning and Memory, 113, 19–24.

Matsumoto, M. and Hikosaka, O. (2007). Lateral habenula as a source of negative reward signals in dopamine neurons. Nature, 447, 1111–1115.

Panksepp, J. (1998). Affective Neuroscience. New York, NY: Oxford University Press.

Porges, S. (2011). The Polyvagal Theory. New York, NY: W.W. Norton and Company.

Raichle, M.E., MacLeod, A.M., Snyder, A.Z., Powers, W.J., Gusnard, D.A. and Shulman, G.L. (2001). A default mode of brain function. Proceedings of the National Academy of Sciences, 98(2), 676–682.

Schlaepfer, T.E., Cohen, M.X., Frick, C., Kosel, M. et al. (2008). Deep brain stimulation to reward circuitry alleviates anhedonia in refractory major depression. Neuropsychopharmacology, 33 (2), 368–177.

Shonkoff, J.P., Boyce, W.T. and McEwen, B.S. (2009). Neuroscience, molecular biology, and the childhood roots of health disparities: Building a new framework for health promotion and disease prevention. Journal of American Medical Association, 301(21), 2252–2259.

Sonuga-Barke, L. (2014). Far from idle: Four ways in which growing knowledge of the 'resting' brain is transforming our understanding of the causes of childhood disorder. Journal of Child Psychology and Psychiatry, 55(12), 1297–1299.

Teicher, M.H., Andersen, S.L., Polcari, A., Anderson, C.M., Navalta, C.P. and Kim, D.M. (2003). The neurobiological consequences of early stress and childhood maltreatment. Neuroscience Biobehaviour Review, 27 (1), 33–44.

Terpou, B. A., Densmore, M., Théberge, J., Thome, J. et al. (2019). The threatful self: Midbrain functional connectivity to cortical midline and parietal regions during subliminal trauma-related processing in PTSD. Chronic Stress, 3, 247054701987136.

Tottenham, N. (2014). The Importance of Early Experiences for Neuro-Affective Development. In S.L. Andersen and D.S. Pine (eds), *The Neurobiology of Childhood* (pp.109–129). London: Springer-Verlag Publishing/Springer Nature.

Vuilleumier, P. (2009). The Role of the Human Amygdala in Perception and Attention. In P. Whalen and E. Phelps (eds), *The Human Amygdala* (pp.220–249). New York, NY: Guilford Press.

Yu, K., Ahrens, S., Zhang, X., Schiff, H. *et al.* (2017). The central amygdala controls learning in the lateral amygdala. *Nature and Neuroscience*, 20, 1680–1685.

CHAPTER 11

Healing Inter- and Transgenerational Trauma Through Indigenous Healing Practices

Judy Atkinson, Margaret Hayes, Carlie Atkinson,
Gerard Webster and Gavin Morris

TRIGGER WARNING: Readers should be aware that this chapter contains potentially disturbing or upsetting content. If only a trigger warning had been issued in 1878.

> Second-Class Inspector Alex Douglas reported an incident that took place around 1878 when he was out on patrol as follows: '(They) captured a female, quite a child, who after being washed by the troopers ... was taken in the camp and ravished by them. My friend hearing her cries and groans during the whole night... That next morning when they saddled up, the child stood dazed and as they moved to leave, staggered towards them apparently not knowing if she were still a prisoner or at liberty: they rode off, leaving her in the bush... (Bottoms, 2013, p.94)

Introduction

We invite you to join a conversation between five colleagues who work in separate but interconnected services responding to the healing needs of Aboriginal and Torres Strait Islander young people, their families, and the communities in which they live. All these groups show symptoms of the impacts of trans- and intergenerational trauma across Australian colonial history. We explore the stories that call for and show the changes we need in our work practices with Aboriginal young people and their families. Together we discuss the historic and continuing racism and layered violence/trauma of Aboriginal lives, and the healing that is required to repair the harm of colonial legacies in the establishment of Australia as a penal colony.

Margaret Hayes, principal of a school for young people with distressed behaviors, in conversation with Gerard Webster, presents the stories of two young people, a young man and a young woman, both allowing us to see the wounding that can happen when we do not protect our youth from harm, and hence label them as 'bad'.

Carlie Atkinson shares the voices and outcomes of Aboriginal men within several Australian correctional centres who volunteered to participate in her PhD research exploring the relationship between Aboriginal male violence and generational post-traumatic stress (now known as complex trauma). The Australian Aboriginal version of the Harvard Trauma Questionnaire (AAVHTQ) was developed to ensure the cultural specificity of this research capturing traumatic stressors and cultural idioms of distress that are relevant to Aboriginal peoples. Judy Atkinson then demonstrates the outcomes of educational therapeutic work with women in prison, what she calls *Educaring*, responding to the women's trauma stories and 'offending' patterns.

Gerard Webster describes what we learned from delivering a workshop for workers in the Department of Education who were concerned with finding a pathway forward for the young people attending their schools. This focused interest from educational staff responds to the challenge to further develop skills to work with their students and develop possibilities within educational systems and in schools for trauma-transformative care and practice, instead of an assumed pathway into prison.

Gavin Morris brings into the conversation the demonstration of *Dadirri* (deep listening) in practice, opening our understanding of 'symptom as history,' the pain embedded within the stories when truth-telling is put into action at the community level. Gavin's research also provides the challenge that opens a pathway forward by whole community engagement in their own healing needs, and the concept of the Ancient University as renewal.

This conversational approach is presented in the hope of opening a broader conversation about Indigenous healing practices grounded within Indigenous critical pedagogy as we respond to the generational layered, compounded, complex trauma we work with. There is a need for deep therapeutic work linking Communities of Care with Communities of Practice across all services to help repair the inter- and transgenerational traumatic wounding of colonized populations. The chapter promotes a reclamation through the work of healing such wounds – a return to our cultural and spiritual roots for well-being. It is therapeutic at the deepest level. The challenge is that community, in its diversity and wounded complexity, must be the healer.

Historical context

Psychosocial ills such as severe mental health conditions, juvenile delinquency, drug addiction, the perpetration of physical, sexual, emotional abuse, and neglect of children all have their origins in traumatic events during childhood. Aboriginal survivors of trauma are particularly vulnerable to long-term consequences of traumatic experiences as they are the subjects of additional forms of abuse. Aboriginal Australians, like most First Nations peoples across the globe, are the bearers of inter- and transgenerational trauma as well as the current targets of overt and covert interpersonal and structural racism. This chapter considers the pathway from childhood trauma to dissociation and aggression, to violence and other crimes that perpetuate cycles of abuse across generations, which ultimately lead to imprisonment and other psychosocial consequences. The importance and success of Indigenous healing practices that are changing the lives of children, teenagers, and adults are explored.

Aboriginal peoples experience a significantly greater prevalence of family, domestic, and sexual violence than is the case in non-Indigenous communities (Parliament of the Commonwealth of Australia, 2021). Such violence occurs between immediate and extended family members or by perpetrators either inside or outside Aboriginal communities. Such violence occurs between adults, by adults on children, and sometimes between children. All of these forms of intrafamilial and extrafamilial violence perpetrated against Aboriginal peoples are contextualized by Australia's history of racial violence and all other forms of racism.

The means by which the British dispossessed Aboriginal peoples of the land that was their physical and spiritual home for well over 60,000 years was indefensible, and its impact on Aboriginal culture and well-being has been catastrophic. The non-sanitized version of Australia's colonial and post-colonial history is that the British Empire took Australia through extreme violence. The Empire dispossessed approximately 250 Indigenous nations of their tribal lands by engaging in or allowing mass murder through gunfire and by the poisoning of food and waterholes, by the brutal capture and enslavement of individuals and tribes, by segregation and impoverishment, and by the rape of women and children. Aboriginal populations were decimated, and communities and cultures disintegrated by such violent strategies. It is estimated that somewhere between 300,000 and 1.25 million Aboriginal peoples lived on the Australian continent in 1788. However, there is no question that only 50,000 Aboriginal peoples survived by 1930. Added to the casualties of racist violence described above, many Aboriginal peoples died of previously unknown diseases introduced by white convicts, soldiers, and settlers, including those diseases which were sexually transmitted as a consequence of rape and child sexual assault. The psychosocial costs to Aboriginal peoples through more than two centuries of genocide, domination, and subjugation are immeasurable.

Australia's Aboriginal peoples continue to be the victims of interpersonal and structural racism – the latter being the cumulative and compounding effects of history, culture, ideology, and institutional policies and practices that systemically privilege white people and disadvantage people of colour. The culture of racism that the British exported to Australia plays out in the lives of many individual Aboriginal Australians in the form of daily taunts, physical and sexual assaults, and the deprivation of multiple basic human rights.

The breaking and building of trust: A conversation between Margaret Hayes and Gerard Webster

At the time of writing, 'Timothy'[1] is currently locked up hundreds of kilometres away from his home: away from country (his ancestral and spiritual homeland), and away from his family and those who love him (his relational home). Why? This 13-year-old boy is alleged to have jumped into a stolen vehicle for a few minutes. No one was hurt. The vehicle was not damaged. But, because this is not the first time he has come into conflict with the law, he is likely to be incarcerated for several months. Being Aboriginal, he is far more likely to receive the full weight of the law for his crime.

By entering the juvenile justice system, Timothy has joined the tens of thousands of Aboriginal men, women, and children before him who have spent too many years in prison and juvenile detention centres. Many of these people entered a life of crime as children, starting with petty offences such as those committed by Timothy. What other statistical categories is Timothy now likely to register his membership of? Will he join other Aboriginal peoples as a member of the most socio-economically disadvantaged group in Australia? Will his physical and mental health be well below that of the general community? Will he leave high school well before his non-Aboriginal age-mates? Will he find it harder to secure and maintain employment than other boys and men in the general population? Will he die 10–20 years earlier than non-Aboriginal Australians? To all these questions, according to decades of research, and despite all the programs trialled under the sun and the moon, the sad answer is 'yes.'

Timothy's plight begs answers to two questions:

- How did he get to the point of having his right to freedom withdrawn by the state at his tender age?
- What can be done to get him back on track to become a proud Aboriginal man and to pursue his potential as a natural leader?

---

1   The authors thank Timothy's mother for providing consent for Timothy's story to be used in this publication. 'Timothy' is a pseudonym used for the purpose of protecting the boy's identity.

Timothy was born in a remote rural community scarred by genocide, historical, collective racist abuses. Multiple violations of human rights across two centuries have given rise to transgenerational trauma, not the least of which was the nearby Myall Creek Massacre in 1838. On this occasion, a landowner and his stockmen killed up to 20 Aboriginal people. Other stockmen and settlers were encouraged to murder any Aboriginal person they came across. This war crime was described by the then police magistrate as 'a war of extermination,' but it is far from the most lethal massacre in the country's history. The Myall Creek Massacre, one of at least 304 known frontier massacres in Australia, lives on in the conscious and unconscious memories of the local Aboriginal peoples. Such massacres were also accompanied by the rape of women, girls, and boys. The trauma of such cruelty is not only remembered as a historical artifact, but it is lived out in the very being of each Aboriginal person, and each of their relationships and behaviors. This phenomenon is what is commonly referred to as transgenerational trauma.

Against this historical context, and like many Aboriginal peoples, Timothy was raised in poverty, surrounded by family, domestic, and sexual violence among other chronic social problems. However, his family was doing well until just a few years ago. Timothy was one of several children raised by his single mother with the support of her community. Each of Timothy's siblings demonstrated great potential in the arts, culture, sport, and academia. Timothy was no different. The children were well protected by their mother and extended family from many of the interpersonal harms so common in their community.

Things changed when a close family member was found hanging from a tree. Although officially determined to be suicide, suspicion of something more sinister abounded within the community about the actual cause of death. Timothy's mother had not been the same since the loss. Her despair led her to chronic drug use and her attention increasingly turned inward. The children's loss was multiplied: an absent father, a deceased relative under suspicious circumstances, and now a debilitated mother. Timothy's older siblings tried to compensate for their mother's deteriorating mental health and its impact on the care Timothy needed, but they could not breach the gap left in the wake of family and communal trauma.

It was at this point in the family's history that Timothy entered the school system. He was quickly identified as a highly intelligent child whose pattern of behavior was extremely problematic. Sanctions against his misbehavior quickly escalated to include multiple episodes of exclusion from school for both brief and lengthy periods.

Timothy was referred to a school for children who have chronic behavior problems soon after his sixth birthday. Most if not all the students attending this school are Aboriginal males. The school has a capacity of 20 students and is staffed by both Aboriginal and non-Aboriginal teachers and support workers. The school principal drives around the town each morning before classes begin to talk to parents and other community members for the purpose of building and maintaining relationships and because she genuinely cares for her students. Her personal investment in the children's welfare is obvious to the community and she is well respected as a result. School attendance has improved dramatically under her leadership.

Timothy's behavior stabilized, and he flourished almost from the moment he arrived at the school. Within a short period, he was heard singing out in top voice across the playground, *'I can read! I can read!'* Any time of the day when Timothy was not in class, he could be found in the playground demonstrating his enthusiasm, agility, and sporting prowess. He was highly valued and enjoyed by staff and students, alike, and he basked in the warmth of affirmation that characterized the school environment. He began volunteering for leadership positions as he progressed through the following years.

Sadly, as Timothy moved toward adolescence, his life began to take a turn for the worse outside the safety of the school community. His mother's ability to provide the necessary care and supervision for Timothy continued to deteriorate after she had more children. She continued to be untreated for depression and she maintained her drug use. Timothy began to spend a lot of time out of the family home late at night, with peers and older children who had developed delinquent patterns of behavior. While Timothy continued to attend school and participate well in all the school's activities (school was his safe place), his increasing exposure to a racist and exploitative world increased his risk of being harmed exponentially.

History is currently repeating itself across Australia with opportunistic non-Aboriginal people, almost exclusively men, luring Aboriginal children into the sex trade. Many hungry Aboriginal children have found a way of filling their stomachs by providing opportunistic truck drivers who pass through regional and remote communities with sexual services in return for food and drugs. It is not long before boys and girls, like Timothy, find themselves addicted to illicit substances. The children's desire for drugs is also fuelled by their need to obliterate the thoughts and feelings that have resulted from racism, transgenerational trauma and, more immediately, earlier and contemporary experiences of child abuse that have occurred within their homes or in their local communities. Such children are typically lost to a world of exploitation that inevitably leads to conflict with the law and a life of misery – misery that too often sets the foundations of a pathway to long-term drug addiction, suicide, mental illness, incarceration, and a host of other social and psychological ills.

Soon after his 13th birthday, Timothy was heard screaming in the distance, *'It wasn't me! It wasn't me!'* The school principal, Margaret Hayes, immediately went to assist, hearing the terror and desperation in his voice. After calming down, Timothy explained that some boys from a neighbouring school had thrown rocks at him, and someone had called the police and blamed him. The police arrived and Timothy was arrested and handcuffed without discussion. He was then paraded through the school playground in front of the entire school community and placed in a police vehicle. In the meantime, the principal took the time to talk with a first-hand witness and learned that Timothy's version of events was correct. Timothy did throw a rock, but this took place in the context of returning fire in response to the racist taunts and rocks being thrown at him by a large group of non-Aboriginal students.

Timothy's screams from inside the police van could be heard far and wide: '*Get me out of here! This is so fucking wrong! Get me out of here!* **Hear the fucking story!**' Fortunately, the school principal was able to locate a police inspector and convey the truth of what had occurred. Timothy was the victim of racist violence. He retaliated. Upon seeing Timothy throw a rock, one witness assumed and reported to police that the black kid was the instigator, not the ten or so white boys who were also throwing rocks. Fortunately, another witness came forward who had seen the whole scenario, which vindicated Timothy and resulted in his immediate release without charges being brought.

Sadly, the end of this story is not a happy one. It is understood that the police watched and hounded Timothy from that day on. It did not take long before harassment by police resulted in this 13-year-old boy becoming increasingly angry, resentful, and retaliatory. To make matters worse, Timothy's mother sank further into addiction. According to the school principal, Timothy 'just totally unravelled and was sent to detention.'

Identifying and understanding the problem: A conversation between Judy Atkinson and Caroline Atkinson

Timothy's pathway to the juvenile justice system was paved by the multiple adverse experiences of his childhood and early adolescence. PhD research conducted by Associate Professor Caroline 'Carlie' Atkinson (2008) confirms the established link between multiple adverse experiences during childhood, subsequent criminal behavior, and extensive histories of incarceration. However, Carlie's research is distinguished by its exposition of the extent to which Aboriginal peoples with significant criminal histories have suffered psychosocial trauma throughout their lives.

The Adverse Childhood Experience (ACE) Study in the United States (Felitti *et al.*, 1998) highlighted childhood trauma, including abuse and neglect, as a critical public health challenge (van de Kolk, 2007). The study examined the responses of mainly white American males between 1995 and

1997 to a questionnaire comprising ten items. The questionnaire asked participants if a parent or carer had been abusive toward them, including physical violence; whether an adult had ever forced them to have sex as a child; whether they ever felt as a child that they were not loved or cared for; whether they had gone hungry and or had been neglected; if their parents had separated, divorced or were absent; if a family member had been depressed, mentally ill or suicidal; whether they had witnessed domestic, family, or community violence, including the use of weapons, often fuelled by alcohol or other drugs; and whether a household member had served time in prison. A score of 4 such adverse experiences in a child's lifetime was considered extremely high, and relevant to ongoing health issues on those impacted (Felitti *et al.* (1998)).

Carlie's research compared the findings of the ACE Study with the stories of the Aboriginal men she interviewed in Australian prisons. Not only did she find a correlation between the studies but also the traumatic imprints of colonization as it continues across generations. Carlie developed and administered an Australian Aboriginal version of the Harvard Trauma Questionnaire (AAVHTQ).

Colonization and slavery have ongoing detrimental impacts across generations. There is a clear trail that shows early childhood adverse experiences can lead to future adverse outcomes unless healing pathways are created. Seven out of ten men in Carlie's study reported being highly distressed from '*feelings of shame for being Aboriginal* and experiencing *racism*' (Atkinson, 2008). Carlie found that the men were more likely to experience symptoms of complex post-traumatic stress disorder if they experience any of the following adversities:

- Unwanted sex/assaults – rape and/or sexual abuse.
- Being hungry/having no home, no school or clinic to go to, lack of support structures.
- Not being accepted by own community.
- Feelings of not belonging to anything – any place – feeling lost.
- No support for physical, mental, emotional, or spiritual health problems.

Carlie's research found that, according to the AAVHTQ, over half (58.6%) of the study population had significant PTSD symptomatology, and the majority had been exposed to a significantly high number of traumatic stressors. The more traumatic stressors endorsed, or the greater amount of exposure to traumatic events, the more likely the participants were to experience PTSD symptoms. Research participants who endorsed traumatic stressors associated with low formal and informal social support and/or a lack of personal and social identity, and who had been sexually abused and/or suffered from symptoms associated with precarious mental health, low self-esteem and social isolation were significantly more likely to suffer PTSD symptoms and appeared to resort to violence to express and repeat their trauma.

Qualitative and quantitative data highlighted the endemic nature and normalization of family violence, grief and loss, and alcohol and drug misuse as both symptoms and causes of traumatic stressors for the men in Carlie's study. Traumatic stressors relating to institutional violence, fractured families, acculturation (colonization) and racism were also identified as significant traumatic stressors through the qualitative results. Significant increases in traumatic stressors and dysfunctional behaviors were revealed in the research participants' current and older generational histograms, lending support for the notion of generational trauma and distress. These results suggest that the high rates of Aboriginal men being incarcerated for crimes of violence could be largely due to a history of widespread traumatic stressors that are being transmitted across the generations, and which will continue to increase across successive generations without effective healing interventions.

These findings must influence our understanding that ACEs have a tremendous impact on future violence victimization and perpetration, and lifelong health and social opportunities. The mean rates of family members who have been or are incarcerated, are a perpetrator and/or a victim of sexual assault/rape and physical violence, have committed or attempted suicide, and misused drugs and alcohol are significantly higher in the current generation than in the older generations. Carlie has since progressed her research as a culturally competent measure of specific traumatic stressors and cultural idioms of distress for Aboriginal peoples (Atkinson, 2008).

The link between adversity in childhood, ongoing psychological distress, violence, and incarceration is, of course, not limited to males.

In 2015, Professor Judy Atkinson was invited to apply trauma relevant principles in response to the needs of the Kunga Stopping Violence Program (KSVP). KSVP is a prison-based violence prevention program that aims to respond to the needs of Aboriginal women on remand or serving sentences in the Alice Springs Correctional Centre (ASCC). Between 95 and 100 percent of the women in ASCC were Aboriginal women. Judy designed her education approach in line with her pedagogical framework of *Educaring*. *Educaring* is a 'trauma-specific blend of Aboriginal traditional healing activities and Western educational and therapeutic processes. It uses experiential learning to enable participants to explore their individual and community transgenerational trauma stories' (Atkinson *et al.*, 2014, p.299).

KSVP's title is derived from Pitjantjatjara, one of the Central Australian languages. In the Anangu languages of the Central Desert, the word *kunga* means 'young woman.' The Kunga four-week course is delivered as part of the full program and is run every six months, twice a year. Eligible Aboriginal women with an alleged history of violent offending, who are incarcerated at ASCC at the time the course is run, are offered the opportunity to participate in the Kunga Program.

The women's need for safety was the first consideration in the design phase of the Kunga Program package. Support for the women's psychological safety was considered an essential requirement for them to be able to explore their anger and violence while in a prison environment. This support was offered before and during the court process, while the women were in prison and on release. As Carlie found with the men she interviewed, Judy found that the women's anger and violent behaviors were fed by earlier experiences of lack of support structures, feelings of not belonging and not being heard, and physical and sexual violence – psychological pain that Judy acknowledged as being a colonial legacy.

In October 2015, KSVP commenced the delivery of the first four-week intensive trauma-specific, violence-prevention educational package. The original educational package design was two days of 'recreating the circle of wellbeing' (exploring cultural issues of spirituality, environment, relationships, emotions, physical body, sexuality, stress, and life purpose) to provide self-regulating tools for the women to access skills to feel safe during the educational-therapeutic delivery. The women then began to explore their stories of anger and violence while considering how they could build boundaries and safety into their lives.

The women explored definitions of family and community violence; what is bad anger, the evolution of anger into violence, and cycles of violence; how anger and violence impact children, youth, families, and communities; anger triggers (including hot and cold anger); managing anger, and stopping violence; alcohol, drugs, and gambling use; jealousy; naming and managing feelings and changing behavior. The women practised being assertive, using 'I statements' and learned about Aboriginal cultural processes for clearing up conflict.

The women proceeded to create the violence/non-violence tree which became a silent acknowledgement and means of managing feelings.

The educational package then moved into exploring issues of loss, grief, bereavement, and mourning. The women saw their different responses to victimization and bereavement. Judy noted that the women were often incarcerated as the result of responding to experiences of victimization with rage, of which they had no memory. They explored loss circles that brought into focus inside and outside feelings with increased body awareness. Each woman was supported to construct their own loss history map.

A loss history map is a tool that helps a person describe and record experiences from birth to the present, allowing them in the process to reflect on how those experiences may be continuing to contribute to their present life circumstances. Working with the women on their loss history maps was often a time of shame-filled disclosures of early childhood or early teenage sexual assault, domestic violence, drinking to dull the pain, disassociated self-harm, and violent rages. Trauma often meshed with compounding losses and complex grief in the lives of the women. This was often a time when they would put their hand over the graph and say with conviction: 'So it is not my fault' and, 'It stops with me.' These insights were the single most important deciding factors for their therapeutic change.

One woman had constructed a loss history map with a blank between the years 13 and 16. Judy and the woman worked together over several days until Judy was ready to challenge her. Judy put her hand over the section that addressed that period in the woman's life, and said, 'It is okay if you do not want to talk about this time in your life but look what has happened after this time. You started to drink, and your first offences began.' The woman sat quietly, went away, and painted again for two days, after which she was ready 'to talk about it.' Her pattern of drinking and offending began when she was being subjected to sexual violence. Since exploring the stories and pain of that period of her life, she has not taken up drinking again nor has she re-offended since she returned to the community.

Loss history maps led to the most profound experience for the women and the workers as the women identified emotionally unhealed losses, and constructed healing in seeking to repair relationships with themselves and members of their families, including their children. In response to the findings from the loss history maps, the KSVP increased its use of trauma-specific recovery tools to support the women to focus on their resilience and to build on their strengths. The loss history maps became an important tool in the KSVP for understanding behaviors or actions as trauma responses.

Formal educational morning sessions included painting, along with music-facilitated meditative processes allowing for inner reflection, mindfulness, and integration, while at the same time serving as a therapeutic calming aid. The women painted each afternoon and talked as they created both individual and group art, resulting in deep healing reflection in the conversations as they painted together. It was during these times that deeper therapeutic work occurred.

The ACE study questionnaire was also used with the women. Considering the questions posed in the questionnaire seemed to give permission to the women to talk about issues of which they felt deep shame. After running the questions of the ACE study, Judy found there was not one woman who had a score under 7. A significant number had 10 – the entire number of adverse experiences identified in the ACE study.

After reviewing the first three deliveries of KSVP, it was clear the focus on loss and grief through therapeutic loss history mapping allowed both the workers and the women to recognize the cumulative, compounded complexity of trauma in the childhood lives of the women. Using the process of the loss history maps, combined with the ACE study questions, provided important evidence on which better therapeutic services for the women could be argued. By 2017, the focus of the 'in prison' work of the KSVP moved to the loss history mapping as a therapeutic process.

In an ANROWS-funded research (Bevis *et al.*, 2020), it was found that most of the women who participated in the study had a clear diagnosis of complex trauma and that, nonetheless, the women showed extraordinary resilience. Four interactive complex trauma enablers were identified:

- Fractured historic, generational, mother-child, family, and community relationships.
- Disconnect in communication and in service delivery between services and the women.
- Failures in legal, policing, courts, and government policies, which disadvantaged and created further abuse of the women.
- Substantial barriers to health, housing, and support services.

The cultural tools for healing comprised story mapping, music and dance, individual and collective art, learning through role-plays, theater, and deep extensive communal therapeutic conversations. The Kunga Stopping Violence Program, *Educaring* and relational approach assisted in drawing out the women's life stories and needs, working therapeutically with them in and beyond prison, and advocating for them at all levels of service delivery. The research found that KSVP worked to hold the complexity of the women's trauma and helped start the healing process. KSVP advocated for the women and challenged the failure of the service systems while demonstrating, at the same time, that the service systems failure surrounding the women continues to be a further complex trauma enabler. KSVP continues to assist women to identify and heal from complex trauma and offer a pathway out from a life of violence, crime, and imprisonment. However, the program needs more attention and support if populations of Aboriginal men and women in prison are to be reduced.

The optimal approach for reducing the numbers of Aboriginal men and women in prison is to engage with children who are at risk of following the pathway from trauma into the juvenile justice system or to invite those children who have taken their first steps along that pathway to recognize better alternatives through more positive connections with Aboriginal culture. It should be recognized that the optimal environment to achieve this goal is to engage with children in the system to which they are already engaged, the education system.

Finding a way forward: A conversation between Judy Atkinson and Margaret Hayes

Children, by nature, are dependent on adults for food, clothing, shelter, nurturance, and education so that they grow to be healthy, empowered adults who can navigate the challenges of life drawing on both their personal resources and the support of trusted and trustworthy people. Children like Timothy described above – who grow up in an environment where love and care are mixed with family, domestic, and sexual violence, fuelled by chronic drug use, and contextualized by transgenerational trauma, poverty, and all the social ills accompanying such an environment – need help from those who can give it. Children have the right to protection but when families are no longer able to offer such protection and statutory authorities continually fail to meet the challenge of protecting those identified as being at serious risk of harm, another system needs to step up and meet the need and render assistance. The education system is well placed to do so, and progress toward this goal is currently being made at the local level at the school which Timothy attends.

Margaret Hayes, Timothy's school principal, has a whole-person, whole-of-community approach to achieving the educational goals for which she is responsible. Margaret has commenced each school day over the last ten years driving around the town talking to community Elders, parents, aunties, and children. From these brief interactions, she has the opportunity to gain relevant information about her students, encourage parents to motivate their children to attend school, help parents' problem solve any issues they are having with their children, and, most significantly, build a relationship based on trust and stability. It is from this trusted place that she has come to be recognized as willing and able to help in a way that is connective to the Aboriginal community, rather than disconnected and dominating. Under these circumstances, children come to her when they are in difficulties – when they are hungry, when their shoes no longer fit, when they have injured themselves, and when they are ready to share information about their secret lives of trauma.

Timothy was rescued from the injustice of a harmful court outcome after police had received racially biased information that led to his arrest. Timothy had a relationship based on years of mutual trust and care with his school principal so they could collaborate to set the record straight with police. Timothy is far from being the only one who has relied on and benefited from a relationship with a trusted person in authority.

Two former female students visited Margaret one evening while she and Judy were working on their ideas of taking *Educaring* into the classroom. Overhearing some of Margaret and Judy's conversation and realizing the significance of their work, one girl asked, 'Can you fix me?' Judy asked her to explain further, and the girl shared her story of victimization, of extreme, vicious sexual violence. Worse still, her story extended beyond the sexual assault to expose a complete deficiency of the support structures in her community that should have been available to respond to her emotional, mental, and spiritual needs. When Judy now talks about the conversation that night, she says, 'Yes, the girl had been hospitalized, and stitched up and physically repaired, as hospitals do. But the betrayal, and the lack of skills in the workforces, more particularly for Aboriginal youth, was clear. It was a deep soul wounding.'

As with the majority of most of the adults and children Judy has worked with over the decades, many of whom have experienced similar acts of violence on their bodies and souls, the critical services created to meet their needs fail them. The two young women who visited Margaret and Judy that night knew of one place they would be welcomed and supported. The relationship built between Margaret and the girls went beyond the point at which Margaret was in the role of school principal. When asked how best to work with the young people who attend her school – children who are typically expelled or frequently suspended from mainstream schools – Margaret simply says, 'Just love them unconditionally.'

Judy and Margaret were left with a question following their interaction with the former student: How can anyone 'fix' such pain – the physical and emotional trauma left by the vicious sexual assault the young woman had endured? Both Judy and Margaret are deeply concerned by the fact that most, if not all, of the children attending the school suffer symptoms of complex trauma resulting from family, domestic, and sexual violence within their families and throughout their non-Aboriginal community, both currently and in the past. Most children would tick all boxes of the ACE questionnaire.

Judy and Margaret have continued their collaboration, building *Educaring* into the school's culture and activities. Judy brought what she found to be of benefit when helping Aboriginal women heal from trauma in the KSVP and applied it to traumatized children within the school system to build a culturally safe, school-based, therapeutic, trauma-informed/integrated and trauma-specific educational and practical approach that promotes health and well-being, and sustainable pathways of positive change for students.

The children were increasingly inclined to disclose sexual and other forms of abuse occurring in their homes and in the community as a sense of trust and safety strengthened. Further, children were beginning to display sexualized and sexually aggressive behaviors while at school. The story of their trauma was therefore communicated by both truth-telling in the form of disclosures, and in their behavior as a repetition of the sexual abuse perpetrated on them. Both forms of communication called for a healthy response from the school, often in the face of absent or inadequate interventions by the local child protection agency. Judy proposes that an effective response can only be achieved in two ways: by upskilling staff and by providing children with opportunities for healing with culturally integrated methods.

Judy recognizes that professional development of staff is crucial to creating an engaging and helpful school environment. The initial task, therefore, was to upgrade the knowledge of school staff about the relationship between trauma and behaviors that are deemed problematic. Teaching and support staff were immediately observed to engage differently with the children. With greater understanding came calmer and more reflective responses to behavior that were seen as problematic.

The second dimension of Judy's trauma-informed and culturally integrated healing approach was to introduce six healing modalities within the school that she found helpful to the women healing from their trauma in the KSVP: music, dance, art, theater, bodywork, and nature discovery (connection to country). The children and staff's feedback about the integration of Indigenous healing practices into the life of the school was resoundingly positive:

- Music: *I really like drumming because it makes me feel really calm. I can hit the drum hard and it makes me feel better.*
- Dancing: *I really like dancing because I can feel the music inside me, from my head to my toes.*
- Art: *I really like art because I can draw what I feel. There are no mistakes in art.*
- Theater: *I really like theater because I get to be different characters and act different to me. It makes me feel different and it is really fun.*
- Bodywork: *I like bodywork because it makes me feel calm and relaxed.* The teachers commented: *We have the freedom to teach in the way the children need. They are so excited about learning. They are not angry anymore.*
- Nature discovery (connection to country): *I really like nature discovery because I love going outside and learning new things.*

Making a start: A conversation between Judy Atkinson, Margaret Hayes, and Gerard Webster

The children's sense of safety at school and their trust in the principal and teachers continued to grow with the introduction of Indigenous healing practices. Further, most behavior problems diminished, and school attendance increased. However, the sexualized and harmful sexual behaviors displayed by children attending the school were not eliminated. This is not surprising given that the children continued to be sexually abused and exploited by family members, local community members, and non-Aboriginal individuals passing through the community outside school hours.

The ongoing need to address the children's sexual behavior problems was addressed with teaching and support staff by a second tier of professional education offered by Dr Gerard Webster. Gerard is a forensic and counselling psychologist and psychoanalyst who has worked with both victims and perpetrators of family, domestic, and sexual violence (FDSV) throughout the last four decades. His holistic approach to forensic psychotherapy gives due weight to the traumatizing influences of family, environmental, and historical experiences that typically lead to the perpetration of harmful behaviors.

While Gerard works with people of all ages, it was his work with children and teenagers who engage in problem sexual behavior that led Margaret and Judy to invite him to speak with school staff. After working with school staff for a decade, it was obvious to Judy and Margaret that staff at the school had become confused and exhausted by their attempts to manage the children's problem sexual behavior, and they were at a loss as to what more they could do to help. Professional education revised the information previously provided by Judy about the relationship between trauma, acting-out behaviors such as depression and self-harm, and acting-out behaviors such as physical and sexual aggression.

Gerard provided an overview of research and clinical findings that children's sexual behaviors fall on a spectrum from normal, to problematic, to harmful (Webster and Butcher, 2012). It began to make sense to staff that the problematic and harmful sexual behaviors that they were witnessing and hearing about emerged in a child's behavioral repertoire due to the challenges that they had faced but were yet to be processed healthily. Children need a place of safety or, if you like, a safe relational home, where they can calm down sufficiently to be able to think and put their experiences into healthier actions and, ultimately, words (Webster, 2019).

Gerard spoke with staff more specifically about the relationship between FDSV and the problem sexual behavior of children in Aboriginal communities throughout Australia as contextualized by over two hundred years of racial violence and the transmission of trauma from one generation to the next. The staff seemed surprised to learn that children and adults who engage in sexual violence can be helped and rehabilitated, contrary to misinformation spread by media and ill-informed activists. Gerard reported that he had seen many people throughout his career, mostly men and boys, who had entered forensic psychotherapy and who had come to sincerely accept responsibility for the harms they had caused others, particularly to loved ones. He had seen such men and boys reach a point where they wanted to dedicate the rest of their lives to non-offending, making sure that the people around them who would be their potential victims were safe, and that they engaged only in caring attitudes and behaviours (Webster, 2018). Staff, on hearing this as breaking news, immediately began to sit up and talk among themselves with positivity. They began to ask more questions and were actively engaged in finding ways of moving forward, rather than being locked into hopelessness and exhaustion.

Much to the surprise of everyone, two processes of change began as a direct result of the professional development experience. First, staff became enthusiastic about their achievements. Gerard observed that the combination of trauma and culturally integrated educational approach to healing developed and implemented at the school had been tremendously successful as it continued the process of building a safe relational home for its severely traumatized students. He argued that the trust built with the children and the Aboriginal community by Margaret and her staff formed the foundation for future development and expansion. The teaching and support staff of the school were in a good position to enhance the already existing emotionally holding and healing environment that had been built.

The second and most surprising development was the impact of the training on Aboriginal staff who began to consider ways that they might engage their Elders and community members in conversations about addressing the ongoing problem of FDSV perpetrated by local adults and children. The remainder of this chapter addresses how this might best be achieved.

Change is happening and healing will occur: A conversation between Judy Atkinson and Gavin Morris

Judy has observed that over her years of work in urban, rural, and remote communities, the concept that government has the will and capacity to respond to such critical needs of Aboriginal peoples has been replaced by two objectives for change. Judy proposes the need for the development of two interdependent communities – what she calls 'Communities of Care' and 'Communities of Practice.'

Communities of Care is the name given to groups of people who live together in small communities, and who care for each other. More particularly, those people who live in small communities know who is struggling and who is feeling pain and decide to do something to support them. They may see some school-aged children struggling at school, being blamed because they are not coping, maybe not attending school. They know of children who need care in the school environment – *Educaring* – and they volunteer to help with children who need support. They may know that the mum is struggling at home, and so they reach out to her, setting up a women's talking circle, a healing group for young mums and older women, sharing the support of each other. They may see young people who have lost direction, and work to set up activities, such as youth discos, camps, activities for youth, engaging with the older men in cultural activities and camps. The Community of Care provides guidance to the Community of Practice.

Communities of Practice are the groups of people who work within specific services, with diverse roles and responsibilities, on an ongoing basis in some common endeavour, generally through professional practice. They may be doctors, health workers, mental health workers, teachers, child and family workers, and so on. They may be non-Aboriginal or Aboriginal peoples. Communities of Practice emerge in response to a common interest, or concern, and play an important role in forming their members' participation in, and orientation to, the world around them. The value of the notion of Communities of Practice lies in the fact that it identifies a social grouping, not in virtue of shared abstract characteristics (e.g. class, gender) or simple co-presence (e.g. neighbourhood, workplace), but in virtue of shared practice.

During regular joint activity, a Community of Practice develops ways of doing things, views, values, power relations, ways of talking. The participants engage with these practices in virtue of their place in the Community of Practice, and the place of the Community of Practice in the larger social order. Two conditions of a Community of Practice are crucial in the construction of meaning: shared experience over time and a commitment to shared understanding. A Community of Practice engages people in mutual sense-making – about the life work they're engaged in, about their respective forms of participation, about their orientation to other communities of practice and to the world around them more generally. Communities of Care and Communities of Practice are promoted as the change-makers, in recovery or healing from the impacts of colonial generational trauma.

Dr Gavin Morris followed the journey of a community that was ready to start healing. He documented what can be achieved when people are listened to and feel heard and valued.

He says when he arrived in the Aboriginal community of Nauiyu, located on the Daly River, approximately 225km south of Darwin, he was privileged with the responsibility to hold the stories of a therapeutic response of a community that was ready to listen to itself and work for change. He had developed deep relationships with the community, relationships built on trust, humility, and reciprocity. These relationships have profoundly changed him as a person, but more importantly, provided a safe, trusted space for the community to tell its story. A strengths-based truth-telling was requested, designed and driven by the Daly River community to privilege Aboriginal voices and attend to a community need. This truth-telling formed a community-designed doctoral study which captured the trauma stories associated with the experience of colonization in a manner that would resonate in two worlds.

The Nauiyu community was suffering deeply from the trauma associated with the impact of colonization. Participants gave their accounts of the challenges they faced living in their community, describing how their loss of control, authority and power had impacted their culture. They also shared stories that detailed the terrible effects of colonization, stories of women fleeing violence at home, stories of suicide, stories of cultural wounding, and stories about precariously living between perpetrator and victim. These stories and the trauma associated with them are now being carried by the younger generation; a significant finding of the study is that the frequency and severity of the destructive behaviors compound and escalate as the trauma is transmitted from one generation to the next. We need to heal. However, the collective stories of the participants should not be seen as negative and lacking. The participants did not position themselves as victims. Instead, as one key male Elder described, their truth-telling was a celebration of strength and resilience.

> This is our time for truth telling. We have to name our trauma, what has happened and what continues to happen to our people in this community to oppress, oppose and disintegrate. We know what is happening in our community. They are our problems. We own them. And we have to be the ones who fix them. Not some white fella, or some other well-intentioned outsider. The answers belong to us, but we have some truths to tell first. Then the healing can start. (Participant 11)

Importantly, attempts to counter the effects of colonization had to be strengths-based and associated with feelings of empowerment. Seeking empowerment drew on the strengths that already existed within the community, where participants wanted to take charge of their future and develop a coherence about their life story:

> It is about time that we tell our story, our side of it all. The white fella blew a hole in the floor and everyone fell into it. Destroyed us, ripped our heart out and for what. I haven't seen nothing. What advancement has there been? Nothing. There has always been something that always put us on the back foot. And then they still turn around and say the black folks got to run their own thing. Let him take the bull by the horns. We broke it for you, now you got to run your own thing now. You can't make wood out of ashes. You burned the tree. You're not gonna get those ashes to rise up and grow into a tree again. But they're expecting us to now put our brains together and come up with a solution to self-improve. We will do it again; we have the strength in us to control our destiny. (Participant 5)

Many participants referred to this search for empowerment through enabling a cultural revival and regeneration which re-placed Aboriginal peoples in the centre of transformational change and healing: 'We have to go back to culture, regrow from the ground, there are green shoots... that is where our strength is' (Participant 35); 'Give us the space to find our strength in our culture then in ourselves again, it's still there within us' (Participant 13), and 'We will start healing when we empower ourselves again in our culture, through our voice, in our way' (Participant 11). Their only support network, however, was each other, and with many suffering from the same unresolved trauma behaviors, individual and collective healing had to take place for sustainable empowerment of the community to occur. Some fought, some ended up drinking, using alcohol and drugs, both as a symptom and a cause of trauma, others went into a mental health spiral, or just completely avoided it, disconnected it, and disconnected from it. Within the stories of the participants, it was clear that the place where they used to find support and strength in their culture had been eroded by colonial influences. Participants claimed they lived in a 'place of grey - neither black nor white,' forced to exist in an empty void, where they felt trapped between two worlds, where, in its current state, neither Aboriginal nor non-Indigenous laws firmly existed.

Participants were unanimous that not only did they own their truth-telling, but they also possessed their own solutions and any effective, sustainable healing response to their experience of colonization must come from within the community. These findings reflect previous research which asserts that the governance of the healing journey would profoundly benefit from the skills and experiences possessed by the people who have directly or indirectly suffered the trauma associated with colonization (Clark *et al.*, 2017; Dudgeon, Watson and Holland, 2017). Despite the corrosive colonial influence, the Nauiyu community still have traditional healing practices that support healing trauma. When compared to Western mainstream medical models, traditional healing practices are more effective in providing a healing response to the experience of trauma as they more closely align with the Aboriginal holistic views of health and well-being.

Nauiyu, for example, is home to a powerful Aboriginal healing modality known as *Dadirri*. Internationally renowned, *Dadirri* aims to lessen the effects of trauma and provide a pathway of empowerment and resilience for individuals and the community. Utilizing *Dadirri* within a local Nauiyu community context provides an opportunity for members to re-engage, trust, and value their own cultural practices. Rather than a quick fix or the need to fix and change what arises, *Dadirri* asks of us to allow each moment, each breath, each story to unfold naturally. It gives us the opportunity to accept what is arising for us, or in us, at each successive moment of experience, without the need to fix, fight, or avert what is arising. Empowering people through the learning and application of their traditional healing practices and knowledge is demonstrated to increase their individual and collective health, strength, and well-being (Atkinson *et al.*, 2010). Dr Miriam-Rose Ungunmerr-Baumann, a distinguished educator, artist, and key Elder of the Nauiyu community, first brought *Dadirri* to national attention in 1988. When first addressing a conference in Tasmania, Ungunmerr-Baumann described the value of *Dadirri*:

> What I want to talk about is another special quality of my people. I believe it is the most important. It is perhaps the greatest gift we can give to our fellow Australians. In our language, it is called Dadirri. It is an inner, deep listening, and quiet, still awareness. Dadirri recognises the deep spring inside us. We call on it and it calls on us. This is the gift Australia is thirsting for...and I believe that the spirit of Dadirri that we have to offer will blossom and grow, not just within ourselves, but in our whole nation... (Ungunmerr-Baumann, 1988)

Dadirri is healing from the heart, really listening, not just hearing – heartfelt listening, feeling deeply, having the courage to heal by expressing your grief and pain. It is growing together, healing together through sharing stories from the heart. Participants recognized the value of the contemplative listening to the stories of others, which allowed for healing and increased their sense of connection and community. The therapeutic phases of *Dadirri* are both relational and individual, and to fully appreciate it, one must move from an individual perspective to a collective one. One participant stated, for example, that it was the sense of belonging and of community that allow stories to be shared without fear of judgement. *Dadirri* is a constant renewal of the spirit that brings peace and contemplation to all aspects of life. As the stories of trauma were repeated over time, another participant revealed: 'Your story eventually changes, and the pain of trauma is released and replaced with love and acceptance as the healing process begins.'

The major theme which emerged from the truth-telling was the support of traditional healing practices in response to trauma through an Ancient University. The term Ancient University refers to an Aboriginal, stand-alone healing centre that privileges Aboriginal healing practices and knowledges. According to the community, the Ancient University should be built on country, out of flood zones for accessibility, and well outside the confines of the Nauiyu community. Not only was healing linked to a connection to country, but participants also felt that healing would most likely occur away from violence, drug and alcohol use and day-to-day pressures of life in the community. Much significance was also placed on the Ancient University for healing, which is holistic in nature and more aligned with Aboriginal views of health. People felt that healing through traditional healing practices in an Ancient University would be powerful as it offered more control, self-determination and understanding over their healing journeys.

The Ancient University would also serve an important function in protecting knowledges for the future. Traditional healing practices and knowledges, which have been suffering the corrosive influence of colonization since white settlement, could be maintained and protected in the Ancient University. A key male Elder, interviewed at Flat Rock, overlooking the Daly River, continued:

> I really like the idea of having this Ancient University. It can be a way to protect our healing ways...too much has already been lost, lost to the grave, the clinic, the grog. Lost because we're just not respecting enough of what we know and just thinking that what has been, will always be. Wrong. We have to protect our healing, maintain and protect. Let's start collecting our healing stories, get all our culture ways of healing and put them together, in one place and look after them. Just like our ancestors would expect us to. (Participant 30)

Other participants asserted that the Ancient University would have an educational utility. Key Elders and other holders of sacred knowledge could share this information through a teaching and learning exchange within the Ancient University. This also provides an opportunity for culturally appropriate education and employment opportunities. Several participants spoke about the importance of providing education and employment opportunities for Aboriginal peoples that reflect their own knowledge and specifically attend to community-related issues. Furthermore, these essential features of the Ancient University will also assist in supporting families and community members who are not skilled up to respond to trauma behaviors.

It is essential, however, that the traditional knowledges and healing practices that have been described become accredited; and recently, it is here where there have been two significant, ground-breaking pieces of work. First, the College of Aboriginal and Torres Strait Islander Healing Practices (CATSIHP) has recently been established as a forum to support, develop, and accredit Indigenous healing practices. The newly formed CATSIHP exists as a key Indigenous-led college within the Psychotherapy and Counselling Federation of Australia (PACFA), which is a leading national peak body for counsellors and psychotherapists in Australia. CATSIHP also now promotes pathways for Indigenous leaders to gain qualifications to learn and teach in tertiary settings, and develops training standards and guidelines for Aboriginal and Torres Strait Islander practitioners that support their use of traditional healing practices. Such has been the impact of CATSIHP's work in accrediting Aboriginal and Torres Strait Islander healing practices that some of Australia's largest private health insurers have contacted CATSIHP to inquire into how traditional healing practices can be included in their health schedules.

The second piece of substantial work involves a newly formed partnership between Batchelor Institute of Indigenous Tertiary Education, Charles Darwin University and We Al-li. In what could be a world-first, the partnership will soon be offering a Master's in Indigenous Therapies, which is an accredited qualification promoting Indigenous healing practices at postgraduate level. This joint venture arises out of an identified need for an accredited program that would skill a workforce in Aboriginal communities who are charged with the responsibility of attending to the needs of people who are living with intergenerational trauma. The Master's in Indigenous Therapies (or Healing Practices) is a decolonized qualification involving coursework that is specifically designed for the needs of Indigenous workers through increased access to Indigenous-specific education, based on the principles of an Indigenous critical pedagogy, using academic and cultural tools embodied with Indigenous healing practices. Thus, not only will Indigenous knowledges and healing practices provide a culturally responsive pathway for Indigenous Australians to complete postgraduate qualifications at the tertiary level in Australia, but the course will also receive formal accreditation through the PACFA.

Accrediting Aboriginal knowledges and traditional healing will ensure that Western mainstream health and education structures recognize Aboriginal knowledges which for so long have been suppressed and denied legitimacy. Moreover, accreditation is significant for communities where traditional healing interventions are being used but are not able to become a part of the referral system due to them being unaccredited. As a result, funding goes to the colonial system, outside, non-Indigenous service providers such as counsellors or psychologists, who parachute into communities with a very different set of values and worldviews to those to whom they were sent to heal or educate. This creates barriers to relationship building, promotes resentment, and disempowers the community because they're not getting the funds that are required to undertake the work that is so fruitful.

Once the community has undertaken its healing and been upskilled in providing its own accredited traditional healing practices, the community can then inform the service providers about how, and in what way, support can be offered. Currently, resources are being distributed to non-Indigenous service providers. While current best practice prescribes a 'community-led collaboration,' service providers essentially still have control over how the resources are utilized. With accreditation, the opposite can be true, where the system is literally flipped on its head and the upskilled and empowered community receives the funding directly. Communities can seek the support of non-Indigenous service providers where required, when it is recognized: 'We've got gaps here, we need support there, we need just more strength in this part of whatever it is.'

Conclusion

Family, domestic, and sexual violence is rife in some Aboriginal communities. These patterns of harmful behavior are contextualized by over two hundred years of interpersonal and structural racism. Just as violent experiences of the most grievous kind have been perpetrated by one culture on another, Aboriginal and non-Aboriginal individuals are repeating those very same abuses: murder, physical and sexual abuse, and chronic mistreatment of children. As with all communities, violence begets violence. However, Aboriginal peoples are also strong, smart, and resilient. While the top-down interventions of government continually fail to address the problems of its making, a bottom-up, grounded process of change is emerging at the local level. Aboriginal peoples are becoming increasingly ready to address problems in new ways – by drawing on their own strengths and by inviting the help of others who can engage in respectful ways.

This chapter has described how Indigenous healing practices, predicated on the emergence of an Indigenous critical pedagogy offers hope for the healing of traumatized Aboriginal men, women, and children that taps into over 60,000 years of tradition, culture, and spirituality. Such healing practices respond to the lives of people living within the generational colonized space, with the intention of healing such generational trauma. Aboriginal communities can continue the progress toward healing by building Communities of Care across the country and finding ways of helping individuals suffering complex trauma with the assistance of Communities of Practice that have the skilled professionals to deliver the services they are employed to deliver in a culturally informed manner.

KNOWLEDGE AND PRACTICE REFLECTION

Joe Tucci, Janise Mitchell, Ed Tronick and Stephen W. Porges

It is a powerful collection of conversations that speak for themselves. Professor Judy Atkinson and her colleagues delve into the deep connection between the violent colonization and oppression of First Nations peoples in Australia and the continued effects of such trauma. The form itself, as dialogue, is reflective of a decolonizing approach to understanding trauma that has been the subject of Atkinson's fearless and tireless efforts and writing since 2002 and which is in the tradition of writing expressed by others such as Renee Linklater (2014) and Michael Yellow Bird (Yellow Bird, 2013; Clarke and Yellow Bird, 2022).

In keeping with this reflective practice, we had a conversation with Judy to reflect on what are the key points that come from this chapter. We have described this rich dialogue below. Because of our relationship, we have opted to talk with Judy rather than position her in the Western academic tradition of using of her surname. For Judy and all of us, this work is deeply personal. It is driven by a commitment to effecting change.

First, the chapter is an important act of 'truth-telling' as a form of meaning making that centres the history of brutal violence against First Nations peoples so that it is acknowledged and its ongoing impact on First Nations peoples in Australia is accepted and understood. Such truth-telling expresses the intentional way that the histories of First Nations peoples are deleted and removed in order to render invisible settler discourses of oppression (Kurtiş *et al.*, 2010). Elkins (2022) has recently traced the way that violence was systematically and strategically used by the British Empire to make claim of ownership over large parts of the contemporary world: 'Britain's first empire, as it is often called, was largely a Western one, comprised mostly of free whites, enslaved Black laborers, and indigenous populations dispossessed of land' (Elkins, 2022, p.8).

Truth-telling is the act of remembering the significance of the connection of First Nations peoples to land and in particular how the pain arising from massacres of Aboriginal people reverberates over generations. The story of Timothy is contextualized over time, bringing back into view the link between his experience in the present and the histories of his family and community:

> Timothy was born in a remote rural community scarred by genocide, historical, collective racist abuses. Multiple violations of human rights across two centuries have given rise to transgenerational trauma, not the least of which was the nearby Myall Creek Massacre in 1838. On this occasion, a landowner and his stockmen killed up to 50 Aboriginal people. Other stockmen and settlers were encouraged to murder any Aboriginal person they came across. This war crime was described by the then police magistrate as 'a war of extermination,' but it is far from the most lethal massacre in the country's history. The Myall Creek Massacre, one of at least 304 known frontier massacres in Australia, lives on in the conscious and unconscious memories of the local Aboriginal people. Such massacres were also accompanied by the rape of women, girls, and boys. The trauma of such cruelty is not only remembered as a historical artifact, but it is lived out in the very being of each Aboriginal person, and each of their relationships and behaviors...

Each sentence is a powerful act of resistance to dominant racist frames that have powered colonization, deconstructing the truth that has separated Timothy and his family from the violation of the past. The land is stained with the memories of pain that are held in the collective consciousness of First Nations peoples.

Second, the chapter offers a way to deeply listen to the experiences of pain and trauma of First Nations peoples. Judy and her colleagues describe the ancient indigenous act of *Dadirri* as:

> ...healing from the heart, really listening, not just hearing. Heart-felt listening, feeling deeply, having the courage to heal by expressing your grief and pain. It is growing together, healing together through sharing stories from the heart...

Judy has used this and other forms of 'indigenous pedagogy' as therapeutic practice in the healing process for First Nations peoples she has supported. All of these approaches start with culture as the core and make it fundamental to the process. The activities described in the chapter are strengths-based, acknowledging the capacity of First Nations people to find and enact solutions that make sense for them in their own time. These activities are collective rather than individual, drawing on the central theme of mutuality and collaboration that exists within culture.

The significance of this chapter is that it invites us to consider more centrally the need to include decolonizing practice as a core principle which is missing from the current conceptualization of trauma-informed practice. Decolonizing practice is more than appreciating the importance of different cultural worldviews or a commitment to ensuring inclusiveness of oppressed groups. It is an active recruitment of ways of understanding trauma arising from violation connected to historical dispossession, racist policies and societal structures, the forced separation of children from their families, families from their land, enslavement and human trafficking, and mass murder of whole communities. It also goes further than the goal of increasing understanding – it compels acts which challenge the ongoing effects of colonization through practices that are led by First Nations peoples and support their self-determination. This includes the establishment of First Nations specific services, assessment approaches, and therapeutic processes that adopt indigenous ways of knowing and ways of providing support to those who are struggling.

A first principle of trauma-transformative practice must be the application of decolonizing practices and a commitment to anti-discriminatory and anti-oppressive ways of working. As noted by Wilson and Yellow Bird (2005), 'decolonisation is the intelligent, calculated, and active resistance to the forces of colonialism that perpetuate the subjugation and/or exploitation of our minds, bodies, and lands, (p.2).

Noting it now as a core element, it will be explored in the last chapter in more detail.

References
References for chapter

Atkinson C. (2008). The Violence Continuum: Australian Aboriginal Male Violence and Generational Post-Traumatic Stress (Unpublished PhD thesis). Darwin: Charles Darwin University.

Atkinson, J., Nelson, J. and Atkinson, C. (2010). Trauma, Transgenerational Transfer and Effects on Community Wellbeing. In N. Purdie, P. Dudgeon and R. Walker (eds), *Working Together: Aboriginal and Torres Strait Islander Mental Health and Wellbeing Principles and Practice* (pp.135–144). Canberra: Australian Institute of Health and Welfare.

Atkinson J., Nelson, J., Brooks, R, Atkinson, C. and Ryan, K. (2014). Addressing Individual and Community Transgenerational Trauma. In P, Dudgeon, H. Milroy and R. Walker (eds), *Working Together Aboriginal and Torres Strait Islander Mental Health and Wellbeing Principles and Practice*. Canberra: Commonwealth of Australia.

Bevis, M., Atkinson, J., McCarthy, L. and Sweet, M. (2020). *Kungas' trauma experiences and effects on behaviour in Central Australia* (Research report, 03/2020). Sydney: ANROWS.

Bottoms, T. (2013). *Conspiracy of Silence: Queensland's Frontier Killing Times*. Sydney: Allen and Unwin.

Clark, Y., Augoustinos, M. and Malin, M. (2017). Coping and preventing lateral violence in the Aboriginal community in Adelaide. *Australian Community Psychologist*, 28(2), 105–123.

Dudgeon, P., Watson, M. and Holland, C. (2017). Trauma in the Aboriginal and Torres Strait Islander population. *Australian Clinical Psychologist*, 3(1), 1741.

Felitti, V.J., Anda, R.F., Nordenberg, D., Williamson, D.F. *et al.* (1998). Relationship of childhood abuse and household dysfunction to many of the leading causes of death in adults. The Adverse Childhood Experiences (ACE) Study. *American Journal of Preventative Medicine*, 14(4), 245–258.

Parliament of the Commonwealth of Australia. (2021). *Inquiry into Family, Domestic and Sexual Violence*. Canberra: Commonwealth of Australia.

Ungunmerr-Baumann, M.R. (1988). Dadirri: Inner Deep Listening.

van de Kolk, B.A. (2007) Developmental Impact of Childhood Trauma. In L. Kirmayer, R. Lemelson and M. Barad (eds), *Understanding Trauma, Integrating Biological, Clinical and Cultural Perspectives*. New York, NY: Cambridge University Press.

Webster, G.P. and Butcher, J. (2012). The assessment of problem sexual behaviours among children: A human rights centred approach. *Sexual Abuse in Australia and New Zealand*, 4(1), 22–32.

Webster, G.P. (2018). Psychoanalytic Complexity Theory: An application to the treatment of child sexual offenders. *Psychoanalytic Psychology*, 35(1), 83–92.

Webster, G.P. (2019). The conscious and unconscious procedures, motives and meanings of pre-pubescent problem sexual behaviour. *Psychoanalytic Inquiry*, 39(5), 305–317.

References for Knowledge and Practice Reflection

Atkinson, J. (2002). *Trauma Trails Recreating Song Lines: The Transgenerational Effects of Trauma in Indigenous Australia*. Melbourne: Spinifex Press.

Clarke, K. and Yellow Bird, M. (2022). *Decolonising Pathways towards Integrative Healing in Social Work*. London: Taylor and Francis.

Elkins, E. (2022). *Legacy of Violence: A History of the British Empire*. London: The Bodley Head.

Linklater, R. (2014). *Decolonising Trauma Work – Indigenous Stories and Strategies*. Nova Scotia: Fernwood Publishing.

Kurtiş, T., Adams, G. and Yellow Bird, M. (2010). Generosity or genocide? Identity implications of silence in American Thanksgiving commemorations, *Memory*, 18(2), 208–224.

Wilson, W.A. and Yellow Bird, M. (2005). *For Indigenous Eyes Only: A Decolonising Handbook*. Santa Fe, NM: School of American Research.

Yellow Bird, M. (2013). Neurodecolonisation: Applying Mindfulness Research to Decolonising Social Work. In M. Gray, J. Coates, M. Yellow Bird and T. Hetherington (eds), *Decolonising Social Work*. Hampstead, UK: Ashgate Publishing.

CHAPTER 12

Early Predictors of Infant Disorganized Attachment as Levers for Risk Reduction by Frontline Workforces

Jennifer McIntosh, Jessica Opie and Anna Booth

Introduction

This chapter aims to enhance practitioner capacity for early intervention during the perinatal period to reduce risk for disorganized attachment in early childhood. We concentrate on enhanced recognition of signals that lie in two risk domains: factors in the caregiving context, and behavioural signals the infant gives about relational trust and attachment organization. As with all infant mental health work, the baby's behaviours often are the first invitation practitioners receive that prompt us to look further. To aide this, we describe the key behavioural contexts in which we could begin to notice that the caregiving environment is disorganizing for the baby. We then discuss the all-important context for these behaviours, referring to two recent studies by our research group that describe the established evidence on predictors of disorganized attachment. We focus on the evidence that helps practitioners recognize key risks that often arise in the perinatal window (pregnancy through to one year post-partum). Critically, as disorganized attachment arises in large part from modifiable risk factors, it is therefore malleable and potentially highly responsive to early intervention (Booth *et al.*, 2022a). In that light, we consider what we know about important protective offsets, and give examples of how two frontline interventions have incorporated this knowledge into their service, each supporting at-risk parent-baby dyads in highly complex contexts.

Framing attachment organization

An all-important job for infants by the end of the first year of life is to establish with each of their caregivers a clear pattern for getting and staying close to them, in order to manage fear and threat the infant feels, be that real or imagined. By the end of the first year of life, we recognize these as patterns of attachment. Put simply, attachment in infancy is the observable part of the baby's bond of psychological dependence with their caregiver, which is manifest in patterns of behaviours seen when the infant is stressed, and in need of protection and soothing from that caregiver. Through attachment theory and assessment, Bowlby (1969/1982), Ainsworth *et al.* (1978), and subsequent researchers have given us a reliable lens for observing the baby's current state of trust in their caregiver when in need, and a language for describing it.

Much of the attachment literature is replete with explanations of the sub-types of attachment patterns – secure and insecure, organized and disorganized, and secure, avoidant, resistant and disorganized – and how they are classified. This is useful knowledge for practitioners, which we summarize in a later section. Noting that formal classification is a complex undertaking, requiring training and certification, we support the lay reader to take the view that organized attachment patterns, be they secure or insecure, are adaptive strategies by the baby for 'getting the attachment job done'. And the baby's attachment job is always about achieving proximity – physical and/or psychological – to their attachment figure for the purpose of protection from fear or threat. In this way, the very presence of the attachment figure can be thought of as the potential solution to the baby's anxiety, provided the dyad's signalling and response can make the care 'transaction' work in an organized way.

As the name implies, organized attachment behaviours are more or less efficient in achieving this end goal of psychological and/or physical closeness. In the same light, disorganized attachment behaviours by the baby when stressed and when their attachment figure is nearby are part of a failed solution to the baby's problem of feeling anxious and in need. These behaviours by the baby are often termed 'incoherent' because they show a confused approach by the baby to getting their needs met. Momentarily at least, disorganized behaviours look a little (or a lot) odd, ill-timed, and out of place. They do not make sense if one understands that the baby is stressed and is needing support and soothing from the parent or carer who is right there with them. So, the solution to their problem is in front of them, yet their dilemma is not resolved. An organized way of being together in the face of stress is not evident. Disorganized behaviours suggest a hesitation by the baby, an uncertainty about how or even whether to approach the caregiver for help during a peak state of stress. Such behaviours repeated over time and across situations of need provide important clues to the potential of a deeper collapse of trust in the parent-infant relationship, and the possible emergence of relational trauma.

Attachment classification: Take-aways for frontline practitioners

We briefly describe the major methods and typology behind attachment classifications, as they provide foundational architecture for framing our later discussion of disorganized attachment. Because attachment is a bio-behavioural system, in infancy and preschool it is preferably assessed through behavioural observations of the child in interaction with their caregiver. Many will have heard of the Infant Strange Situation Procedure (SSP) (Ainsworth *et al.*, 1978), which is the most highly validated approach to formal classification of attachment in the infant and preschool years. In its official form, it is a 21-minute laboratory-based observation consisting of eight episodes involving the infant and parent in play in a new environment, the introduction of a stranger, two separations of the infant and parent, and two reunions. Each episode is designed to slowly increase the child's level of stress to progressively activate their attachment system. The Cassidy and Marvin (1992) Preschool Attachment Classification System is an adaptation of the SSP infant classification system for three- to four-year-olds, and it remains the gold standard observational method for assessment of this age group. In both, the young child's response to their parent's return is of particular importance, revealing how the child uses their attachment figure in times of stress to regulate their emotions.

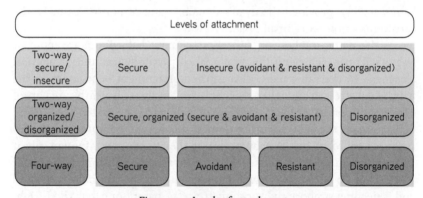

Figure 12.1: Levels of attachment.

Using such observational systems, attachment classifications define the pattern of behaviours in three ways: 1) as either secure or insecure, 2) as secure or one of the three forms of insecure attachment (i.e. avoidant, resistant or disorganized), or 3) as organized or disorganized. Figure 12.1 shows these levels of description. Importantly, we would never refer to a baby as 'secure' or 'disorganized'. The attachment classification always refers to a quality of the dyad being observed. Attachment patterns are unique one-to-one relationships, shaped by the blueprint of responsiveness shown by a particular caregiver in response to the baby's need states, particularly when the baby is frightened, tired or ill. In this way, the baby's attachment behaviours can and do differ between different parents or carers in the same family.

Secure attachment

In dyads where attachment is classified as 'secure', the young child is active and direct in seeking physical or psychological proximity to their caregiver on reunion. And the hallmark of security is that the child's behaviour works to solve their problem of feeling anxious. The child is relatively easily soothed by the parent within a matter of moments to minutes. The child's behaviour is straightforward – they show very little if any avoidance or anger with their parent in these moments; they get what they need by knowing how to efficiently solve their problem (Berlin *et al.*, 2008; Lyons-Ruth and Jacobvitz, 2008).

Insecure/Avoidant attachment

In dyads classified as 'insecure/avoidant', the child typically shows minimal emotion, and may ignore or simply be neutral with respect to the caregiver, actively directing attention away from their own emotional state rather than seeking restoration through proximity.

Insecure/Ambivalent attachment

The 'insecure/ambivalent' or 'insecure/resistant' classification is the second insecure grouping. Children in these dyads often show a lot of upset or anger on separation and also on reunion, when they are not readily soothed by the return of the parent. Typically, these young children show a mix of proximity-seeking and angry behaviours towards the parent. Although both the avoidant and ambivalent groups are regarded as suboptimal to the secure group, the strategies in dealing with stress are nonetheless regarded as organized and predictable. These dyads have adapted to each other, and have a way of working it out, which is more or less organized.

Disorganized attachment

The above is probably well enough known to most early childhood practitioners. Here we'll go into more details on the behaviours that typify a disorganized classification. Perhaps typify is a misleading word, for indeed as the name implies, disorganized attachment does not show itself as a clear pattern. Instead of or in addition to any of the above, the infant will have key moments in being with their parent where they are in clear need of care but go about solving that problem in a rather oblique way. That can include simultaneously approaching and avoiding the parent and giving incongruous or very unclear and misdirected signals about their need. Sometimes we see the baby doing 'incomplete' things, like moving towards the parent when upset then rapidly turning away, or giving odd body or facial expressions which seem very slowed down or disoriented. In the SSP, some babies will redirect their need away from the attachment figure to the stranger in the room, and some will show clear apprehension of the parent, such as stumbling, freezing or falling when near the parent (Main and Solomon, 1990). In this light, a good umbrella word for the practitioner to hold onto about disorganized signals from the baby is 'paradoxical' behaviour. The behaviour does not make sense and lacks organization.

Origins of disorganized behaviours

The origins of these paradoxical behaviours are believed to emerge from a confusion of the evolutionary drive to seek closeness and comfort from a caregiver to maximize survival of the helpless infant, with the baby's actual experience of the attachment figure as a source of alarm, uncertainty, fear and/or threat. In other words, the baby has learned through experience that their caregiver may – inadvertently or otherwise – be an additional source of uncertainty or threat during moments of need. This places the child in a seemingly unresolvable dilemma; their attachment figure is dually and concurrently a needed source of safety yet their presence is confusing or feared for the infant. Understandably, this leaves the infant apprehensive, driven to simultaneously approach and avoid their attachment figure, with both behaviours serving to promote survival of the infant. The situation often exceeds the infant's capacity to make sense of these contradictions, so their behaviour, when in need of care, appears anomalous, bizarre, mistimed or otherwise incongruous (Duschinsky, 2018).

Formally recognized behavioural markers of disorganization

The certification process to become a reliable coder of infant attachment and especially of disorganization takes hundreds of hours. For research purposes, certification is imperative. For clinical purposes, it remains important for frontline workers to be aware of the tone and tenor of disorganized behaviours and affects, to make effective referrals for support to specialist infant mental health services. Equally important are the skills to distinguish disorganization from momentary behaviours arising from transient circumstances, such as infant ill-health and maternal exhaustion.

Formally recognized behavioural markers of disorganization can be plainly obvious (e.g. appearing fearful of the parent) while at other times hidden in plain sight (e.g. using avoidant and ambivalent strategies in the same attempt to get support). Such infant behaviours with the parent include (Main and Solomon, 1990):

- starkly opposing behaviours, such as being upset and approaching the parent facing backwards
- trying secure, avoidant and ambivalent behaviours, all at once or in rapid succession
- appearing disoriented, confused or fearful of the parent
- looking extremely disengaged from the parent, or dazed and confused
- freezing, stilling, and/or using strange body postures
- not seeking the parent out when they are visibly frightened
- stuffing in their emotions
- displaying jerky, tension movements
- hiding from the attachment figure after a brief separation.

The key context to hold in mind when observing a baby and their caregiver together is to do so when the baby is a little stressed and needs a response from the parent. A key behaviour to hold in mind is the paradoxical way the infant goes about signalling that need. Some of these behaviours parallel hyperactivation of the sympathetic nervous system, while others reflect hypoactivation of the parasympathetic nervous system in trauma responses seen in young babies, showing the baby is overstressed without a way to manage these emotions. If we return to the idea that the baby has a problem and their solution (i.e. their attachment figure) is right there in front of them, either way, their behaviours do not make sense in the moment. And in this very paradox, these are important attempts at communications from the baby.

Why attachment disorganization matters

Disorganized attachment behaviours give us an important clue about a significant level of confusion in the parent-infant relationship that can over time be very draining for multiple aspects of the baby's social-emotional development, and of the parent's enjoyment in parenting. Now, 60 years on from Bowlby's (1969/1982) seminal thinking, the science of attachment in early childhood is reasonably well settled. We know that, for optimal development, the dependent baby must learn over time that their strong affective need states will be seen, validated and responded to well enough by their caregiver, and thus overwhelming emotions will be well managed, together. This assurance that emotional states can be co-regulated in turn creates optimal impacts on emerging brain structures and circuitry associated with regulatory capacity and a lasting and positive developmental legacy for social and emotional functioning (Feldman, 2017; Granqvist *et al.*, 2017; Madigan *et al.*, 2013). Although associated with some adverse outcomes, avoidant and ambivalent-resistant attachment patterns in infancy are nonetheless organized ways of 'getting the attachment job done'. Likely a result of their predictability, they appear less taxing on the developmental resources of the young child than disorganized pathways, and usually less consequential for mental health trajectories.

Also reasonably well settled is the science of attachment-related trauma. Disorganized attachment may be transitory, reflecting, for example, a profound but temporary emotional challenge for the caregiver, which is readily responsive to support. Of concern, early disorganized attachment endures for about 37 per cent of infants and parents throughout the early childhood years (Opie et al., 2021). As a pathway of developmental confusion, disorganized attachment tends towards a pattern of controlling behaviour in preschool, and is a known a precursor to poor cognitive and socio-emotional outcomes in middle childhood, later psychopathology including dissociative and borderline personality symptoms, and suicidal ideation in adolescence and early adulthood (Lyons-Ruth and Jacobvitz, 2008; van IJzendoorn et al., 1999; Verhage et al., 2016).

Of note, disorganization is not uncommon at low levels in the general population, and is about 15 per cent in low-risk samples (van IJzendoorn et al., 1999). Some children, otherwise secure in their attachment, show disorganized behaviours following traumatic events, such as accidents, but most would not meet the formal criteria for disorganization. If the infant can use their caregiver to help co-regulate and support them to manage, short-term distressed attachment behaviours soon subside.

In high-risk maltreated samples, proportions of disorganization are much higher, at up to 77–90 per cent in child protection and family violence populations (Barnett et al., 1999; Carlson et al., 1989; Cicchetti et al., 2006; van IJzendoorn, 1995).

Here, we emphasize a critical caveat. For some time, researchers in the attachment tradition have rightly been careful not to equate disorganized attachment in the parent-infant relationship with disorders of attachment seen in abusive relationships (e.g. van IJzendoorn and Bakermans-Kranenberg, 2003). We fully support this view. Infant disorganized behaviours provide us with an important visual clue that, in a moment of need, when afraid or anxious, the infant behaves as if they are confused about trusting their parent to respond in the way they need. So, while it is true that attachment disorganization is over-represented in maltreating parent-child samples (Barnett et al., 1999; Cicchetti et al., 2006; Van IJzendoorn, 1995), disorganized behaviours from the infant do not tell us anything about why this infant is confused about their relationship with this particular parent. And context matters. Little is also known about differential susceptibility, yet it is clear that some infants are particularly sensitive to disorganized attachment behaviours in the absence of an alarming environment (Duschinsky, 2018). It is for the practitioner to come to understand whether the parent-infant relationship is strained from a blend of temporary challenging circumstances, or indicative of a more chronic interpersonal trauma dynamic.

Attachment theory hypothesizes that, once formed, patterns of attachment become increasingly resistant to change. The meta-analytic evidence shows that across early childhood (from 12 to 72 months), disorganization is maintained for 36.59 per cent of parent-infant dyads (Opie *et al.*, 2021). Attachment patterns are both responsive to change (i.e. the introduction or reduction of environmental threat) and have decreasing malleability with age (Fraley, 2002; Opie *et al.*, 2021). As a result, self-protective, maladaptive forms of attachment that are consolidated early in life may persist, despite no longer being functional, due to the ongoing nature of early-formed models of relating (Sroufe *et al.*, 1990).

Risk pathways for disorganized attachment

In recent years, our research group set out to help universal health services and specialist clinicians alike to notice early signs of disorganized attachment in the infant and, critically, the risk and protective factors in the surrounding caregiving environment. We translated that research into a professional development programme, called MERTIL (My Early Relational Trauma Informed Learning: www.mertil.com.au). We first set out to find and synthesize the best longitudinal research available about associations between suboptimal attachment development and perinatal risk exposure. In focusing on well-conducted longitudinal studies, our systematic search of the literature (McIntosh *et al.*, 2021) shone a spotlight on this group of significant yet modifiable risks:

- Parent's low socio-economic status.
- Severe maternal depression.
- Perinatal loss of a child (miscarriage, stillbirth or early death of a newborn).
- Caregiving intrusiveness.
- Couple/Parent conflict.

We also confirmed two major protective factors: maternal sensitivity and high metacognition during pregnancy (i.e. the ability to differentiate one's feelings from another's, and capacity for reflective functioning).

In this first study, we confirmed the need to avoid a singular view of the origins of disorganized relationships. Impoverished socio-economic circumstance, marginalization and contextual stresses of unemployment, unstable living arrangements, family disruption, severe marital conflict and time constraints of sole-carer provision all sit in pathways towards infant attachment disorganization. With respect to specific assaults on the caregiver's capacity to be present, loss of a prior pregnancy or a stillbirth also increased the risk of disorganized attachment for the next-born child.

Intimate partner violence and infant disorganized attachment

In a second meta-analytic study, we confirmed the additional unique contribution of intimate partner violence (IPV) to infant disorganized attachment. We examined the evidence from all available longitudinal studies of mother's IPV victimization and the subsequent offspring attachment relationship for children aged one to five years (McIntosh et al., 2019). We confirmed that mothers' experience of IPV during pregnancy was significantly associated with later attachment disorganization in children aged one to five years. We found that mothers' emotionally and physically based experiences of violence are a stronger predictor of offspring attachment disorganization than maternal depression or socio-economic stressors. These effects are comparable to the effects found for non-IPV inter-parental conflict and are similar to those found for general caregiver insensitivity.

How can a parent's grief and violence victimization derail infant attachment organization?

In summary, recent evidence from our two large-scale studies shows that maternal adverse experiences impact on critical emotional aspects of caregiving, to a degree that can derail attachment organization for the baby. How? There are many suggestions from the clinical literature about this. First, it is likely that unresolved grief and trauma may generate a potent sense of helplessness in making meaning from these events. In other words, if the way the mother conceives of her role when the baby is in need of care remains damaged post trauma, the risks of disorganization are higher (Huth-Bocks et al., 2004). We also know that traumatic preoccupation and depression interfere with the accuracy of the mother's interpretation of her infant's distress cues and damage her caregiving representations. In a climate of domestic violence or unresolved grief, the mother who is preoccupied, frightened or poorly supported can behave towards her baby in either a subtle or overt manner that is confusing and disorganizing.

Enactments of unresolved feelings likely occur in parenting behaviours and are perceived as alarming to the infant. This includes transmission of alarm, fear, numbing and helplessness to her infant, together with impeded capacity to recognize and respond to her child's attachment needs. In this context, IPV and similar traumas are understood not only as 'an assault on women, but on the caregiving system as a whole' (Levendosky et al., 2012, p.402).

Diversity

Clearly, there is no reason to believe that the mechanisms would differ by gender, specifically for fathers. It's just that the studies are not there yet. Noting that male IPV victimization is different from that of women in degree and type in both Eastern and Western societies (Australian Bureau of Statistics, 2017; Garcia-Moreno *et al.*, 2006; Smith *et al.*, 2018), when fathers are bereaved or are victims of IPV, the attendant strain may also impact mental health and the infant-father attachment relationship. Our research also considered socio-economic, racial, ethnic and gender diversity, but this level of diversity is still not well represented in longitudinal research. Sexual orientation, religion, ability and culture are particularly under-represented to date in studies examining the connections between attachment and IPV experiences. Cross-culturally, there do not appear to be differences in the core finding that a mother's experience of IPV victimization or loss during pregnancy increases risk of disorganized attachment for the next-born offspring.

Translation into preventative efforts

In this light, we suggest the science of antenatal trauma and loss and attendant risk to offspring attachment organization is well settled. So, what would we do about it? We first noted that clinical treatments for interpersonal trauma are now pervasive, from psycho-educative materials (McIntosh and Tan, 2017) through to dyadic relationship-based interventions for infants and parents, such as Attachment and Biobehavioural Catch-up (ABC) (Dozier, 2003; Dozier and Bernard, 2017; Dozier *et al.*, 2017) and Child-Parent Psychotherapy (CPP) (Cicchetti *et al.*, 2006; Lieberman *et al.*, 2005; Lieberman *et al.*, 2006). The latter interventions are focused on ameliorating attachment disorganization and share common goals, including supporting parents to recognize the baby's need for nurturance, expanding the parent's empathic responsiveness to their child, altering distorted perceptions of their child, developing skills to minimize frightening behaviour, and managing difficult moments.

Beyond the well-published efficacy of these intensive mental health interventions lies the problem of their accessibility. These are expensive, intensive interventions for targeted clinical groups. In our view, a clear gap lies in frontline services that meet the population of concern well in advance of clinical status being established. We felt that our research into pathways towards disorganization translated into opportunity for frontline practitioners to be:

- trained in recognition of predisposing contexts of trauma
- trained in recognition of the attachment behaviours in infancy that might alert us to caregiving stress

- upskilled in partnering with the parent from the first interaction, to counter use of non-relational and non-reflective approaches that may parallel aspects of the trauma experienced.

Our team's initiatives have focused on frontline workforces and their unique opportunities to influence the attachment course of at-risk babies and their parents. We summarize two examples here.

MERTIL: Training frontline practitioners in recognition of and response to relational trauma

In 2018, our group developed a specialist training programme for this workforce, called MERTIL (My Early Relational Trauma-Informed Learning). We began with state-wide delivery to the Maternal and Child Health workforce in Victoria, Australia, which provides universal healthcare to families and their children from birth to preschool age. MERTIL, which has since been expanded to multiple early childhood services, translates attachment and caregiving theory and evidence into application for frontline early childhood settings, with a focus on contexts of family violence and intergenerational attachment trauma. The 20-hour programme is delivered via multimedia online learning and face-to-face clinical workshops. The course content emphasizes recognition of infant disorganized behaviours, and of traumatized interactions by the parent with the baby. Training in rapid frontline response emphasizes early support through direct, warm and strengths-based conversations. Practical resources to support this work now include the MERTIL for Parents online psycho-education parent programme, about building and repairing early relational trust (Opie et al., in press).

A unique qualitative study of nurses' encounters with relational trauma highlighted a clear need for this specialist training (Booth et al., 2022a). Programme evaluation has repeatedly shown very high satisfaction with the course and significant gains in practitioner confidence and capacity to respond to early relational trauma, sustained and reinforced with each step of a three-tiered exposure to MERTIL content across three months (Clancy et al., 2020). We suggest such workforce-wide training initiatives are key to the earliest detection of troubled relationships, with translation potential across many early childhood settings.

An early assessment and referral service for at-risk mothers and infants

In a second programme, we helped to translate some tangible prevention levers into action, for a highly vulnerable group of women, victimized by IPV and homelessness during pregnancy (Booth et al., 2022b). This example of a targeted response to at-risk client groups is the Western Child and Family Assessment and Referral Network (WCFARN) in the state of South

Australia, led by a community organization, Relationships Australia South Australia (RASA). The programme is part of the South Australian government's strategy to prevent the need for children to enter the statutory child protection system by providing a protective, proactive, integrated referral service to support prevention pathways for parent-infant dyads during the first thousand days of life. Unique to the WCFARN model, the programme provides a collaborative approach between the parent and practitioner to shaping an understanding of the mother-baby needs for safety and security, and to establishing a proactive referral network that honors the caregiving intention of the parent. Together, worker and parent elucidate the infant's core attachment needs, at the centre of the family risk picture, using well-validated assessment tools such as the Maternal Postnatal Attachment Scale (MPAS) (Condon and Corkindale, 1998) and Detection of Overall Risk Screen (DOORS) (McIntosh and Ralfs, 2012) in transparent mapping conversations. Based on the philosophy of restorative practice, these conversations are designed to engage the parent authentically in new hope for understanding their relationship with their baby, through a therapeutic balance between challenge and empowerment (Pennell, 2006). Throughout, the relationship between workers and clients is central to creating a nurturing environment for change (Lauridsen and Munkejord, 2022).

WCFARN service involvement with a family spans six months on average, with at least weekly contact with a family for the first six to eight weeks of service involvement, planning of the referral, kinship, and support network, followed by a warm handover to a broader team for longer-term care, with all these relationships enlisted as part of the newly evolving network of shared responsibility for the baby's security. In cases where a mother's trauma has overwhelmed her capacity to keep her baby safe, typically where concurrent family violence concerns exist, care is taken to make transparent and helpful referrals to child protection, negotiated with mother and her allies.

Summary

This chapter summarizes the disorganized attachment construct, origins and behaviours, and their collective importance for alerting us to contexts of care that may signal early relational trauma between infant and parent. Our latest evidence highlights key modifiable risk factors in the pregnancy and perinatal pathways towards infant attachment disorganization, and their interaction with socio-economic and family violence risks. Each factor and the pattern they sit within provides a useful prevention target. Our findings have since informed both the development of skills training (e.g. MERTIL) and service structures (e.g. WCFARN) to support frontline practitioners in recognizing potentially disorganizing pathways, and with them, opportunities for response and early prevention. Beyond this, we suggest that arising from this collection of research is a broader social imperative to give increasing attention to the baby's communications and resources and to the support of parents who have experienced loss and trauma in the perinatal period, to improve the social-emotional health of generations to come.

KNOWLEDGE AND PRACTICE REFLECTION

Janise Mitchell, Joe Tucci, Ed Tronick and Stephen W. Porges

In a timely reminder, McIntosh, Opie and Booth note that attachment is not an individual characteristic held by children or their carers on their own. The nature of the attachment between children and their carers is experienced in the quality of the relationship between them.

> Attachment patterns are unique one-to-one relationships, shaped by the blueprint of responsiveness shown by a particular caregiver in response to the baby's need states, particularly when the baby is frightened, tired or ill. In this way, the baby's attachment behaviours can and do differ between different parents or carers in the same family...

Disorganized attachment patterns occur when an infant is confused by the intentions and behaviour of their carer. It is reflected in experiences which lack predictability and are particularly taxing on the developmental resources of the infant, and the capacity of the carer at times as well. It leaves the child not able to collaboratively generate meaning through which the world is assembled into consistent form, preventing them from establishing the internal models of expectancies that they need to communicate and have their needs met by others important to their care.

The significance of disorganized attachment between child and carer is that it becomes amplified in scenarios where mothers are subject to domestic and family violence and the traumatic impacts associated with the experience, in particular when it occurs during pregnancy. Here, McIntosh, Opie and Booth point to the loss felt by mothers which ripples through their lives and serves to break down their 'caregiving systems'. The violence itself tears apart the mothers' capacity to be present, attend to and identify the needs of their children, and have the energy to act to address their needs. The perpetrator causes an escalation of stress to both the mother and the children, requiring the mother to protect herself and her children. She may be so overwhelmed with the danger she faces that her defensive mechanisms for herself and her children are deeply compromised. In that toxic whirlwind of violence and violation, mothers and children can lose connection to each other, feeling the pain of ever-increasing isolation and separation.

Accountability for such impact rests with the perpetrator of the violence. It is the men in these situations who make vulnerable the integrity of the women and children. They defy orders to stay away and stop the violence. They intimidate and use oppressive tactics to their own advantage. It occurs within the broad context of gendered violence in which constructs of male dominance are realized.

In recent times, there is growing recognition that coercive control is a fundamental strategy used by perpetrators to manipulate and distort the experience of reality, which is in itself a violation. It also forms the basis for ongoing threatened and real physical violence. For children and young people, being forced to live in environments in which relational resources are weaponized as abusive dynamics is a form of emotional and psychological maltreatment (Tomison and Tucci, 1997; Tucci and Mitchell, 2017).

Disorganized attachment does not seem significant enough a construct to capture the severity of the experience for mothers and infants in these contexts. They are both traumatized. They are both the target of a coordinated and deliberate attack on themselves as individuals as well as their experience of each other in relationship.

The very real problem, as McIntosh, Opie and Booth highlight from their research is that:

> ...once formed, patterns of attachment become increasingly resistant to change. The meta-analytic evidence shows that across early childhood (from 12 to 72 months), disorganization is maintained for 36.59 per cent of parent-infant dyads...

Adverse childhood experiences start in utero. The unsettled physiology of a child arising from the increased stress before birth only intensifies as the violence towards their mother and them continues. As Tronick and others have already pointed to in earlier chapters, the neurosomatic meaning making of the infant is damaged by the experiences of violation. The messages they receive from such violence reaffirm that they are not safe, that the world is dangerous, that there is very little predictability they can rely on, that their needs will not be acknowledged, that they are on their own when they are desperately in need of someone else to experience their experiences and validate them. This sets them up for patterns of interactions which are confusing for the very people whom they seek out for comfort and support.

However, as a construct, disorganized attachment offers a sense of the continuity of trauma and adversity in the lives of children across their lifespan. This is not meant to be a deterministic frame that says that relational templates cannot be changed. Instead, it highlights the very need to attend to the complexity of influences which over time shape the ways that individuals interact with each other and the relational environment they live in. It delineates the meaning making systems highlighted by Tronick in his chapter. Even more importantly, it emphasizes how internal states and external relationships are organized – coordinated, mobilized and reinforced. These dynamics give us insight into how the responses of victims and survivors are organized within different contexts by their history and the context themselves.

Trauma-transformative practice carries with it multiple frames through which it tries to understand the lived and living experience of victims and survivors of violence. It recognizes the intricacy of such experience and resists the temptation to bring order by finding unitary explanations for how trauma takes hold in the lives of individuals, families and communities. Attachment theory is one such frame of reference that can be used to stay open to finding helpful insights that offer resources for change. It is not the only frame, but it is one with a long pedigree of research across ages and developmental stages of children, family constellations, geographical areas and cultures of origin.

It is the nexus between practice and complexity that trauma-transformative practice finds its utility. It is confident in its use of different perspectives and integrates with the philosophical and value underpinning of organizations which offer a range of diverse services. It challenges violence by ensuring that victims and survivors are not blamed for their own violation. It ensures that historical and cultural ways of understanding violation and healing are privileged over what is the favoured evidence of the time. It holds a long-term view of knowledge, enabling points of connection to be supported and competition to be avoided.

An anti-reductionist orientation gives trauma-transformative practitioners, organizations and systems the legitimacy with which unique experiences of victims and survivors can be traced with curiosity and without judgement.

References
References for chapter

Ainsworth, M.D.S., Blehar, M.C., Waters, E. and Wall, S. (1978). *Patterns of Attachment: A Psychological Study of the Strange Situation*. Hillsdale, NJ: Lawrence Erlbaum Associates.

Australian Bureau of Statistics. (2017). *Personal Safety, Australia, 2016 (No. 4906.0)*. Canberra, Australia: Author.

Barnett, D., Ganiban, J. and Cicchetti, D. (1999). Maltreatment, negative expressivity, and the development of Type D attachments from 12 to 24 months of age. *Monographs of the Society for Research in Child Development*, 64, 97–118.

Berlin, L.J., Zeanah, C.H. and Lieberman, A.F. (2008). Prevention and Intervention Programs for Supporting Early Attachment Security. In J. Cassidy and P.R. Shaver (eds), *Handbook of Attachment: Theory, Research, and Clinical Applications* (second edition) (pp.745–761). New York, NY: Guilford Press.

Booth, A.T., McIntosh, J., Clancy, E., Hartley, E. *et al.* (2022a). Australian community nurses' encounters with early relational trauma: A qualitative study of lived experiences and the impact of specialist training. *Australian Journal of Advanced Nursing*, 39(3).

Booth, A.T., McIntosh, J.E., Sri, L., Decrea, S., Lee, J. and Ralfs, C. (2022b). A culturally safe referral service for at-risk mothers and infants in marginalised, Aboriginal, and culturally and linguistically diverse families. *Australian Health Review: A Publication of the Australian Hospital Association*, 47(1), 58–63.

Bowlby, J. (1969/1982). *Attachment and Loss: Vol. 1. Attachment*. New York, NY: Basic Books.

Carlson, V., Cicchetti, D., Barnett, D. and Braunwald, K. (1989). Disorganized/disoriented attachment relationships in maltreated infants. *Developmental Psychology*, 25, 525–531.

Cassidy, J. and Marvin, R.S. (1992). Attachment Organization in Three and Four Year Olds: Procedures and Coding Manual (Unpublished manuscript). University of Virginia, Charlottesville.

Cicchetti, D., Rogosch, F.A. and Toth, S.L. (2006). Fostering secure attachment in infants in maltreating families through preventive interventions. *Development and Psychopathology*, 18, 623–649.

Clancy, E.M., McIntosh, J., Booth, A.T., Sheen, J. *et al.* (2020). Training maternal and child health nurses in early relational trauma: An evaluation of the MERTIL workforce training. *Nurse Education Today*, 89, 104390.

Condon, J.T. and Corkindale, C.J. (1998). The assessment of parent-to-infant attachment: Development of a self-report questionnaire instrument. *Journal of Reproductive and Infant Psychology*, 16(1), 57–76.

Dozier, M. (2003). Attachment-based treatment for vulnerable children. *Attachment and Human Development*, 5, 253–257.

Dozier, M. and Bernard, K. (2017). Attachment and biobehavioural catch-up: Addressing the needs of infants and toddlers exposed to inadequate or problematic caregiving. *Current Opinion in Psychology*, 15, 111–117.

Dozier, M., Bernard, K. and Roben, C. (2017). Attachment and Biobehavioural Catch-up. In H. Steele and M. Steele (eds), *Handbook of Attachment-Based Interventions*. New York, NY: Guilford Press.

Duschinsky, R. (2018). Disorganization, fear, and attachment: Working towards clarification. *Infant Mental Health Journal*, 39, 17–29.

Feldman, R. (2017). The neurobiology of human attachments. *Trends in Cognitive Sciences*, 21, 80–99.

Fraley, R.C. (2002). Attachment stability from infancy to adulthood: Meta-analysis and dynamic modeling of developmental mechanisms. *Personality and Social Psychology Review*, 6(2), 123–151.

Garcia-Moreno, C., Jansen, H.A.F.M., Ellsberg, M., Heise, L. and Watts, C.H. (2006). WHO Multi-country Study on Women's Health and Domestic Violence Against Women Study Team. Prevalence of intimate partner violence: Findings from the WHO multi-country study on women's health and domestic violence. *Lancet*, 368, 1260–1269.

Granqvist, P., Sroufe, L.A., Dozier, M., Hesse, E. *et al.* (2017). Disorganized attachment in infancy: A review of the phenomenon and its implications for clinicians and policy-makers. *Attachment and Human Development*, 19(6), 534–558.

Huth-Bocks, A.C., Levendosky, A.A., Theran, S.A. and Bogat, G.A. (2004). The impact of domestic violence on mothers' prenatal representations of their infants. *Infant Mental Health Journal*, 25, 79–98.

Lauridsen, M.B. and Munkejord, M.C. (2022). Creating conditions for professional development through a trauma-informed and restorative practice. *Social Work*, 67(2), 135–144.

Levendosky, A.A., Lannert, B. and Yalch, M. (2012). The effects of intimate partner violence on women and child survivors: An attachment perspective. *Psychodynamic Psychiatry*, 40, 397–433.

Lieberman, A.F., Ghosh Ippen, C. and Van Horn, P. (2006). Child-parent psychotherapy: 6-month follow-up of a randomised controlled trial. *Journal of the American Academy of Child and Adolescent Psychiatry*, 45(8), 913–918.

Lieberman, A.F., Van Horn, P. and Gosh Ippen, C. (2005). Toward evidence-based treatment: Child-parent psychotherapy with preschoolers exposed to marital violence. *Journal of the American Academy of Child and Adolescent Psychiatry*, 44(12), 1241–1248.

Lyons-Ruth, K. and Jacobvitz, D. (2008). Attachment Disorganization: Genetic Factors, Parenting Contexts, and Developmental Transformation from Infancy to Adulthood.

In J. Cassidy and P. Shaver (eds), *Handbook of Attachment: Theory, Research, and Clinical Applications* (second edition) (pp.666–697). New York, NY: Guilford Press.

Madigan, S., Atkinson, L., Laurin, K. and Benoit, D. (2013). Attachment and internalising behaviour in early childhood: A meta-analysis. *Developmental Psychology*, 49, 672–689.

Main, M. and Solomon, J. (1990). Procedures for Identifying Infants as Disorganized/Disoriented During the Ainsworth Strange Situation. In M.T. Greenberg, D. Cicchetti, and E.M. Cummings (eds), *Attachment in the Preschool Years: Theory, Research, and Intervention* (pp.121–160). Chicago, IL: The University of Chicago Press.

McIntosh, J.E., Olsson, C.A., Schuijers, M. Tan, E.S. *et al.* (2021). Exploring perinatal indicators of infant social-emotional development: A review of the replicated evidence. *Clinical Child and Family Psychology Review*, 24, 450–483.

McIntosh, J.E. and Ralfs, C. (2012). *The DOORS Detection of Overall Risk Screen Framework.* Canberra, Australia: Australian Government Attorney-General's Department.

McIntosh, J.E. and Tan, E.S. (2017). Young children in divorce and separation. Pilot study of a mediation-based parent education program. *Family Court Review*, 55, 329–344.

McIntosh, J.E., Tan, E.S., Levendosky, A.A. and Holtzworth-Munroe, A. (2019). Mothers' experience of intimate partner violence and subsequent offspring attachment security ages 1–5 Years: A meta-analysis. *Trauma, Violence, and Abuse*, 22(4), 885–899.

Opie, J.E., Hooker, L., Gibson, T. and McIntosh, J.E. (in press). My Early Relational Trust-Informed Learning (MERTIL) for Parents: A study protocol for a brief, universal, online, preventative parenting program to enhance relational health. *PLoS ONE.*

Opie, J.E., McIntosh, J.E., Esler, T.B., Duschinsky, R. *et al.* (2021). Early childhood attachment stability and change: A meta-analysis. *Attachment and Human Development*, 23(6), 897–930.

Pennell, J. (2006). Restorative practices and child welfare: Toward an inclusive civil society. *Journal of Social Issues*, 62(2), 259–279.

Smith, S.G., Zhang, X., Basile, K.C., Merrick, M.T. *et al.* (2018). *The National Intimate Partner and Sexual Violence Survey (NISVS): 2015 Data Brief – Updated Release.* Atlanta, GA: National Center for Injury Prevention and Control, Centers for Disease Control and Prevention.

Sroufe, L.A., Egeland, B. and Kreutzer, T. (1990). The fate of early experience following developmental change: Longitudinal approaches to individual adaptation in childhood. *Child Development*, 61(5), 1363–1373.

van IJzendoorn, M.H. (1995). Adult attachment representations, parental responsiveness, and infant attachment: A meta-analysis on the predictive validity of the adult attachment interview. *Psychological Bulletin*, 117, 387–403.

van IJzendoorn, M.H. and Bakermans-Kranenburg, M.J. (2003). Attachment disorders and disorganized attachment: Similar and different. *Attachment and Human Development*, 5(3), 313–320.

van IJzendoorn, M.H., Schuengel, C., and Bakermans–Kranenburg, M.J. (1999). Disorganized attachment in early childhood: Meta-analysis of precursors, concomitants, and sequelae. *Development and Psychopathology*, 11, 225–250.

Verhage, M.L., Schuengel, C., Madigan, S., Fearon, R.M.P. *et al.* (2016). Narrowing the transmission gap: A synthesis of three decades of research on intergenerational transmission of attachment. *Psychological Bulletin*, 142, 337–366.

References for Knowledge and Practice Reflection

Tomison, A. and Tucci, J. (1997). *Emotional Child Abuse.* Child Abuse Prevention, National Child Protection Clearing House Discussion Paper.

Tucci, J. and Mitchell, J. (2017). *Safe and Secure – A Trauma Informed Model for Responding to Children Forced to Live with Family Violence.* Melbourne: Australian Childhood Foundation.

CHAPTER 13

Endowed with Play Circuitry

Theresa Kestly

It started with a Friendship Group for children

When the school counselor and I told the fifth-grade boys about the Friendship Group[1] we were forming at school based on playing together for an hour each week, Tommy said, 'You mean, you're just going to let us play?' 'Yes,' we replied, 'because we know that children develop friendships when they play together, so that is what we are going to do...'

We did not spell out to the boys that they had been referred to the Friendship Group by the school principal due to behavioral issues. The principal personally knew each boy because they were either frequent visitors to her office for disciplinary reasons, or they were having serious academic problems.

All the boys were eager to be in the playgroup.

Although school systems are not generally able to gather in-depth family histories, we soon learned during the play sessions that most of the boys in our initial group had significant trauma and abuse histories. We could see and hear the underlying trauma in the stories they created with the miniature figurines and the small trays of sand we provided for their play sessions. Our structure for their time together was simple: 40 minutes for free play with sand and miniatures, and 20 minutes for telling the stories about their sand worlds. Each boy could tell his story during the last 20 minutes, or he could choose to pass with no judgment or coercion from us. During the storytelling time, the other boys who were listening continued to play actively in their own individual sand trays. Occasionally, we needed to prompt them to play quietly enough so we could all hear the storyteller's words. We simply witnessed and reflected their stories back to them with genuine interest and respect. As facilitators, we intentionally modeled and showed them how to witness each other during the storytelling time as well as the free play time. Even during the 40 minutes of play time, we

---

1   The clinical examples in this chapter are based on composite material drawn from several clinical situations. I have done it this way to protect the confidentiality of clients while preserving the authenticity of the material.

sat next to the children, offering reflection, quiet focus, and availability if they needed anything. We wanted them to feel our presence and genuine interest in their play and storytelling.

We organized the playgroup so that we could meet for ten sessions during regular school hours. It was not surprising to us that the boys eagerly looked forward to their weekly play time or that they quickly opened to the idea of telling metaphorical stories about the scenes they had created in the sand. What did surprise us was the school principal's request, about six weeks after we completed the ten play sessions, to explore the possibility of expanding our project during the next school year. Noting the surprised expressions on our faces, she quickly explained, 'Not one of the nine boys who were in your group has been sent to my office since your play sessions ended.' She realized that some kind of positive behavioral change had occurred that allowed these boys to refocus their energies toward more appropriate and productive behavior in the school environment. The principal wanted more of that, and she helped us obtain a small grant so that we could expand our project significantly during the following school year.

With additional resources and several talented interns, we were able to see over 250 children in various combinations of 12-week playgroups. At the end of the school year, the school principal again reported similar improvement in the children's behavior and academic success. She often came to us during the expanded project to say, 'This child needs to be in one of your playgroups.' She was so confident in the changes she was observing that she would simply assign a child to a playgroup whenever we could work him or her into our schedule, even if it meant pulling that child out of a core academic class. She could see that the behavioral changes leading to academic improvement were more than making up for the lost class time.

At the close of our expanded Friendship Group project, I began a serious quest to understand the power of play that we had witnessed within these groups. What were the primary elements that prompted these children to change their behaviors, allowing them to improve socially and academically? For example, how could we explain 11-year-old Jack's reversal of troubling behaviors on the playground (throwing stones at other children) and lack of motivation to complete his classroom tasks? Although Jack's teacher was reluctant to release him from his academic work to participate in a playgroup because he was so far behind in his schoolwork, the principal convinced her, and so Jack joined one of our groups. As with all the other children, we said nothing to Jack about his academic problems or his poor behavior on the playground.

About midway through our 12-week group, Jack and I had an interesting encounter at the close of school one day. Though usually quiet and somewhat withdrawn, he came up to me and asked, 'What's a school counselor for?' I began explaining to him about children sometimes feeling better when they have a chance to talk about their feelings. Barely waiting for me to finish he said, 'Yeah, since I've been in this group, I haven't been in no more trouble.' About a month later, Jack saw me in the school hallway. Catching up with me, he said, 'I caught up with all my work.' He said it with such pride. I was delighted, and yet puzzled. I had never spoken to Jack about his poor playground behavior or his lagging schoolwork. I decided to check with his teacher just to see if she saw it the same way. She said (also with great pride), 'Yes, indeed. He has completely caught up.'

This exploratory play project took place before the development of trauma-informed treatment protocols and right before the decade of the brain in the 1990s. Jaak Panksepp, renowned researcher, was still in his animal laboratory studying mammalian emotional and motivational systems in the brain. At the close of our project with the Friendship Groups, we were just getting glimpses into the coming neuroscience information explosion. Panksepp (1998) was referring to it as the new integrative form of psychobiology. I had just completed a dissertation on a research study about brain asymmetry, so I had a foundation in concepts of hemispheric differentiation and integration. I could see that the design of our Friendship Groups, based on safe, relational play, had given children opportunities to play in a way that collaborated with the brain's natural tendency to push toward wholeness. First, the children were drawing from their right hemispheres with their sensory systems as they created visual images in the sand, and then flowing into their left hemispheres when telling their stories to articulate their life experiences. We were also getting some good information about the importance of being reflected with warmth and care from attachment research, so I attributed some of our project success to our focus on witnessing the play activities in a way that would encourage bonds of connection among the children and with us as facilitators. In a way, we became small, healthy families in each group. It seemed that even such a short experience was able to seed new relational possibilities in these young brains.

I needed to know more, much more, and so I began researching, writing, exploring, teaching, and focusing my energies on everything I could find on relational play. Over time, this focus led me to several related fields of study: interpersonal neurobiology (IPNB) (Siegel, Schore, and Cozolino, 2021) deepens our understanding of attachment and how we are shaping one another's brains from moment to moment; the laboratory studies of Jaak Panksepp (1998, 2009, 2011) show how play circuitry is inborn and activated when we feel connected; Polyvagal Theory, developed by Stephen Porges (2011, 2015), helps us understand the autonomic nervous system and how safe play is a regulating neural exercise; and the neurosequential model of therapeutics by Bruce Perry (Perry, 2009; Perry and Winfrey, 2021) directs us to attend to brainstem dysregulation which can be harmonized through the rhythms of play, particularly in the company of others.

This convergence of interdisciplinary fields of study was helping me understand more clearly what happened with Jack and the other children who participated in our playgroups. Equally important, my studies of IPNB and relational neuroscience were priming me to recognize more easily what my patients were reaching for in their desire to heal. I was learning that when we are wounded, there is a disruption in the systems of our embodied brains. Our right and left hemispheres are not able to collaborate, our autonomic nervous system is dysregulated, and often our attachment system is disturbed. The neural circuits between aspects of our brain that are impacted by trauma do not integrate in order to protect us from feeling the effects of trauma every moment (Badenoch, 2018). While this segregation of trauma is important for us to be able to continue our daily lives, it also leaves fragility and suffering in its wake.

At the same time, the neuroscience was assuring me that our body/mind/brain system is constantly pushing toward more optimal integration. With the support of caring others, this inherent capacity can be activated. This was so hopeful that I was able to carry that sense into the counseling room with my children and adults. Drawing from this principle as I both observed and participated in relational play for purposes of healing, I could see more easily that the play of children (and in more sophisticated ways, the play of adults) was offering me a wonderful opportunity to see how the two hemispheres were integrating and collaborating, how the autonomic nervous system was gaining the capacity for regulation, and how the signs of more secure attachment were emerging. Play is an experience-rich, bottom-up process that provides what is needed for trauma to be integrated, paving the way for widespread neural integration. As participant-observer in relational play, I realized that I had a front row seat to an unfolding and moving drama of one of life's strategies for making whole and healthy what has been split apart and disturbed due to unfortunate experiences of trauma and neglect. I had a lot to learn not only from IPNB, but also from the children at play.

In this chapter, I want to explore how relational play can weave together our right and left hemisphere modes of processing and reunite the circuits that have been split apart by trauma. One of the keys to how this process unfolds is leading with our right relational hemisphere as we witness children's play. This cultivates a safe space in which the neural circuitry that holds their traumas can open to receive healing. I believe this is possible without abandoning the left, but instead inviting its capacity to understand what is unfolding to provide balance for opening into the fluid right. Through our caring presence, regulation and attachment are being nurtured. We will also see that sensory-based play is a necessary foundation for developing the top layers of the sophisticated cognitive brain, so it facilitates academic learning as well.

Children at play

I sometimes use 'storytelling play' to describe what happened in our Friend-ship Groups. Prior to our group sand tray project, I had noticed in my ther-apy practice with individual children that sensory play with images in the sand seemed to open their language systems for telling stories that were metaphorically consistent with the clinical histories I had gathered from parents or other significant caregivers. I could see that play and storytelling were making it possible for the children to relieve the pain and fear their young brains had been holding and to make sense of their life experiences.

Additionally, the sand tray process and storytelling brought them the pleasure that arises naturally from play and the positive feelings that come when we can articulate our inner experiences to interested and caring lis-teners. From these clinical observations with our clients, we opted to give the children in our Friendship Groups opportunities to tell stories about the sand trays they had generated through sensory play. Our decision to structure our playgroup with 40 minutes for play and 20 minutes for story-telling was based on our belief that children's sensory play was opening the door to the imaginal/conceptual world that gave them the ability to express their thoughts and experiences. We told the boys they could pass on tell-ing their stories, and during the first session most of them did pass, but a few boys wanted to share. As soon as the rest of the boys realized that we were eager to hear their stories and that we would not judge, edit, or direct them, they all wanted to participate. We soon had to use egg timers to give every boy a chance to be heard within our 20 minutes of storytelling time. Clearly, the articulation of the stories while we listened was as powerful as the deep motivation to play together. Being received at every stage of the process is powerful healing medicine.

We did not set an intention at the beginning of the project to help chil-dren integrate the two halves of their brains through the storytelling play. We only articulated to the children with words and group structure the idea of developing friendships through relational play and sharing stories. In retrospect, I can now see that we were prioritizing the motivations of children over academic protocols in a way that allowed us to design and lead the playgroup from the perspective of right-mode awareness. Children love to play and tell their stories, and friendships are a priority for them. We wanted to connect with them, and so we started there. I think now we were lucky to have the freedom from any preconceived notions of what we needed to accomplish with these children. We were free to explore and learn from the 'children at play.' Given that the right hemisphere specializes in relationships and creativity, we were right where we needed to be to lead from a right-mode perspective. We had entered the field of play.

The 'children at play' gave us a new way to look at the power of play to heal trauma. It stood in contrast to a left-mode perspective that begins with setting treatment goals that can be measured and evaluated at the end of treatment. Instead, we were collaborating with the children's intrinsic motivation to play and heal within community bonds, a relational and bottom-up approach. With the help of neuroscience studies and research, I began to understand what happened to the children in our group (Kestly, 2014). It is now clear to me from the laboratory discoveries of Jaak Panksepp (Panksepp, 1998; Panksepp and Biven, 2012) that the children had given us a real-world example of how the midbrain circuitry dedicated to PLAY[2] (discovered by Panksepp in the mammalian brain) emerges when we feel connected to others. This sense of being accompanied makes room for the person playing to feel safe enough to move into the difficult realm of trauma. In addition to the PLAY circuitry, Panksepp was also able to locate and identify six other emotional-motivational systems in the midbrain:

1. Care
2. Panic
3. Separation distress
4. Fear
5. Rage
6. Lust.

According to Panksepp and Biven (2012), these systems are present at birth. We do not have to learn them. Mother nature did not bestow the circuitry of play on us just because she wanted us to have fun, although it is a wonderful, life-enhancing gift as well. The circuitry of play has been conserved through the course of mammalian evolution because play confers positive survival benefits. What follows is just a small sample. Physically, coordination and motor skills improve. Emotionally, children are exposed to emotions like fear, frustration, and anger, and, with support, learn how to regulate them. Socially, they are learning to collaborate, negotiate, and participate with others. Empathy grows. Cognition develops because children are paying attention, reasoning, and remembering. In free, unstructured play, creativity blossoms, too. The joy of it also releases hormones and neurotransmitters that contribute to curiosity and well-being. Because of the opportunity for the children to bond to one another and to us, the midbrain attachment system (combination of CARE, PANIC, and SEPARATION DISTRESS) was also being activated and associated with memories of caring connection. Because many of our children had not experienced this in their homes, these times with us were rewiring their body/mind/

---

2   To be consistent with Panksepp, I am using all caps when writing about these seven motivational systems, to remind us that we are talking about the specific core circuits that Panksepp identified as being intrinsic to all mammals.

brain in a direction that helped them relate more peacefully with their peers, even after the group concluded.

Relational play, Allan Schore (2019) suggests, is fundamental to the development of regulation during infancy:

> Attachment is not just the reestablishment of security after a dysregulating experience and a stressful negative state. It is also the interactive amplification of positive affects, as in play states. Play calms and soothes infants, and it modulates their stressful states of negative arousal, replacing stress with intense joy and excitement. The dual regulatory processes of affect synchrony embedded in play states, and interactive repair, embedded in soothing and calming moments that modulate states of negative arousal, are the fundamental building blocks of attachment and its associated emotions. Synchrony and repair promote resilience and security... (p.226)

What Schore says here may seem as if this kind of play is something that happens primarily during infancy, but he goes on to say that this psychobiological attachment dynamic is expressed in all later development. Schore (2019) continues:

> Homeostatic regulation between members of a dyad is a stable aspect of all intimate relationships throughout the life-span. In all ensuing periods of human development, attachment dynamics find expression in right brain-to-right brain communications of affect and the interactive regulation of affective arousal. The evolutionary mechanism of attachment is, fundamentally, the biological synchronicity between and within organisms. This mechanism occurs most prominently at later points of shared, spontaneous, improvised, and emotionally rewarding moments of intimate contact, including intersubjective play... (p.230)

Schore's reference to the nature of play in later stages of development captures what we were seeing in the 'children at play' – the eagerness and capacity to play creatively and spontaneously, as they improvized and shared with one another while held in the embrace of our attentive care. It was visible in their expressions of joy and satisfaction, followed by improved attitudes and behaviors in the school setting. Through this sensory and relationally rich experience, children were integrating traumas, moving toward secure attachment, and developing their capacity for emotional regulation.

The circuits that activate when we feel disconnected (PANIC, SEPARATION DISTRESS, FEAR, and RAGE) help us with short-term survival strategies that are primarily for the purpose of getting reconnected with caring others. However, PLAY helps us with long-term survival by supporting physical and emotional well-being and freeing our curiosity to run wild. This last aspect no doubt partly accounts for the improved academic performance our children were experiencing. In the video, *The Primal Power of Play*, Panksepp says, 'I like to think of PLAY as the science of joy' (Phillips, 2010). For the sheer pleasure of being alive, there is nothing quite like play, and while this aliveness cannot be measured, it can be felt and delighted in.

Prior to Panksepp's laboratory work on PLAY, it was difficult to explain to parents, teachers, and colleagues why play is essential to healthy human beings or why it can have such a pivotal role in healing. Neuroscience now gives us the foundation to proceed with confidence about the role of play, even in the context of Western cultures that have dismissed it as being frivolous and unworthy of a place in the education and development of children beyond the early years, much less for adults throughout the lifespan. As we have seen, Panksepp placed PLAY among the seven emo-tional-motivational circuits that are inborn and crucial for human survival alongside attachment (CARE, PANIC, and SEPARATION DISTRESS) and procreation (LUST). For evolution to have preserved these circuits speaks to the importance of each of them. Play also provides us with a beautiful example of what it means to fully engage the right hemisphere for purposes of exploring and making sense of novel ideas. In short, play and storytelling show us how to lead with our right hemispheres without losing our capac-ity to incorporate what the left knows due to its ability to analyze, dissect, digitize, and then organize information.

Recently I found a beautiful passage in the prologue to Judy Atkinson's book, *Trauma Trails: Recreating Song Lines* (Atkinson, 2002) about the power of storytelling for healing trauma and pain:

> ...during a time of great pain and crisis in my life, my great grannie came to me and gave me a gift. She sent me a dream...I asked 'what do we do now?' And the answer came 'We come here, and we sit with each other. We tell our stories. We grieve together. And we dance and we sing together. If we do this, as we listen to each other's stories, in our grieving, in our singing, in our dancing, we give power to each other for the healing to begin...' (Atkin-son, 2002, p.1)

For me, this passage summarizes deeply and beautifully what children seem to know instinctively if they are accompanied and given a safe place to play, tell stories, and heal together. Play often leads to storytelling, and they heal from belonging and from being able to make sense of their lives in the pres-ence of peers and adults who want to know what happened to them. They do the storytelling play metaphorically because it provides them with the ability to put a symbolical veil over their deep pain and hurt while also being able to reveal intimately what happened to them and who they truly are. Children have a deep desire to be seen in a safe and nurturing environment.

This idea of telling others about what happened to us in a way that leads to healing has been captured beautifully in a book by neuroscientist Bruce Perry and talk show host Oprah Winfrey called *What Happened to You?* (Perry and Winfrey, 2021). They wrote the book to help change the usual accusatory question, 'What's wrong with you?' to a more supportive (and accurate) question, 'What happened to you?' which can support healing instead of shame and defensiveness. Asking about 'what's wrong' implies that a person is defective, often leading to dorsal vagal shutdown or to states of fight or flight, taking away the possibility of co-regulation (Porges, 2011). 'What happened to you' invites a story and potentially provides a safe listener.

Perry and Winfrey draw from the healing methods of Indigenous people the world over to propose that connection and a supportive community are core to healing. Storytelling – the invitation to talk about what happened to you (and/or your clan) – is one example of an Indigenous healing practice. It is universal and as ancient as humankind. These healing practices also include dramatic enactment, poems, rhythmic chanting, rhymes, humor, play, songs, and more. Perry (Perry and Winfrey, 2021) points out that Indigenous and traditional healing practices create total mind-body experiences that impact multiple brain systems. He says:

> Remember, trauma 'memories' span multiple brain areas. So these traditional practices will have cognitive, relational-based, and sensory elements. You retell the story; create images of the battle, hunt, death; hold each other; massage; dance; sing. You reconnect to loved ones – to community. You celebrate, eat, and share. Aboriginal healing practices are repetitive, rhythmic, relevant, relational, respectful, and rewarding – experiences known to be effective in altering neural systems involved in the stress response. The practices emerged because they worked. People felt better and functioned better, and the core elements of the healing process were reinforced and passed on. Cultures separated by time and space converged on the same principles for healing… (p.230)

Using an upside-down triangle divided into four parts, Perry describes the four levels of the neurosequential[3] brain (Perry, 2009; Perry and Winfrey, 2021). Our brains develop and organize from the bottom (brainstem) to the top (cortex), moving sequentially from the brainstem to the diencephalon, then the limbic, and finally the cortex. Panksepp's midbrain circuitry is at the very top of the brainstem where it interfaces with the diencephalon, so

3   Numerous visual diagrams of Perry's neurosequential model may be found with an internet search.

is part of the flow of information moving upward to the limbic and cortical regions. The lower parts (brainstem, diencephalon) receive input from the five senses (touch, taste, smell, hearing, and sight) and from the internal (interoception) experiences of our bodies. Sequentially these incoming signals are processed first in the lower brain (brainstem, diencephalon), where they are sorted and organized in the service of regulating ourselves in relationship to our immediate environments.

Perry emphasizes the importance of paying attention to this sequential order that begins in the brainstem, which is particularly attending to the rhythms of experience. It is the gateway to bodily and social functioning, and it is essential for the regulatory processes that allow us to eventually influence the cortex, the highest part of the brain where reasoning can take place. He calls this hierarchical process the 'sequence of engagement.' If our core regulatory networks (originating in the brainstem and diencephalon and spreading up throughout the entire brain) are not functioning optimally due to trauma, abuse, or neglect, they will always affect the higher parts of the brain (limbic, cortex), influencing how we relate and think. Perry says that if we want to reason (cortex) with another person, it is necessary to proceed first with 1) regulation, and then 2) relationship, followed by 3) reasoning. It is always this order, whether you are talking with a child or an adult: regulation, relationship, reason. If the core regulatory networks are dysregulated for any reason, our autonomic nervous system responds by automatically initiating the protective states of sympathetic fight/flight and dorsal parasympathetic shutdown or collapse. The neuroendocrine system also responds by sending cortisol throughout our bodies to help us protect ourselves.

Fortunately, as Porges (2009, 2011) points out, our bodies evolved to engage when safe and to disengage – turning to protective states – when threatened. Protective states are often continuously online when we are carrying trauma, abuse, and neglect. The relational and academic difficulties in school that sent children to our playgroups reflect struggles with the three areas that Perry speaks about: regulation, relationship, and reasoning. It is important to notice that regulation comes first. The ability to return to the connected state of social engagement depends on the detection of cues of safety, which we were providing in abundance in our groups. Prolonged and repetitive trauma often results in the loss of resilience in the nervous system. This was true of our sand tray storytelling crew because they had so little opportunity for the social engagement system to be strengthened in their unsafe families or even in school. Sympathetic and dorsal states had become their baseline, making relationships chaotic and leaving them with little interest in or capacity for learning. Physical and emotional health requires us to maximize our time in social engagement because that is the state where health, growth, and restoration take place (Porges and Dana, 2018). Social engagement is the state where secure attachment happens, where we are able to co-regulate with each other, and is required for academic learning to be successful. Once again, 'the children at play' demonstrated to us that academic success follows a sense of belonging and connection.

Returning to Perry's list of the Rs of aboriginal healing practices – **R**epetitive, **R**hythmic, **R**elational, **R**espectful, and **R**ewarding (experiences known to be effective in altering neural systems involved in the stress response) – we can see what happened with the 'children at play.' All the Rs were evident in their group play. You could see the **R**hythmic and **R**epetitive movements of their bodies as they formed landscapes in the sand – patting, sweeping, stirring, and pounding it to get it just the way they needed it. Activating the PLAY circuitry with the simple invitation to play was clearly **R**elevant to them, especially by inviting them into **R**elationship with their peers as a way of promoting friendships. **R**espect easily came most of the time because we developed a structure for group play that created safety. When conflicts emerged, as they often do in play, we were able to help them as facilitators to resolve their differences in a way that deepened their **R**espect for one another. We were also able to model **R**espect and to nurture their **R**elationships with us and with one another. Finally, play is its own **R**eward. We had it all – the pathway to altering the neural systems that allowed these children to feel better about themselves and to function better socially and academically.

What does all of this mean for trauma-informed and trauma-integrated care? Further, how might we move forward to weave play in as one of the major processes that the body/mind/brain can engage to transform traumatic experiences that tend to live on in the body's memory? Finally, how do we invite the integration of both the vertical and lateral processes of the body/mind/brain?

Supporting integration

Vertical integration, bringing information from the body up to the limbic region, happens naturally in the sensory and relational environment of play. Without thought, scenes emerge in the sand, often shifting rapidly as a visual story unfolds. Often, story in words follows spontaneously as the newly released swirling energies of the right make their way to the left hemisphere to find their voice. With the release of trauma, the brain's ongoing push toward integration unfolds on its own, especially when assisted by the presence of someone warm and safe who listens without judgments.

How do we best facilitate this integration? Relational exploratory play requires us to be fully present to one another, open to the rapid shifts we need to navigate in an environment that is presenting us with a lot of choices and unknowns. In addition, it invites us to listen to metaphorical thinking, image thinking, and concrete thinking (thinking with our fingers by constructing things) in contrast to only logical or abstract thinking. In other words, we are invited to witness a fully embodied practice that is following the inherent paths of integration by moving from the bottom up so that language and concepts follow what is emerging, often unexpectedly and always dynamically, from the right hemisphere. We are invited to do this without judgments or meaning making of our own. Being fully present during relational play (or any kind of relational task) gives us an advantage that the left hemisphere alone cannot give us. If clinicians have a robust knowledge base about trauma but they proceed without relational presence, they risk being coercive in the clinical setting as they follow the patterns of particular protocols. Relying on full presence alone without the clarity of a scientific knowledge base, however, can easily lead clinicians to underestimate and underuse the power of play for healing purposes. Without being able to rest on the solid ground of knowledge, they may also feel dysregulated by the intensity of energies that arise. We need both hemispheres to be engaged in a particular way to be of greatest support as traumas come forward to heal. How do we embrace both the left and right simultaneously to activate the flow of energy back and forth between the two hemispheres, supporting healing integration through play?

Being fully present during relational play requires us to temporarily suspend our cognitive focus on left-centric ideas, allowing the right hemisphere to integrate rapidly and seamlessly what is coming from the left so we can offer what is needed, moment by moment, in the play environment. It may be necessary to read this sentence slowly a few times because it can seem contradictory. This movement back and forth between the hemispheres happens very rapidly which requires us to let go of the slower process of conscious focus on what the left is offering. Because of the speed, the interplay unfolds below the level of awareness. People sometimes refer to this as intuitive clinical experience. It *is* intuitive, but it is not void of scientific knowledge and study. It is what can happen when we lead with our right brain relational presence while being supported by the flow of information from the rich storehouse of left-mode details and knowledge. When what the left hemisphere knows is supportive of the value of the right hemisphere taking the lead, the collaboration provides powerful support for healing (McGilchrist, 2009).

Jung's idea of transcending differences in the service of higher levels of integration (Jung, 1991) guides us toward understanding this process more clearly, as does Siegel's idea of differentiation and integration being the means to a more robust brain and healthier attachment relationships (Siegel, 2020). We can appreciate the separate contribution of the differentiated hemispheres while sensing the deep value of their supportive integration. Schore's *Right Brain Psychotherapy* (2019) also points us to this phenomenon. The idea of leading with the right while temporarily withdrawing our focus from the left may seem counter to the notion that only evidence-based modalities are permissible in clinical treatment. This is a left-hemisphere viewpoint that leaves out the unmeasurable component of the relationship. Based on neuroscience studies, however, we can make a case that not factoring in the many ways that warm, safe connection is the foundation for healing means that evidence-based interventions are insufficient. How do we include both the right and left hemispheres? How can we learn to hold both/and rather than either/or?

Turning to metaphor

Embracing differences is an age-old challenge, especially in Western cultures where we have made so many scientific advances by shifting toward left-mode dominance, which sees the world through an either/or lens and puts everything in strict categories. Iain McGilchrist (2009) speaks about the blindness of the left hemisphere once it is in charge. Because it makes the world line up according to its values, a mechanical model emerges that devalues relationship and individuality in favour of procedures for getting things done properly. Evidence-based practice arises from this way of seeing the world.

Even though our neurobiology is inherently inclined toward integration, it is difficult to embrace the relationship between both modes of thinking simultaneously in contexts where linear thinking is so highly rewarded, sometimes to the exclusion of right-mode wholeness. This struggle to simultaneously hold scientific *and* intuitive processes in clinical settings is well illustrated by what it means to practice from a trauma-integrated position as well as a trauma-informed one. The latter invites us to gain knowledge about trauma and healing, while the former suggests the possibility of a relationally grounded application of this knowledge in the relationship between therapist and client. Informed *and* integrated invites us to heal the split. Words alone may not be adequate to accomplish this task, and it may help to turn toward metaphor to get a different perspective.

One of the first recognized play therapists, Margaret Lowenfeld (1993) wrestled with this task of explaining the power of play to heal when she tried to describe the theory behind the sand tray play process that she was using in her clinic to treat traumatized children. Lowenfeld served in Poland during World War I as a paediatrician, where she encountered children in orphanages who had experienced severe trauma. These experiences had a deep impact on her, and when she returned to London after the war in the late 1920s, she organized a clinic for children with the conviction that words alone could not heal trauma. Intuitively, she reasoned that there must be a nonverbal region in the brain that operated apart from the reality-based areas that supported logical thinking. Lowenfeld believed that she would need to give children a means to express with images and sensory-based play the feelings associated with their trauma experiences without having to use words. She set up a play environment of small trays of sand and water, with small figurines that would allow children to use their sensory systems to express what had happened to them. The clinic lent itself to the sometimes-messy play of children, and so very naturally the children began to combine the sand, water, and small figurines in their trays. When the children began identifying the scenes in the sand as their 'worlds,' Lowenfeld[4] recognized that with the help of the children, she had found a method that could support young ones in healing through play.

Lowenfeld called it 'The World Technique,' and after her death in 1973, a book was published with her writings (Lowenfeld, 1993). In this book, she identified her difficulty in finding a way to describe the theory she was trying to develop, and so she turned to metaphor. She pointed to the well-known 'Secret Garden' stories of childhood. In the many different versions of these stories, there is always a key to a secret door that leads to a world of magic and wonder inside a beautiful garden. The key is invisible to most people, especially grown-ups, but if you are courageous enough to find the key, you will be able to unlock a hidden door giving you access to a magical kingdom. Children who have the key (and most do!) know that the door can only be opened, in the dark, at midnight when their parents are asleep, enabling them to leave their ordinary homes undetected to play for a little while inside the magic garden where all things are possible. They can play to their heart's content, find new friends, and make wishes come true. In the garden, there are good fairies and wise gnomes to help. There are also ogres, wicked spells, and other dangers. Everything is welcome here. If you know the rules of the magic kingdom and are virtuous, you will not get hurt. There are wondrous treasures of gold, jewels, and other precious gems. Best of all, when it is time to return to your ordinary world right before your parents wake up, you will have special energies, gifts, and new discoveries that you can take with you and keep forever. This metaphorical description reveals to us the healing field of sensory-based relational play.

Part of the reason Lowenfeld had difficulty articulating the play theory within the tradition of her rigorous training in the physical and biological sciences was that her intuitive sense of a region in the brain that operated differently from the ordinary logical part was ahead of her time scientifically, and it emerged before the development of the instruments needed to measure and verify it. We know now that she was pointing to the right hemisphere before scientists even understood its role in the brain. She used

---

4   Lowenfeld (1993) noted that this apparatus that she called the world came into existence in 1929.

the Secret Garden metaphor to draw a contrast between the magical realm and the ordinary garden, two realms that children know so well. They can navigate easily between these two places, and they are quite capable of combining them for purposes of healing and working with novel ideas. Lowenfeld (1993) described the Secret Garden as a 'well-defined region' with a 'wall' separating it from the house garden. She elaborated:

> The rules of conduct and the type of event that occurs on one side of the wall are different from those on the other side. What is expected in one garden does not happen in the other, and in the magic garden almost anything can come about... (p.17)

Inside the garden, time and space are essentially limitless, creating possibilities for transformation. If you had the courage (or the innocence of childhood), you could venture in, encounter whatever was there to be found, and access treasures and desired changes that you could incorporate into your ordinary home garden to transform daily life.

The two areas Lowenfeld described are remarkably like the way Iain McGilchrist (2009) differentiates the two hemispheres of the brain. Even though each hemisphere perceives the world in its own unique way, they are both essential and complementary to one another. McGilchrist suggests that a strong relationship between the hemispheres involving deep respect for the uniqueness and independence of each is key to solving many of the current problems of Western cultures that have emerged because of separation and mistrust. His insights are as applicable to the individual mind as to the culture. Metaphorically, Lowenfeld delivered to us one of the keys to understanding that relational exploratory play helps children heal from trauma. She was, perhaps, the first trauma-informed *and* trauma-integrated play therapist.

Learning to trust the play spiral

Setting the intention to engage in relational play with vulnerable children, families, and communities requires us to show up, being fully present to the emotional-motivational system of PLAY. We must begin with the innate desire of play rather than our list of trauma-informed practices. It is not helpful, however, to disregard the left-hemisphere-based list. We can study it, understand it, value it, and bring it to our practices, but leading with the list is almost certain to override the intrinsic emotional-motivational system of PLAY that helps to heal trauma in the deepest reaches of the body/brain/mind. For a trauma-integrated practice, we must reach beyond the information alone in the same way that Lowenfeld knew that she had to offer something that reached the whole brain, not just the linguistic part.

True PLAY, as Panksepp (1998, 2009, 2011) describes it, has no agenda. It has no list. It trusts that the child's whole system, already in a state of connection, will know how to respond to this opportunity in this moment.

The research on PLAY by Panksepp has helped us to develop a scientific foundation for the integrating/healing functions of play. One of the challenges seems to be trusting that this knowledge base, rooted in our left hemispheres, will not disappear when we venture into the realm of the right where relational play seems to arise spontaneously with little regard for agendas, predictable order, or lists of things to be accomplished. Play is facilitated by us being fully present in the moment, something the right hemisphere does well. The left, however, being concerned with the logical order of things, finds it difficult to suspend, even temporarily, its sure-footed, predictable, and methodical way of viewing the world (McGilchrist, 2009). It fears being lost and disregarded.

Once the left hemisphere is well fed with an understanding of the principles that suggest the right hemisphere takes the lead and the left acts as support staff, it can come to peace with its natural role and be a valuable part of a whole. Immersing ourselves in relational neuroscience until it becomes who we are seems to be one pathway for the two hemispheres to get into relationship in this healthy way (Badenoch, 2018).

While the left on its own seems to be incapable of understanding the metaphorical Secret Garden where movement between the two worlds (left and right, or magic and reality) is natural, easily accomplished, and even cherished, the right seems to know that temporary suspension of conscious attention to the left is necessary for meaningful integration to occur. The truth is, as in the Secret Garden, we (children and adults) can enter the unknown realm (magical, spiritual, creative, non-linear, or illusive), deal with monsters and find treasures and new ways of being, and then return to ordinary reality bringing the jewels (new levels of integration) with us, enabling us to experience an enhanced and more meaningful ordinary reality. The new level of right-hemispheric integration now becomes knowledge that is transmitted to the left, where once again, the left can sort, digitize, and organize. Stabilizing this new state is part of the rightful and essential role of the left. As McGilchrist suggests, in spiral form, this 'worked through' data of the left then returns to the right through metaphor for another round of integration at ever higher levels. I call it the 'spiral of play' (Kestly, 2014). We can imagine that our playgroup children were moving along this spiral week by week, returning to the daily world of school with new ways of being together and an active interest in learning.

When we weave together Siegel's insight about the importance of differentiation and integration in the healing process, Schore's idea of the amplification of the positive affect of play states increasing secure attachment, Panksepp's identification of PLAY circuitry in the brain, and Porges' theory of play as a neural exercise that expands regulation, we can begin to visualize a scientific foundation for the healing power of play. We can make the case for the benefits of play throughout the lifespan, not only for a sense of well-being (physically and emotionally), but also for providing a direct avenue into healing and reconnecting what has been split apart during trauma and abuse.

We can learn to trust the spiral nature of our brains, but perhaps we must do that in a conscious, intentional way. Lowenfeld did just that by inviting children to enter the magical garden of exploratory play where words could be uttered, or not. The children could create, form deep bonds with others and with nature, and give meaningful and satisfying form to their trauma experiences. The children did it metaphorically and with abundant support, transforming the painful reality of what had happened to them to find new visions of how to be. Lowenfeld recognized that the children had the key. It was their inheritance. She simply needed to create the wondrous, safe, and protected garden space where she could nurture their healing and growth. Endowed with PLAY circuitry, the children knew exactly what they needed to do.

KNOWLEDGE AND PRACTICE REFLECTION

Joe Tucci, Janise Mitchell, Ed Tronick and Stephen W. Porges

Kestly's chapter casts its own magical spell over the reader, warmly and expertly integrating the joy of play with an in-depth knowledge of the neuroscience of trauma, relationships and healing. She brings together her own experience as a pioneer of play with the reflections of an even earlier pioneer of play therapy – Margaret Lowenfeld.

It honours the power of children using their embedded circuitry as resources that are enlivened in the embrace of an adult who cares, attends and explores their experience and meaning making with curiosity and compassion.

This chapter is hope. It cherishes hope. It allows hope to feel real and not some idealized objective that is unlikely to be reached. It locates hope in the strengths that children hold in the face of overwhelming violence. It finds it in the relationships which are offered to children when the power to lead is offered genuinely with the view to it being taken up. Hope is a form of knowledge that results from the integration of science, practice and embodied experience.

Kestly finds herself needing to use trauma integrated to add definitional aspects to trauma informed. This is an example of the limitation of the current construct of trauma-informed practice. On its own, it does not hold the conceptual resources that are needed to communicate the ways in which it can make a difference. Just as Siegel (2015) applies integration as the paramount function of the brain-body system, Kestly raises integration as a way of bringing together evidence and practice, as the experience of children as they engage in play and storytelling and as a metaphor for the way that change is empowered in the lives of those affected by trauma.

Trauma-integrated care responds to the importance of including strengths-based orientation that celebrates the wonder of transformation.

For trauma-transformative practitioners, organizations and systems, the significance of play and the hope that comes with it cannot be underestimated. Play is a rich resource for children and adults. It is restorative and reparative. It is an inbuilt endowment for humanity when it grapples with the hurt and pain caused by others. It is gently evoked by engaging in it. It coaxes the physiology of the brain/body system to reorganize itself away from states of self-protection towards states of creativity, appreciation and connectedness. In these states, it is more likely that children, adults, families and communities become open to possibility and growth.

Maintaining an orientation that change is possible builds hope into trauma-transformative practice if for no other reason that in the face of despair and pain arising from violence, hope is critically needed.

References

References for chapter

Atkinson, J. (2002). *Trauma Trails Recreating Song Lines: The Transgenerational Effects of Trauma in Indigenous Australia*. Melbourne: Spinifex Press.

Badenoch, B. (2018). *The Heart of Trauma: Healing the Embodied Brain in the Context of Relationships*. New York, NY: W.W. Norton and Company.

Jung, C.G. (1991). *Psyche and Symbol*. Princeton, NJ: Princeton University Press.

Kestly, T. (2014). *The Interpersonal Neurobiology of Play: Brain-building Interventions for Emotional Well-being*. New York, NY: W.W. Norton and Company.

Lowenfeld, M. (1993). *Understanding Children's Sand Play: The World Technique*. Cambridge: Margaret Lowenfeld Trust.

McGilchrist, I. (2009). *The Master and his Emissary: The Divided Brain and the Making of the Western World*. New Haven, CT: Yale University Press.

Panksepp, J. (1998). *Affective Neuroscience: The Foundations of Human and Animal Emotions*. New York, NY: Oxford University Press.

Panksepp, J. (2009). Brain Emotional Systems and Qualities of Mental Life: From Animal Models of Affect to Implications for Psychotherapeutics. In D. Fosha, D. Siegel and M. Solomon (eds), *The Healing Power of Emotion: Affective Neuroscience, Development and Clinical Practice* (pp.1–26). New York, NY: W.W. Norton and Company.

Panksepp, J. (2011). Cross-species affective neuroscience decoding of the primal affective experiences of humans and related animals. *PLoS ONE*, 6(9): e21236. doi:10.1371/journal.pone.0021236.

Panksepp, J. and Biven, L. (2012). *The Archaeology of Mind: Neuroevolutionary Origins of Human Emotions*. New York, NY: W.W. Norton and Company.

Perry, B. (2009). Examining child maltreatment through a neurodevelopmental lens: Clinical applications of the neurosequential model of therapeutics. *Journal of Loss and Trauma*, 14, 240–255.

Perry, B. and Winfrey, O. (2021). *What Happened to You? Conversations on Trauma, Resilience, and Healing*. New York, NY: Flatiron Books.

Phillips, B. (2010, June 16). *The Primal Power of Play*. [Video] YouTube. https://youtu.be/3KanfLqKXYg.

Porges, S. (2009). Reciprocal Influences Between Body and Brain in the Perception and Expression of Affect: A Polyvagal Perspective. In D. Fosha, D. Siegel and M. Solomon (eds), *The Healing Power of Emotion: Affective Neuroscience, Development, and Clinical Practice* (pp.27–54). New York, NY: W.W. Norton and Company.

Porges, S. (2011). *The Polyvagal Theory: Neurophysiological Foundations of Emotions, Attachment, Communication, and Self-regulation*. New York, NY: W.W. Norton and Company.

Porges, S.W. (2015). Play as a Neural Exercise: Insights from the Polyvagal Theory. In D. Pearce-McCall (ed.), *The Power of Play for Mind Brain Health* (pp.3–7). Available from http://mindgains.org.

Porges, S. and Dana, D. (eds) (2018). *Clinical Applications of the Polyvagal Theory: The Emergence of Polyvagal-informed Therapies*. New York, NY: W.W. Norton and Company.

Schore, A.N. (2019). *Right Brain Psychotherapy*. New York, NY: W.W. Norton and Company.

Siegel, D.J. (2020). *The Developing Mind: How Relationships and the Brain Interact to Shape Who We Are* (third edition). New York, NY: Guilford Press.

Siegel, D.J., Schore, A.N. and Cozolino, L. (eds) (2021). *Interpersonal Neurobiology and Clinical Practice*. New York, NY: W.W. Norton and Company.

References for Knowledge and Practice Reflection

Siegel, D.J. (2015). Interpersonal neurobiology as a lens into the development of wellbeing and reslience. *Children Australia*, 40(2), 160–164.

CHAPTER 14

Trauma-Informed Practice with Children and Young People Who Engage in Harmful Sexual Behavior

Kevin Creeden

Introduction

We have seen an increased understanding of the immediate and long-term impact of childhood adversity, maltreatment, and trauma experiences on the emotional, behavioral, intellectual, and physical well-being of children and adolescents (Felitti *et al.*, 1998; Anda *et al.*, 2006; De Bellis *et al.*, 2013). Subsequently, there has been a focus on integrating our increased understanding of the developmental effect of these experiences into the treatment approaches, interventions, and environments formulated to meet the needs of these youth. These efforts have generally fallen under the umbrella of what has become known as trauma-informed care.

While not all children and adolescents who engage in problematic or harmful sexual behaviors have histories of adversity or trauma, research has indicated that these histories are a central feature in the lives of the majority of youth we see presenting with these problems and especially those youth who present with serious and persistent harmful sexual behaviors (HSB) (Baglivio and Epps, 2015; Dillard and Beaujolais, 2019; Chouinard-Thivierge *et al.*, 2022). This chapter aims to examine how well this *trauma-informed* awareness has been incorporated into our understanding and treatment of problematic and harmful sexual behaviors and ways that we might better utilize the research on the impact of trauma to broaden our interventions and enhance our effectiveness.

Trauma-informed care/treatment

Trauma-informed care (TIC) is a systemic approach to working with individuals suffering from the impact of adverse or traumatic experiences. Broadly speaking, TIC is a strengths-based approach to intervention that is grounded in an understanding and responsiveness to the developmental impact of trauma, and focuses on safety, empowerment, resilience, and growth (Bloom, 2013; Hopper *et al.*, 2009).

How a TIC perspective is operationalized into policy, protocols, treatment, and interventions can be quite varied, depending on the type of setting, institution, context, and individuals involved, and significantly on education, training, and a persistent attention to the principles of TIC in the everyday interactions we engage in with clients. Specifically, the five core elements of TIC have been identified as safety, trustworthiness, choice, collaboration, and empowerment (Harris and Fallot, 2001). However, these core elements are frequently in conflict with the concerns raised by HSB and the manner in which the primary social institutions involved with youth (families, schools, social services, juvenile justice) conceive of and respond to HSB engaged in by children and adolescents. Indeed, how we operationalize the principles of choice, collaboration, and empowerment with children at different developmental stages is subject to a variety of diverse views and approaches.

Specifically addressing TIC in relation to HSB, Levenson and her colleagues (2020) note that trauma-informed practices address the connection between past experiences and presenting problems through a process that recognizes the client's early adverse experiences and delivers treatment interventions in a 'relational context that considers how early adversities shape thinking, feeling, and behaviour' (p.199). She suggests that TIC for HSB relies more heavily on the therapeutic process than on the content for addressing issues of self-regulation and healthy relational skills (Levenson *et al.*, 2017).

The challenge for clinicians who work with these youth is to be able to articulate the *process* to the child, their family, and any other involved members of the child's service system in a manner that promotes respect, safety, trust, competency, and optimism for change and growth. This is not a *one size fits all* endeavor and can vary greatly depending on (among a range of factors) the individual child's presenting behavior, developmental level, learning style, and life experiences, including their previous experience in treatment settings. The facilitation of family engagement will be similarly varied depending on family members' own history of trauma, prior experiences in treatment, level of resources and supports, and other emotional and social stressors. Finally, involved systems such as schools, social services, court systems, and so on, each have their own perspectives and priorities when it comes to their understanding of trauma, harmful sexual behavior, and their definition of what constitutes a successful outcome for the youth. This requires that as treatment providers, we not only consider how early life adversities have shaped or impacted the presenting issue of HSB but also how they shape the ways in which the child or adolescent perceives themselves, their relationships to adults and peers, their response to reward and punishment, their interests, the ways in which they learn and remember, and their hopefulness regarding future life outcomes. Our capacity as treatment providers to integrate a broad understanding of the potential impacts of trauma into our consideration of problematic sexual behavior and the formulation of a comprehensive treatment approach enhances the possibility that the involved systems respond in a coherent and consistent manner and that the youth and their family receive the different types of resources and interventions that support posttraumatic growth (Tedeschi and Moore, 2021).

Safety and the importance of attachment relationships

The primary foundation for addressing trauma-related issues is establishing a sense of safety and stability in the lives of the clients we treat, and the central element for acquiring and maintaining a sense of safety for humans lies in the availability of secure attachment relationships. John Bowlby (1973, 1982) contended that humans were biologically wired to develop attachment systems principally as a means for detecting threat and enhancing survival. Bowlby describes the key components of the attachment system as: 1) the individual's monitoring and appraising for potential threat; 2) monitoring and appraising the availability of a responsive person who can provide comfort and safety; and 3) monitoring and appraising the likelihood that seeking this person for comfort and safety can be achieved.

Bowlby (1982) saw the importance of attachment relationships in providing for the care, nurturance, and safety that allowed children to increasingly explore the world around them. These relationships provided a 'safe base' to return to, thereby enhancing positive growth and development. Sroufe (2000) notes that if we consider attachment in this manner, it becomes the chief organizing feature of the infant's early social environment and that the outcomes of these experiences provide the basis for the child's sense of safety and for their capacity to engage in social relationships. The presence of secure attachment relationships has been shown to be a protective factor against the effects of physical and emotional distress (Porges, 2011; Sachser et al., 1998). Conversely, the absence of a secure and attuned child/caretaker relationship can negatively affect the child's capacity to regulate their emotional and behavioral responses to stress and may disrupt their ability to engage in future social relationships (Bales and Carter, 2009; Chen and Baram, 2016; Harms et al., 2018; Sroufe 2000).

Attachment, trauma and neurodevelopment

An increasing amount of neurodevelopmental research indicates that the emotion regulation processes that develop from consistent and positive child/caregiver interactions create a regulatory system that is both social/emotional and neurological (Hart, 2011; Schore, 2001). Therefore, a clinical understanding of the impact of trauma and in turn trauma-informed care must take into account what the neurological and neurodevelopmental research tells us about how trauma impacts the brain development and the broader neurological responses of the individuals who come to us for care and treatment (Crittenden, 1997; Seigel, 1999; Creeden, 2017; Creeden, 2004).

These consistent and reciprocal interactions between the caretaker and the child have been referred to as 'serve and return' behaviors (Center on the Developing Child, 2012) and these behaviors shape the formation of neural circuits which respond to the type and intensity of sensory stimuli in a developmentally progressive manner. Neurodevelopmental research would suggest that:

> ...because responsive relationships are developmentally expected and biologically essential, their absence signals a serious threat to child well-being, particularly during the earliest years, and this absence activates the body's stress response systems... (Center on the Developing Child, 2012, p.1)

These 'serve and return' responsive relationships in childhood operate as the basis for what is often referred to as 'co-regulation' (Fogel and Garvey, 2007) and while the neurological structures of co-regulation develop in early childhood, we continue to utilize co-regulation processes throughout our lives through the relationships and social supports we develop.

A lack of responsiveness to the child's needs, either through persistent overstimulation or understimulation of the sensory signals that relay to the child a sense of stability and safety, is at the very basis of disrupted attachment relationships and the types of emotional regulation difficulties that can accompany them. These regulatory struggles are impacted by the differential assessments that the child makes in response to the emotional information associated with facial cues and other sensory stimuli and the ways in which this information is interpreted with regard to safety versus threat, and approach versus avoidance (Opendak et al., 2016).

Attachment styles may actually reflect the underlying neurological systems that develop in an effort to maintain stability and safety. Vrtička and Vuilleumier (2012) have suggested that avoidant attachment is characterized by a blunted response of the emotional activation system (amygdala, stratium, insula, cingulate, hippocampus) and serves to deactivate attachment needs and utilize a greater reliance on more cortically based suppression responses to achieve regulation and safety. Conversely, they would view anxious attachment as being correlated with enhanced responsiveness to information signaling threat and precipitating a hyperactivation of attachment needs but this hyperactivation creates difficulties in perspective-taking that allow for accurate appraisal and effective problem-solving.

Adversity, cognition and self-regulation

There is a growing body of evidence indicating that the experience of child maltreatment places a child at risk for a range of frequently overlapping neurodevelopmental issues that can affect cognitive functioning and self-regulation specifically, and several aspects of executive functioning more broadly (Cicchetti, 2016; Hostinar and Gunnar, 2013.

In their study comparing maltreated children with and without PTSD to a control group, De Bellis, Wooley, and Hooper (2013) found lower IQ scores, academic achievement, and neurocognitive abilities in the maltreated groups regardless of whether they had been diagnosed with PTSD or not. Child maltreatment places children at greater risk for developing language-based learning problems, including receptive-expressive language disorders and central auditory processing disorders (Snow, 2009; De Bellis *et al.*, 2009; Teicher *et al.*, 2002). De Bellis and his colleagues also found that childhood experiences of abuse and neglect led to a wide range of learning problems in reading, mathematics, complex visual attention, visual memory, verbal memory, and planning and problem-solving (De Bellis *et al.*, 2009). These learning difficulties appear to be directly related to brain structures impacted by child maltreatment and the connectivity of brain regions that facilitate the effective processing, attention, retrieval, organization, and integration of sensory-based, language-based, and emotionally relevant stimuli (Hart and Rubia, 2012). It is important to recognize that these learning problems not only impact experiences like academic performance or vocational achievement but they also create risk factors for future behavioral difficulties and obstacles to developing resilience in response to early adverse experiences (Perkins *et al.*, 2014; Sylvestre *et al.*, 2016.)

Karoly (1993) defined self-regulation as an integrated set of skills that draw from executive function and emotion regulation capacities which are invoked to accomplish short-term and long-term goals – while also noting that it was the central skill required to cope with stress in an adaptive manner. Emotional and behavioral regulation require the activation and coordination of the parasympathetic and sympathetic nervous systems, the neuroendocrine system, and brain regions in the limbic, lower brain, and higher cortical region (Thompson *et al.*, 2013; Porges, 2011). Differences in individual capacities for self-regulation arise from the complex interaction of biological, environmental, and experiential factors (Deater-Deckard and Mullineaux, 2010; Gross and Thompson, 2007).

Self-regulation difficulties have been associated with a range of social, behavioral, and emotional problems including increased risk for aggression (especially in males), learning problems, poor academic performance, social difficulties, and mood disorders (McLaughlin and Lambert, 2017; Shackman and Pollak, 2014; Kim and Cicchetti, 2010; De Bellis *et al.*, 2009). Difficulties in self-regulation are often identified as a central feature among individuals engaged in harmful sexual behavior (Stinson and Becker, 2013; Joyal *et al.*, 2018; Marshall and Barbaree, 1990).

As we try to integrate the research on childhood adversities, attachment, and self-regulation into our understanding and treatment of our clients there appear to be clear connections between the presence (or absence) of consistent and available responses from caregivers; the importance of these responses in buffering children from stress and adversity; the neurodevelopmental consequences of adversity when these relationships and buffers are absent; and the subsequent cognitive, behavioral, and emotional difficulties that can emerge. However, in our work, we are consistently made aware of the complexity and variation of outcomes we see in our clients in response to adversity and trauma even when it appears that the experiences are very similar.

Research seems to indicate that the type of stress or adversity that an individual experiences does not fundamentally alter the neurological response (Smith and Pollak, 2020; McEwen, 2012). Consistent with the research on ACEs, this would suggest that what is likely to define our client's experience of adversity and maltreatment is the frequency with which these experiences occur (Feletti *et al.*, 1998; Dong *et al.*, 2004). Yet we know that different individuals can view the same experience very differently and that the impact of some experiences seems to have greater effect than the impact of others. These individual differences could be shaped by a variety of factors, including genetics, the availability of support, the stability of the home, the individual's perception of the intensity of the experience, and the level of threat posed by the experience.

There is accumulating evidence that different types of maltreatment and stress experienced at different stages of child development can result in notably different neurological impacts. This alone can make research regarding the effects of trauma hard to compare and integrate and make the symptoms or behaviors presented by the youth we treat difficult to link to specific types of adverse experiences. However, it also highlights the importance of taking a more individualized, developmental, and contextual perspective to understanding the complex responses our clients have to trauma (Cohodes *et al.*, 2020; Smith and Pollak, 2020) and should dissuade us from seeking a 'one size fits all' approach to trauma treatment (Creeden, 2020).

Teicher and Samson (2016), in a review of the current research involving the neurobiological effects of child maltreatment, propose two different hypotheses for understanding how structural and functional neurological changes emerge from the experience of child maltreatment. The first is that abusive experiences induce a 'cascade of stress-mediated effects on hormones and neurotransmitters that would affect the development of vulnerable brain regions' (p.4). Evidence indicates that these effects would largely be witnessed in 'stress-susceptible regions' such as the amygdala, hippocampus, cerebellum, and neocortex. This hypothesis proposes that persistent experiences of stress are harmful for the brain and that these stressful experiences can be especially problematic or damaging when they occur early in the neurodevelopmental process. The second hypothesis is that the changes seen in brain structure and function in individuals exposed to early child maltreatment are adaptive responses (largely geared to promoting survival) to experiences that present the world as a dangerous, stress-filled environment and the lack of available supports/resources necessary to modulate those stressors. This hypothesis views the difficulties precipitated by these responses as emerging 'due to the mismatch between the world the brain was modified to survive in and the world it finds itself in during subsequent developmental stages' (Teicher and Samson, 2016, p.5).

In considering a trauma-informed approach to treatment, this perspective that views the presenting issues as emerging from an adaptive rather than a pathological response can shift the focus of our interventions from solely addressing the difficulties reflected by the symptoms and behaviour of the child, to creating safer environments where reliable adults support and guide the child to develop a range of adaptive responses that are consistent with a world that poses less threatening environmental demands.

The different phases of treatment

A consensus seems to have emerged that trauma-focused treatment is most effective when approached in phases or stages (Cook *et al.*, 2005; Saxe *et al.*, 2007). The phase-oriented approaches can be defined somewhat differently but all have common elements of safety, attachment, self-regulation, and developing a different understanding and narrative regarding the traumatic experiences that promotes a change in the individual's view of themselves, their sense of competency and agency, and their sense of hopefulness moving forward. The youth we treat can face obstacles in each of these treatment phases, and treatment providers need to recognize those obstacles and then teach, promote, or facilitate ways in which the process can move forward.

Integrating trauma knowledge into the treatment of harmful sexual behaviors

Theories addressing the etiology of harmful sexual behaviors frequently identify the importance of developmental variables and developmental experiences (Lussier and Chouinard-Thivierge, 2017; Elkovitch *et al.*, 2009; Smallbone, 2006; Marshall and Marshall, 2000) but this perspective does not always filter into how we implement our treatment process (Creeden, 2017). Conceptually, a developmental process moves from simple to complex, from foundational needs and capacities to more varied, nuanced, and complicated operations. One view of the impact of trauma on development and behavior would be to see the experience of trauma as disrupting the development of these foundational skills and capacities and consequently, altering the child's developmental trajectory neurologically, emotionally, and behaviorally in ways that are less adaptive, flexible, and responsive to new experiences that can promote safety, personal growth, and positive relationships. This requires that we not only recognize the presence of adverse experiences and traumatic events in our clients' lives but also understand when they occurred in the developmental process and what that might mean for certain skills that are acquired in developmentally sensitive periods (Perry, 2009; Pechtel *et al.*, 2014; Teicher and Parriger, 2015).

Viewed from this perspective, a trauma-informed developmental approach to treating HSB seeks to identify the ways in which adverse experiences interfered with or disrupted these foundational skills (e.g. attunement, attachment, self-regulation, attention, working memory) and how these experiences precipitated, shaped, or motivated the child or adolescent's engagement in HSB. This perspective also encourages us to identify the individual strengths and resources available to support resiliency and growth because the goal of a developmentally focused approach is not only to eliminate harmful or problematic behavior, but also to promote and facilitate:

- the presence of stable and supportive family relationships
- a stable and safe living environment
- the youth's ability for self-regulation,
- the ability to engage in adaptive, prosocial problem solving
- the development of academic and/or vocational competence
- the capacity to make and sustain positive prosocial relationships
- the capacity for intimacy and an understanding of healthy sexuality.

Trauma-informed developmental treatment
Safety and stabilization: The environment
Since the experience of trauma essentially incorporates vulnerability to threat and danger, finding ways to create safe environments becomes an essential feature of the treatment process (Allen, 2001; Briere and Scott, 2006). Ideally, we would be able to ensure safety in all the environments in which our clients operate (e.g. home, community, school, work) but given the various difficulties these children and families face and the histories of complex trauma that they frequently enter treatment with, such broad assurance is generally beyond our control. What we can impact is the child

and family's experience of safety in the treatment environment and the treatment relationship.

Establishing safety in the therapeutic environment and relationship is an active endeavor that requires attention in several different areas. Built into our thinking is an understanding that the youth and family are concurrently dealing with the anxiety of entering treatment in addition to stressors that may be stemming from conflicted family relationships, social service involvement, school difficulties, court involvement, and the traumatic experience itself. From a trauma-informed perspective we know that individuals are typically less anxious when there is a greater level of predictability and while novelty can precipitate interest, exploration, and growth in well-regulated children and adolescents, it can be initially overwhelming for many of the youth we treat. We also recognize that anxious and overwhelmed individuals who have been impacted by trauma have a tendency to flee, withdraw, or become actively defensive. The youth who come to us for treatment tend to be acutely aware of environmental cues that suggest threat or safety.

With this in mind, treatment providers should attend to the nature of the treatment space and, to the degree possible, adapt things like the lighting, sound, furniture, and available materials (e.g. pillows, drawing materials, fidget toys, exercise bands) to fit with the sensory needs and style of the youth. Another important element of safety in any environment is the establishment of a consistent and predictable structure. This includes basics such as the frequency and length of the meetings, who will attend, how information will be shared and with whom, transportation, childcare, work and school schedules, and any other issues that might create a barrier to treatment. Establishing a safe treatment environment also includes addressing the different concerns and expectations of all participants and making sure that these are integrated into treatment planning. For the clinician, conveying a consistent stance of respect, attunement, acceptance, and openness allows for an environment where anxiety and shame can diminish and trust and safety can develop (Bergman and Creeden, 2011). This initial process of establishing safety highlights all five elements of trauma-informed care: safety, trustworthiness, choice, collaboration, and empowerment.

Practical considerations

In many of the settings that we work in, we may have only limited control and influence over things like furnishings, sound, and lighting but our awareness of the physical environment as contributing to or diminishing a sense of safety for our clients means that we attend to those elements that we can adjust or control, acknowledge the existence of problematic environmental cues, and work collaboratively with our clients to make the treatment environment as safe as possible. There have been instances where simply marking out a section of the office with masking tape on the floor and establishing that as the child's space where different items (pillows, weighted blankets, a rocking chair) can be placed has made a remarkable difference in the child's sense of control and safety. If treatment is provided in a family's home, establishing, in collaboration with the family, consistent expectations around space, noise, lighting, and privacy at the start of the treatment process is an important element that should not be overlooked and must be attended to on a persistent basis.

Porges (2015) suggests that it may be helpful to consider that our client's may not only be hypervigilant to cues suggesting threat, but they may also struggle with the ability to 'feel safe.' While we are often aware of the types of situations, experiences, and environments that might trigger traumatic responses, paying attention to the somatic and sensory experiences that can promote safety may prove to be equally valuable.

Attunement and attachment (safety, skill building, self-regulation)

We have noted already the importance of attachment in promoting a sense of safety and enhancing self-regulation but how do we go about fostering attachment and the capacities for attachment in treatment? I believe there is a general agreement among clinicians working with children and adolescents that attachment relationships are important for positive treatment outcomes both in terms of facilitating safe and consistent relationships between the child and the supportive adults around them and between the child and the clinician. However, I also find that many clinicians struggle with identifying those elements that might enable or assist those relationships to develop.

If we consider attachment as a developmental process, it may make sense for us to initiate interventions that seek to address attachment difficulties by focusing on attunement. I think of attunement as those 'serve and return' interactions that were discussed earlier where the participants attend to, respond to, and adjust their responses in a mutual and continuous manner. The difficulty for many of the youth we treat is that they frequently enter treatment with genuine obstacles in their abilities to accurately attune to others in their environment due to early experiences of threat and early disruptions in their attachment relationships. These disruptions result in them misinterpreting cues related to understanding the motivations and intentions of others and more broadly to accurately appraising threat and safety in the environment.

We have already mentioned how consistency in the treatment environment, the session structure, scheduling, length of sessions, and so on can lay a foundation for promoting a sense of safety. A central element of this treatment structure is, of course, the clinician. The therapist's capacity for self-regulation, attention, and engagement allows for the development of a consistent and safe relationship. Persistent attention to those 'serve and return' interactions with a focus on posture, tone of voice, facial expression, and energy enables the clinician to provide the co-regulation that not only allows the child or adolescent to feel safe but can serve as a basis to developing greater self-regulation skills moving forward.

Practical considerations

In individual sessions, the therapist might use simple, structured activities to promote the serve and return process, like bouncing a ball back and forth while talking (or not), by taking turns in a game, or by simply walking 'in sync' with the child or adolescent outside. The actual activity will depend on the interests, developmental level, sensory style, and level of engagement of the individual youth. What the therapist is looking to create is the opportunity for continuous, mutually adjusted interaction that is the product of being attuned, and that the regular experience of these interactions also enhances greater capacities for attunement.

When youth struggle with accurately reading social cues, I find it helpful to practice these skills regularly for short segments of our individual treatment sessions. I find brief video clips of one to three individuals in a scene. I initially play the clip with the sound off, asking the child or adolescent to 'tell me the story' about what is going on in the scene regarding the nature of the relationships, the emotions, the outcome and what they are seeing in the scene that informs their version of the story. We will then go back and review the scene, this time with the dialogue, and discuss whether they feel their initial understanding of the scene was accurate or not and why. This activity allows the youth to practice reading social cues and environmental cues as a 'third party' observer without the interpersonal demands and dynamics that come into play during a family therapy session or a group therapy session. It also provides the clinician with a sense of what the youth is focused on in interpreting these social interactions and how this might be affecting their understanding and response to others. We might continue to teach and reinforce attunement through mirroring exercises, drumming, and other activities that highlight the experience of being 'in sync' with those around you. Obviously, we are then looking to see the youth be able to internalize and apply these skills to their interactions with family and peers.

The families that we work with can frequently present with multigenerational histories of trauma and disrupted attachment relationships (DeGregorio, 2013; Worley *et al.*, 2012). In these cases, the clinician needs to foster attunement not only with the child but also with the parent. In the earlier phases of treatment, these sessions might be done separately, with attention paid to helping the parent to develop a sense of trust as well as enhancing their sense of agency and control through education and skill building (Cohen *et al.*, 2006; St. Amand *et al.*, 2008). Parents, like their children, often enter treatment defensive, ashamed, and overwhelmed by the variety of demands being placed on them. Being attuned to the perspective, needs, and the challenges facing these parents can create a treatment environment where they feel supported rather than judged, and empowered rather than helpless. Often, I find, treatment providers can become more easily frustrated and critical of the attitudes and behaviors of the parents than they are of the children and adolescents they treat. This may indicate that we have failed to develop that attuned and collaborative relationship that facilitates the parent being open to learning new skills and then utilizing those skills to adjust or repair the attachment relationship they have with their child. It may also indicate that we need to focus more directly on the parent's ability to attend to and accurately interpret social cues in the environment, especially in relation to their understanding and responsiveness to their child.

In joint sessions with parents and their children, I try to start each session with a structured 'serve and return' activity that promotes the experience of being 'in sync' through interactions that are simple, playful, and engaging in a sensory or physical manner. Especially when working with adolescents and their parents, reminding them that they can actually enjoy their interactions with one another creates space for addressing more difficult issues that can emerge in the treatment process.

Self-regulation

What brings our clients to treatment is typically the observation or discovery of concerning, problematic, or harmful behavior. In the case of treating youth engaged in HSB, the primary presenting issue is likely to be sexual behavior, but these behaviors frequently co-exist with other concerning behaviors like aggression, elopement, stealing, and a range of oppositional behaviors at home or school. It is not unusual, especially if the client is male, for them to have been identified with an attention disorder with or without hyperactivity.

Schore (2003) has noted that the most significant impact of early relational trauma is the loss of ability to regulate the intensity and duration of affects, while van der Kolk (2005) identifies the core of traumatic stress as the breakdown in the capacity to regulate internal states such as fear, anger, and sexual impulses.

As we have already noted the developmental process of self-regulation for children starts with co-regulation, which stems from an attuned and consistently available adult attachment figure. But the capacity to self-regulate also requires the individual to internalize and integrate certain skills that allow them to modulate their emotional and behavioral response while accurately appraising social and situational stimuli and responding in a manner that directs them toward identified goals and outcomes (Berkman, 2016).

Neurological research has shown evidence of two distinct functional-anatomical executive functioning networks engaged in these processes – one involved in coordinating and controlling emotional behavior and the other involved in complex cognitions such as planning and problem-solving. When we discuss self-regulation as a focus of treatment it is important that we recognize that we are really discussing a variety of functions that include: emotional activation, attention, appraisal, emotional regulation, behavioral control, and adaptive problem-solving (Ardila, 2013; Jazaieri *et al.*, 2013).

For a number of our clients one of the genuine obstacles to self-regulation is simply being 'out of touch' with their own bodies and sensations. Enhancing accurate interoception from a developmental perspective requires a 'bottom-up' approach where the youth is directed to attend to their own movement, posture, and breath. This goes beyond simply talking about how you stand, walk, balance, and move but actually engaging in and processing somatic and sensory experiences as an aspect of treatment.

The importance of sensory-based, body-based, and experiential learning for the youth we treat cannot be over-stated. First, we know that early trauma experiences can impact left-hemisphere brain development, resulting in language-based learning difficulties (Sylvestre *et al.*, 2018; Teicher and Sampson, 2016). This therefore makes a reliance on 'talking therapy' inconsistent with principles of responsivity that encourage treatment interventions that take into account the learning styles or learning difficulties presented by their clients. Second, developmentally we know that play is central to how children learn and how they acquire a sense of mastery and competency (Russell, 2018) and that the experience of competency is a core element to building resilience (Masten, 2014). Interventions borrowed from sensory-based occupational therapy or utilized in sensorimotor psychotherapy illustrate how important this aspect of treatment is, not only for developing self-regulation but also for understanding how we have somatically incorporated our trauma experiences (Ogden and Fisher, 2015; Champagne, 2008).

Along with improved interoception, our clients and their families are often in need of developing an expanded emotional vocabulary. This allows these youth and their families to appraise and understand their sensory, somatic, and emotional experiences with higher degrees of distinction and clarity. My experience with my clients is that they frequently enter treatment with a very dichotomous way of viewing their experiences and emotions: things are either 'good' or they are 'bad,' they are either 'happy' or 'angry.' Expanding the emotional vocabulary means that feelings like excited, interested, satisfied, calm, and hopeful can now be labeled more accurately. It means that 'anxious' can be experienced and understood as both a 'good' and a 'bad' feeling.

And it means that the feeling of anger might be accurately understood and responded to as disappointed, embarrassed, sad, hurt, or rejected. Being able to recognize and label how we feel is a necessary component to organizing responses that move us toward desired outcomes and goals. Far too often, we are working with youth whose emotional and behavioral dysregulation regularly reinforces and compounds negative responses and places them at greater risk for harming others or being harmed themselves.

Finally, to improve self-regulation we need to assess and enhance executive-functioning skills related to organizing, planning, and implementing adaptive problem-solving. Neurodevelopmental research has identified several factors that appear to be highly influential in adolescent decision-making, including: the importance of peer acceptance, hypersensitivity to rejection, and different responses than either younger children or adults to risk/reward outcomes and responses to threat cues (Dreyfuss *et al.*, 2014; Sebastian, 2015; van Duijvenvoorde *et al.*, 2015). Understanding the individual differences our client's may exhibit based on their developmental stage and past experiences can help us identify specific areas for treatment intervention and more effective approaches to behavior management for parents, schools, and other involved treatment providers.

Practical considerations

For youth engaged in HSB, difficulties in self-regulation often present as the primary consideration in treatment from the perspective of parents, schools, social service agencies, and the juvenile courts. While from a personal safety and community safety frame this makes sense, there is frequently a rush to behavior management approaches that prove ineffective because they do not take into account all of the elements necessary to improve self-regulation (safety, structure, attunement, attachment, interoception, executive functioning) and move instead to a regimen of rewards and punishments, with a strong emphasis on the punishment end, that they hope will motivate better/safer decision-making and behavior.

Creating environments that provide the necessary level of structure and supervision to meet the child's and community's need for safety establishes the context for self-regulation but does not develop or integrate the necessary skills required for increased regulatory abilities. Interventions that address the brain/body processes involved in self-regulation need to be available to the therapist treating HSB and are especially important in the treatment of adolescents. We have already noted the role of sensory-based and body-based treatment interventions but therapists should also consider research-supported interventions such as EMDR, biofeedback, and neurofeedback when addressing trauma-related difficulties in self-regulation (van der Kolk *et al.*, 2016; Johnston *et al.*, 2010)

Re-thinking our understanding of trauma: A new narrative

The final phase of treatment is facilitating a re-formulating of the client's understanding of their trauma experiences integrated with an acknowledgment of the impact that their harmful sexual behavior has had on others. Because of their early, and frequently persistent, adverse experiences the clients we work with often present without a clear narrative of their personal or family history. Instead, we hear fragmented or compartmentalized versions of their past with notable gaps in time frames and understanding. In these instances, traumatic events can become the focal points of their history, blurring any positive relationships or personal strengths. Their traumatic experiences are blocked out and avoided in their narrative are then filled in with often repeated phrases like, 'don't know,' 'can't remember,' 'no clue.' These difficulties in narrative emerge not only as efforts to somehow manage traumatic memories but also because of the impact of trauma on neurodevelopment. A lack of left-hemisphere development and reduced hippocampal volume has been noticed in individuals with early trauma histories (McLaughlin *et al.*, 2019; Teicher and Sampson, 2016; Teicher *et al.*, 2002) with the potential to impact language development, verbal memory, and sequencing. These neurodevelopmental issues can create obstacles to remembering, organizing, and conveying a coherent personal narrative that also serves as the basis to formulating a future narrative of resilience, hopefulness, and growth.

Allowing for the development of a narrative through a variety of modalities (visual images, drawing, music, journaling, raps, poems) allows for different ways to access emotions and memories while also building on the client's preferred style of expression and learning. Focusing on the underlying themes of the narrative rather than specific events allows for the exploration and re-formulation of how traumatic experiences relate to the adolescent's current functioning (Cohen *et al.*, 2012).

An important element in creating a narrative of resilience, competency, and growth for youth engaged in HSB is the recognition of how their own trauma histories are connected to the harm they have caused to others. To move beyond feelings of guilt, shame, embarrassment, and resentment we need to expand the adolescent's view of the consequences of their behavior as not only impacting themselves but also affecting others. Frequently, the motivation for desisting from HSB is framed by and for the adolescent as the avoidance of onerous personal consequences (rejection by family and peers, incarceration, sex offender registration) but this focus suggests a very limited view of the adolescent's motivations and their capacity for broader moral development. An approach to 'accountability' for one's behavior that not only moves beyond self-focus but also promotes competence, development, and desistence can be found in restorative justice practices (Dillard *et al.*, 2019; Ward *et al.*, 2015; Mercer and Sten Madsen, 2011). The utilization of restorative justice practices accentuates that the goal of treatment is not just desistence or the 'avoidance of bad' but the empowerment of the youth and their families to move beyond the experience of trauma to a place of personal agency, competence, and emotional, physical, and spiritual health.

Practical considerations

Helping these young people to organize and structure a narrative can sometimes be facilitated using explicit organizing tools or narrative templates that are already available to them. During the course of treatment, I will take material from different exercises or interventions and keep them in a scrapbook. These might include collages, drawings, poems, raps, song lyrics, family photos and other materials generated during sessions. At different intervals, we will take the different pages of the scrapbook out and sequence them in a manner that allows for a more coherent narrative or a reformulation of the youth's current understanding and assumptions. This process of physically 'controlling' the narrative of one's life has proven very powerful for some clients.

Another approach has been to take narratives that the youth is already familiar with through movies or books and use those as a means for understanding the impact of trauma and the pathways to resilience. I have found that for many youths, these stories have frequently involved 'superheroes', with Batman and Spiderman frequently appearing in these narratives and providing a metaphor for not only discussing trauma but also framing the development of one's own superpowers as an important element of treatment.

Conclusion

Youth who engage in harmful or problematic sexual behaviors are a heterogenous group frequently presenting with family histories and personal experiences that are full of adversity, complexity, and obstacles. There is no one treatment approach or set of treatment interventions that will meet the needs of all these clients. Instead, we need to remain open to new ways of understanding the impact of trauma and the variety of ways that this impact can be manifested in the clients that come to us. If we work from an understanding that the relationship in therapy is ultimately the 'engine that drives the train,' this puts us in the best place to be helpful to these young people and the communities in which they live.

KNOWLEDGE AND PRACTICE REFLECTION

Janise Mitchell, Joe Tucci, Ed Tronick and Stephen W. Porges

Kevin Creeden's chapter showcases the importance of applying trauma knowledge for children and young people who have engaged in harmful sexual behaviour because it maintains a focus on the background experiences and needs of these children. Way too often, they are cast as perpetrators of sexual abuse, equating them with the same motivations and capabilities as adult predators. In this context, their vulnerabilities are pushed into the background, and their behaviour, which is significant in its impact, is emphasized. They can be ostracized quickly. They carry with them the apprehension that those important to them hold as a result of the sexual behaviour being exposed. They are excluded almost immediately from congregate settings such as school and sport because they are deemed to pose too much of a risk to others. The underlying needs which drive these behaviours are overlooked and can be minimized altogether. They feel the harsh criticism of their peers. They lose support from people who they need the most at the very time that such support is critical.

Retaining a focus on the lived experience of trauma of these children and young people enables practitioners, systems and communities to recognize the very strong association between the abuse and disadvantage that these children have suffered, and its expression in the behaviour they engage in.

Creeden shows how compassion, openness and curiosity about the children and young people themselves, their unique circumstances and their individual life stories offer them the resources through which they can separate a little from the intensity of the shame that debilitates them even further. In doing so, there is the hope that the young person will change their behaviour not only to avoid punishment, but also because they begin to engage in relationships in novel ways that are respectful of others, building their own agency and commitment to behaviour that is more fulfilling and prosocial.

> Frequently, the motivation for desisting from HSB is framed by and for the adolescent as the avoidance of onerous personal consequences (rejection by family and peers, incarceration, sex offender registration) but this focus suggests a very limited view of the adolescent's motivations and their capacity for broader moral development. An approach to 'accountability' for one's behavior that not only moves beyond self-focus but also promotes competence, development, and desistence can be found in restorative justice practices... The utilization of restorative justice practices accentuates that the goal of treatment is not just desistence or the 'avoidance of bad' but the empowerment of the youth and their families to move beyond the

experience of trauma to a place of personal agency, competence, and emotional, physical, and spiritual health…

A deeper analysis of the text highlights that the way in which Creeden is operationalizing trauma-informed practice or care in ways that, while continuing to use the terminology of trauma-informed approaches, we consider him to have usefully evolved its conceptualization beyond its original definitional boundaries.

Like Kestly, in her earlier chapter, who used trauma integrative as her preferred construct, the fact that Creeden must add the use of *developmental* to bolster the meaning of *trauma informed* in this context acknowledges the fraying edges of the construct of *trauma informed* as the basis on which practice and organizational change can be supported. For example, in the early part of the chapter, he sets out clearly the need for a trauma-informed developmental approach to treating HSB which goes beyond the notion of traditional one-to-one treatment and is inclusive of the relational and physical environments as contributing to the therapeutic effort:

> …seeks to identify the ways in which adverse experiences interfered with or disrupted these foundational skills (e.g. attunement, attachment, self-regulation, attention, working memory) and how these experiences precipitated, shaped, or motivated the child or adolescent's engagement in HSB. This perspective also encourages us to identify the individual strengths and resources available to support resiliency and growth because the goal of a developmentally focused approach is not only to eliminate harmful or problematic behaviour, but also to promote and facilitate:

- the presence of stable and supportive family relationships
- a stable and safe living environment
- the youth's ability for self-regulation,
- the ability to engage in adaptive, prosocial problem solving
- the development of academic and/or vocational competence
- the capacity to make and sustain positive prosocial relationships
- the capacity for intimacy and an understanding of healthy sexuality.

As such, he argues for the need to:

> …shift the focus of our interventions from solely addressing the difficulties reflected by the symptoms and behaviour of the child, to creating safer environments where reliable adults support and guide the child to develop a range of adaptive responses that are consistent with a world that poses less threatening environmental demands.

Trauma informed is certainly a helpful orientation. It offers a variety of ideas that a practitioner can consider as goals for the work they undertake to support children and young people who engage in harmful sexual behaviour. It certainly serves to remove excessively punitive elements which would characterize intervention if it were to be based solely on accountability and rehabilitation of the young person as *a sex offender*. It also looks to the future. It orients the practitioner to building the capabilities of the young person, using their strengths as the starting point.

However, the use of *trauma informed* in this chapter is not the same as it is used by Harris and Fallot (2001) or SAMSHA (2014). In Creeden's text, it is used as the vehicle through which trauma knowledge is integrated with practice wisdom to create an approach to intervention. And in so doing, the use of trauma informed goes well beyond having an awareness of the impact of trauma as advocated by current conceptualizations of *trauma-informed practice or care*.

Trauma-informed care needs to blend together with a range of other frames to deliver a wider amalgam of ideas, strategies and modalities. On its own, it is not enough. When trauma knowledge and other knowledge domains are integrated, they become part of an intentionally put together constellation of principles that make most sense for the context and the overarching goals of the support. Creeden highlights how successful and essential this analysis is for children, young people and their families with whom he works.

Of course, many of the chapters in this book find themselves dealing with these language and conceptual conundrums. These same issues are present in other literature. These themes will be explored in more detail in the final chapter.

However, it supports the need for a stronger and clearer frame of reference that can be used to hold together all of the different terms such as trauma sensitive, trauma aware, trauma informed, trauma specific and others, within a change arc whose descriptor signifies more effectively its fundamental purpose. As Tucci and Mitchell have argued previously (2019), it is the move to *trauma transformative* that may hold the most potential to achieve the original intent of the *trauma-informed movement*.

References
References for chapter

Allen, J.G. (2001). *Traumatic Relationships and Serious Mental Disorders*. New York, NY: Wiley and Sons.

Anda, R.F., Felitti, V.J., Bremner, J.D., Walker, J.D. *et al.* (2006). The enduring effects of abuse and related adverse experiences in childhood: A convergence of evidence from neurobiology and epidemiology. *European Archives of Psychiatry and Clinical Neuroscience*, 256, 174–186.

Ardila, A. (2013). Development of metacognitive and emotional executive functions in children. *Applied Neuropsychology of Children*, 2(2), 82–87.

Bales, K. and Carter, C.S. (2009). Neuroendocrine Mechanisms of Social Bonds and Child-Parent Attachment, from the Child's Perspective. In M. DeHann and M. Gunnar (eds), *Handbook of Developmental Social Neuroscience* (pp.246–264). New York, NY: Guilford Press.

Baglivio, M.T. and Epps, N. (2015). The interrelatedness of adverse childhood experiences among high-risk juvenile offenders. *Youth Violence and Juvenile Justice*, 14(3), 1–20.

Bergman, J. and Creeden, K. (2011). Attachment is a Verb. In C. Haen (ed.), *Engaging Boys in Treatment: Creative Approaches to the Therapy Process* (pp.241–264). New York, NY: Routledge.

Berkman, E.T. (2016). Self-Regulation Training. In K.D. Vohs and R.F. Baumeister (eds), *Handbook of Self-Regulation: Research, Theory and Applications* (third edition). New York, NY: Guilford Press.

Bloom, S. (2013). *Creating Sanctuary: Toward the Evolution of Sane Societies*. New York, NY: Routledge.

Bowlby, J. (1973). *Attachment and Loss. Vol. 2: Separation: Anxiety and Anger*. New York, NY: Basic Books.

Bowlby, J. (1982). *Attachment and Loss. Vol. 1: Attachment* (second edition). New York, NY: Basic Books.

Briere, J. and Scott, C. (2006). *Principles of Trauma Therapy*. Thousand Oaks, CA: Sage Publications.

Center on the Developing Child at Harvard University (2012). *The Science of Neglect: The Persistent Absence of Responsive Care Disrupts the Developing Brain: Working Paper No. 12*. Retrieved from www.developingchild.harvard.edu.

Champagne, T. (2008). *Sensory Modulation and Environment: Essential Elements of Occupation* (third edition). Southampton, MA: Champagne Conferences and Consultation.

Chen, Y. and Baram, T.Z. (2016). Toward understanding how early-life stress reprograms cognitive and emotional brain networks. *Neuropsychopharmacology*, 41, 197–206.

Chouinard-Thivierge, S., Lussier, P. and Daignault, I.V. (2022). A longitudinal examination of developmental covariates of sexual behavior problems among youth referred to child protection services. *Sexual Abuse*, 34(5), 537–567.

Cicchetti, D. (2016). Socioemotional, personality, and biological development: Illustrations from a multilevel developmental psychopathology perspective on child maltreatment. *Annual Review of Psychology*, 67(1), 187–211.

Cohen, J., Mandarina, A. and Dellinger, E. (2006). *Treating Trauma and Traumatic Grief in Children and Adolescents*. New York, NY: Guilford Press.

Cohodes, E., Kitt, E., Baskin-Sommers, A. and Gee, D. (2020). Influences of early-life stress on frontolimbic circuitry: Harnessing a dimensional approach to elucidate the effects of heterogeneity in stress exposure. *Developmental Psychology*, 1–20.

Cook, A., Spinazzola, J., Ford, J., Lanktree, C. *et al.* (2005). Complex trauma in children and adolescents. *Psychiatric Annals*.

Creeden, K. (2004). The neurodevelopmental impact of early trauma and insecure attachment: Rethinking our understanding and treatment of sexual behaviour problems. *Sexual Addiction and Compulsivity*, 11(4), 223–247.

Creeden, K. (2017). How Neuroscience Can Inform Our Understanding of Sexually Harmful Behaviour by Youth. In B. Schwartz (ed.), *Handbook on Youth Who Engage in Sexually Abusive Behaviour*. Kingston, NJ: Civic Research Institute.

Creeden, K. (2020). Trauma and Young People Who Display Sexually Harmful Behaviour. In H. Swaby, B. Winder, R. Lievesley, K. Hocken and N. Blagden (eds), *Sexual Crime and Trauma* (pp.85–112). London: Palgrave.

Crittenden, P.M. (1997). Toward an Integrative Theory of Trauma: A Dynamic Maturation Approach. In D. Cicchetti and S. Toth (eds), *Rochester Symposium on Developmental Psychopathology* (Vol. 8, pp.33–84). Rochester, NY: University of Rochester Press.

Deater-Deckard, K. and Mullineaux, P.Y. (2010). Cognition and Emotion: A Behavioural Genetic Perspective. In S.D. Calkins and M.A. Bell (eds), *Child Development at the*

Intersection of Emotion and Cognition (pp.133–152). Washington, DC: American Psychological Association.

De Bellis, M.D., Woolley, D.P. and Hooper, S.R. (2013). Neuropsychological findings in pediatric maltreatment: Relationship of PTSD, dissociative symptoms, and abuse/neglect indices to neurocognitive outcomes. *Child Maltreatment*, 18(3), 171–183.

DeGregorio, L.J. (2013). Intergenerational transmission of abuse: Implications for parenting interventions from a neuropsychological perspective. *Traumatology*, 19(2), 158–166.

Dillard, R. and Beaujolais, B. (2019). Trauma and adolescents who engage in sexually abusive behaviour: A review of the literature. *Journal of Child Sexual Abuse*, 28(6), 629–648.

Dillard, R., Newman, T. and Kim, M. (2019). Promoting youth competence through balanced and restorative justice: A community-based PYD approach. *Journal of Youth Development*, 14(4), 14–35.

Dong, M., Anda, R.F., Felitti, V.J., Dube, S.R. *et al.* (2004). The interrelatedness of multiple forms of childhood abuse, neglect, and household dysfunction. *Child Abuse and Neglect*, 28(7), 771–784.

Dreyfuss, M., Caudle, K., Drysdale, A.T., Johnston, N.E. *et al.* (2014). Teens impulsively react rather than retreat from threat. *Developmental Neuroscience*, 36(3–4), 220–227.

Elkovitch, N., Latzman, R.D., Hansen, D.J. and Flood, M.F. (2009). Understanding child sexual behaviour problems: A developmental psychopathology framework. *Clinical Psychology Review*, 29(7), 586–598.

Felitti, V.J., Anda, R.F., Nordenberg, D., Williamson, D.F. *et al.* (1998). Relationship of childhood abuse and household dysfunction to many of the leading causes of death in adults: The Adverse Childhood Experiences (ACE) Study. *American Journal of Preventive Medicine*, 14(4), 245–258.

Fogel, A. and Garvey, A. (2007). Alive communication. *Infant Behavioural Development*, 30(2), 251–257.

Gross, J.J. and Thompson, R.A. (2007). Emotion Regulation: Conceptual Foundations. In J.J. Gross (ed.), *Handbook of Emotion Regulation* (pp.3–17). New York, NY: Guilford Press.

Harms, M.B., Shannon Bowen, K.E., Hanson, J.L. and Pollak, S.D. (2018). Instrumental learning and cognitive flexibility processes are impaired in children exposed to early life stress. *Developmental Science*, 21(4), Article e12596.

Harris, M. and Fallot, R. (2001). *Using Trauma Theory to Design Service Systems*. San Francisco, CA: Jossey-Bass/Wiley.

Hart, H. and Rubia, K. (2012). Neuroimaging of child abuse: A critical review. *Frontiers in Human Neuroscience*, 6, 52.

Hart, S. (2011). *The Impact of Attachment*. New York, NY: Norton Press.

Hopper, E., Bassuk, E. and Olivet, J. (2009). Shelter from the storm: Trauma-informed care in homelessness services. *The Open Health Services and Policy Journal*, 2, 133.

Hostinar, C.E. and Gunnar, M.R. (2013). The developmental effects of early life stress. *Current Directions in Psychological Science*, 22, 400–406.

Jazaieri, H., Urry, H. and Gross, J. (2013). Affective disturbance and psychopathology: An emotion regulation perspective. *Journal of Experimental Psychopathology*, 4(5), 1–16.

Johnston, S., Boehm, S., Healy, D., Goebel, R. and Linden, D. (2010). Neurofeedback: A promising tool for the self-regulation of emotion networks. *NeuroImage*, 49, 1066–1072.

Joyal, C.C., Tardif, M. and Spearson-Goulet, J.A. (2018). Executive functions and social cognition in juveniles who have sexually offended. *Sexual Abuse: Journal of Research and Treatment*, 32, 2.

Karoly, P. (1993). Mechanisms of self-regulation: A systems view. *Annual Review of Psychology*, 44, 23–52.

Kim, J. and Cicchetti, D. (2010). Longitudinal pathways linking child maltreatment, emotion regulation, peer relations, and psychopathology. *Journal of Child Psychiatry and Psychology*, 51(6), 706–716.

Levenson, J., Willis, G. and Prescott, D. (2017). *Trauma-Informed Care: Transforming Treatment for People who have Sexually Offended*. Brandon, VT: Safer Society Press.

Levenson, J., Willis, G. and Prescott, D. (2020). Evidence Based Practice and the Role of Trauma-Informed Care in Sex Offending Treatment. In H. Swaby, B. Winder, R. Lievesley,

K. Hocken, N. Blagden, and P. Banyard (eds), *Sexual Crime and Trauma* (pp.197–224). London: Palgrave.

Lussier, P. and Chouinard-Thivierge, S. (2017). A Developmental Life Course View of Juvenile Sex Offending. In W.D. Murphy and S. Righthand (eds), *The Safer Society Handbook of Assessment and Treatment of Adolescents Who Have Sexually Abused* (pp.77–106). Brandon, VT: Safer Society Press.

Marshall, W.L. and Barbaree, H.E. (1990). An Integrated Theory of the Etiology of Sexual Offending. In W.L. Marshall, D.R. Laws and H.E. Barbaree (eds), *Handbook of Sexual Assault* (pp.257–275). New York, NY: Springer.

Marshall, W.L. and Marshall, L.E. (2000). The origins of sexual offending. *Trauma, Violence, and Abuse: A Review Journal*, 1, 250–263.

McEwen, B.S. (2012). Brain on stress: How the social environment gets under the skin. *Proceedings of the National Academy of Sciences*, 109 (Suppl. 2), 17180–17185.

McLaughlin, K.A. and Lambert, H.K. (2017). Child trauma exposure and psychopathology: Mechanisms of risk and resilience. *Current Opinion in Psychology*, 14, 29–34.

McLaughlin, K.A., Weissman, D. and Bitrán, D. (2019). Childhood adversity and neural development: A systematic review. *Annual Review of Developmental Psychology*, 1, 277–312.

Mercer, V. and Sten Madsen, K. (2011). *Doing Restorative Justice in Cases of Sexual Violence: A Practice Guide*. The International Journal for Restorative Justice View Project. Leuven Institute of Criminology.

Masten, A.S. (2014). Global perspectives on resilience in children and youth. *Child Development*, 85(1), 6–20.

Ogden, P. and Fisher, J. (2015). *Sensorimotor Psychotherapy: Interventions for Trauma and Attachment*. New York, NY: W.W. Norton.

Opendak, M. and Sullivan, R.M. (2016). Unique neurobiology during the sensitive period for attachment produces distinctive infant trauma processing. *European Journal of Psychotraumatology*, 7(1), 31276.

Pechtel, P., Lyons-Ruth, K., Anderson, C. and Teicher, M.H. (2014). Sensitive periods of amygdala development: The role of maltreatment in preadolescence. *NeuroImage*, 97, 236–244.

Perkins, S.C., Smith-Darden, J., Ametrano, R.M. and Graham-Bermann, S. (2014). Typologies of violence exposure and cognitive processing in incarcerated male adolescents. *Journal of Family Violence*, 29(4), 439–451.

Perry, B.D. (2009). Examining child maltreatment through a neurodevelopmental lens: Clinical application of the Neurosequential Model of Therapeutics. *Journal of Loss and Trauma*, 14, 240–255.

Porges, S. (2011). *The Polyvagal Theory: Neurological Foundations of Emotion, Attachment, Communication, and Self-Regulation*. New York, NY: W.W. Norton and Company.

Porges SW (2015). Making the world safe for our children: Down-regulating defence and up-regulating social engagement to 'optimise' the human experience. *Children Australia*, 40, 114–123.

Russell, W. (2018). Thinking a Little Differently about Resilience and Play. In W. Russell and K. Schuur (eds), *The Strength of European Diversity for Building Children's Resilience through Play and Drama: A collection of articles from the EU Erasmus Plus ARTPAD project 2015–2018*. Gloucester: University of Gloucestershire.

Sachser, N., Dürschlag, M. and Hirzel, D. (1998). Social relationships and the management of stress. *Psychoneuroendocrinology*, 23(8), 891–904.

Saxe, G., Ellis, B.H. and Kaplow, J. (2007). *Collaborative Treatment of Traumatised Children and Teens: The Trauma Systems Therapy Approach*. New York, NY: Guilford Press.

Schore, A. (2001). The effects of early relational trauma on right brain development, affect regulation, and infant mental health. *Infant Mental Health Journal*, 22, 201–269.

Schore, A.N. (2003). *Affect Dysregulation and Disorders of the Self*. New York, NY: W.W. Norton and Company.

Sebastian, C.L. (2015). Social cognition in adolescence: Social rejection and theory of mind. *Psicología Educativa*, 21(2), 125–131.

Seigel, D. (1999). *The Developing Mind: Toward a Neurobiology of Interpersonal Experience.* New York, NY: Guilford Press.

Shackman, J.E. and Pollak, S.D. (2014). Impact of physical maltreatment on the regulation of negative affect and aggression. *Development and Psychopathology*, 26(4pt1), 1021–1033.

Smallbone, S. (2006). Social and psychological factors in the development of delinquency and sexual deviance. In H.E. Barbaree and W.L. Marshall (eds), *The Juvenile Sex Offender* (pp.105–127). New York, NY: Guilford Press.

Smith, K.E. and Pollak, S.D. (2020). Rethinking concepts and categories for understanding the neurodevelopmental effects of childhood adversity. *Perspectives on Psychological Science*, 16(1), 67–93.

Snow, P.C. (2009). Child maltreatment, mental health and oral language competence: Inviting speech-language pathology to the prevention table. *International Journal of Speech-Language Pathology*, 11(2), 95–103.

St. Amand, A., Bard, D. and Silovsky, J. (2008). Meta-analysis of treatment for child sexual behaviour problems: Practice elements and outcomes. *Child Maltreatment*, 13(2), 145–166.

Sroufe, L.A. (2000). Early relationships and the development of children. *Infant Mental Health Journal*, 21(2), 67–74.

Stinson, J.D. and Becker, J.V. (2013). Pedophilia: A Case Study in Empirically Supported Treatment. In W. O'Donohue and S.O. Lilienfeld (eds), *Case Studies in Clinical Psychological Science: Bridging the Gap from Science to Practice* (pp.425–456). New York, NY: Oxford University Press.

Sylvestre, A., Bussières, È.L. and Bouchard, C. (2016). Language problems among abused and neglected children. *Child Maltreatment*, 21(1), 47–5.

Tedeschi, R.G. and Moore, B.A. (2021). Posttraumatic growth as an integrative therapeutic philosophy. *Journal of Psychotherapy Integration*, 31(2), 180–194.

Teicher, M., Andersen, S., Polcari, A., Andersen, C. and Navalta, C. (2002). Developmental neurobiology of childhood stress and trauma. *Psychiatric Clinics of North America*, 25, 397–426.

Teicher, M.H. and Parigger, A. (2015). The 'Maltreatment and Abuse Chronology of Exposure' (MACE) Scale for the retrospective assessment of abuse and neglect during development. *PLoS ONE*, 10(2), e0117423.

Teicher, M.H. and Samson, J.A. (2016). Annual Research Review: Enduring neurobiological effects of childhood abuse and neglect. *Journal of Child Psychology and Psychiatry and Allied Disciplines*, 57(3), 241–266.

Thompson, R.A., Virmani, E., Waters, S.F., Meyer, S. and Raikes, A. (2013). The Development of Emotion Self-Regulation: The Whole and the Sum of the Parts. In K. Barrett, N.A. Fox, G.A. Morgan, D.J. Fidler and L.A. Daunhauer (eds), *Handbook of Self-Regulatory Processes in Development* (pp.5–26). New York, NY: Taylor and Francis.

Vrtička, P. and Vuilleumier, P. (2012). Neuroscience of human social interactions and adult attachment style. *Frontiers in Human Neuroscience*, 6. doi.org/10.3389/fnhum.2012.00212.

van der Kolk, B.A. (2005). Developmental trauma disorder: Toward a rational diagnosis for children with complex trauma histories. *Psychiatric Annals*, 35, 401–408.

van der Kolk, B.A., Hodgdon, H., Gapen, M., Musicaro, R., Suvak, M. and Hamlin E. (2016). A randomised controlled study of neurofeedback for chronic PTSD. *PLoS ONE*, 11(12), e0166752.

van Duijvenvoorde, A.C.K., Huizenga, H.M., Somerville, L.H., Delgado, M.R. *et al.* (2015). Neural correlates of expected risks and returns in risky choice across development. *The Journal of Neuroscience: The Official Journal of the Society for Neuroscience*, 35(4), 1549–1560.

Ward, T., Gannon, T. and Fortune, C.A. (2015). Restorative justice-informed moral acquaintance: Resolving the dual role problem in correctional and forensic practice. *Criminal Justice and Behaviour*, 42(1), 45–57.

Worley, K., Church, J. and Clemmons, J. (2012). Parents of adolescents who have committed sexual offenses: Characteristics, challenges, and interventions. *Clinical Child Psychology and Psychiatry*, 17(3), 433–448.

References for Knowledge and Practice Reflection

Harris, M. and Fallot, R.D. (2001). Envisioning a Trauma-Informed Service System: A Vital Paradigm Shift. In M. Harris, and R.D. Fallot (eds), *Using Trauma Theory to Design Service Systems* (pp.3–22). San Francisco, CA: Jossey-Bass/Wiley.

Substance Abuse and Mental Health Services Administration (SAMHSA) (2014). *Trauma-informed Care in Behavioural Health Services – Treatment Improvement Protocol (TIP) Series 57* (HHS Publication no. (SMA) 13-4801).

Tucci, J. and Mitchell, J. (2019). Therapeutic Services for Traumatised Children and Young People Healing. In R. Benjamin, J. Haliburn and S. King (eds), *Humanising Mental Health Care in Australia: A Guide to Trauma-Informed Approaches* (pp.319–320). London: Routledge.

CHAPTER 15

A Resilience Roadmap Model Combining Somatic Experiencing, Secure Attachment, and Embodied Mindfulness Principles for Systemic Change in Schools and Community Mental Health

Maggie Kline

Introduction

In my early life as a teacher, counselor, and school psychologist working in diverse and poverty-stricken neighborhoods of Long Beach, California, I observed far too many students in strife. Some were hyperactive or angry, others depressed, others aggressive and/or underachieving and unfocused. Still others were returning from juvenile jail for convictions of assault with a deadly weapon, substance abuse, selling drugs, and theft. Despite becoming a marriage and family psychotherapist in private practice, trauma specialist, and Somatic Experiencing® faculty member, I never lost my desire to be a change-maker for schools. By offering practical ideas for adults to help children in the classroom, my intention is to also give stressed-out teachers tools to replace their exhaustive attempts to 'manage' the increasing numbers of youngsters with academic, behavioral, and social issues. The vast majority of mental health workers (within and outside school) have had zero training in transforming trauma. At best, they do recognize and empathize with suffering students. Of those who have attended 'trauma-sensitive' workshops, it is rare to find knowledgeable professionals addressing the physiological root cause of traumatic re-enactment or implementing classroom activities or a school-wide program that makes social-emotional health as important a priority as academic achievement.

Out of a wish to start a movement within schools to ensure that all children (with or without trauma histories) have both a resilient sense of self and a sense of belonging as a valued community member, my Resilience

Roadmap Model was born. The first step is in helping school staff and community agencies to understand how trauma affects the brain and the body. Next is to share the concrete dual-path laid out in the Resilience Roadmap. One path builds resilience through daily development of internal resources by teaching kids (and their adults) about their brains and bodies, with guided practice in tracking their own arousal/settling cycles. This builds interoceptive intelligence using basics skills from Somatic Experiencing®. Embodied meditation practices also build sensation awareness of the body/brain connection. The other path is through external resources provided by adults using the 'Eight Essentials of Healthy Attachment' to repair relationship deficits suffered during the formative years. The nurturing attitudes and activities create an environment in which children can feel safe, nurtured, secure, and valued, and develop pleasurable relationships. The eight essentials tone the ventral vagal branch of the autonomic nervous system necessary for both co- and self-regulation. These lay the foundation for emotional health and increase the protective factors associated with addiction prevention.

What is trauma?

While the magnitude of an event such as abuse, abandonment, accident, medical procedure, natural or man-made catastrophe is an important factor, it does not define trauma. Dr. Peter Levine, originator of Somatic Experiencing®, teaches that trauma resides not in the event itself, but rather in its effect on the nervous system. Infants and children, therefore, are the most vulnerable as their brains and bodies are still developing, and their ability to defend themselves is limited to crying out followed by shutting down. Whether witnessing an egregious act, such as an assault or a catastrophic event, like an accident, fire or flood or directly experiencing an attack or the urgency to quickly evacuate, the shock is primarily physiological rather than psychological (Levine 1997). This is, of course, in contrast to ongoing familial neglect and abuse and/or intergenerational trauma from societal marginalization. Trauma from being chronically bullied or denied opportunities due to race, religion, ethnicity, socio-economic status, or suffering discriminatory bias due to gender, neurodivergence, or a disability (or in whatever way) impedes belonging and opportunities, and requires systemic change. Being abused or scapegoated within one's family, school, or community creates cumulative chronic stress, which deeply affects children psychologically, as well, as causing physiological problems. These interfere with sleep, digestion, respiration, and immune functions exacerbating their mental health issues. It is, therefore, imperative to go beyond cognitive-emotional and behavioral paradigms to bring forth a universal understanding of how to help children, teens, and their parents and teachers reset physiology that has been distorted by either shock trauma, accumulated toxic stress, or both.

The impact of trauma on the body

When a child senses danger, whether real or perceived, an alarm is set off by the amygdala in the midbrain, bypassing the prefrontal cortex. The threat response activates an extraordinary amount of energy to prepare for spontaneous self-defense, even when impossible. Infants and children are the most impacted as they are exquisitely sensitive beings who absorb overwhelming sights, sounds, smells, tastes, and touch like a sponge. Quick responses are orchestrated by the oldest and deepest structures of the brain for the sole purpose of survival. Physiological responses are instinctual, even in the very young who are unable to defend themselves. Yet, when danger is perceived, the threat response automatically mobilizes energy to escape just as it does in older children, adolescents, and adults. Along with a pounding heart, more than 20 other physiological responses are unleased in preparation for protective movements. These rapid involuntary shifts include physical dynamics, for example, the redirection of blood flow (away from the digestive and skin organs and into the large motor muscles of flight) along with rapid respiration and a decrease in the normal output of saliva. These prepare the body to defend itself by fighting, running, jumping, hiding, or some other means of escape. The key to avoid being traumatized is to 'use up' (slowly and consciously) the excess energy evoked for self-protection. This resets the autonomic nervous system to a state of alert relaxation afterwards.

Alternatively, muscles may collapse as the body shuts down and goes into an altered state of consciousness. This protects us from pain when we cannot defend ourselves, making kids the most vulnerable to freeze and dissociated states. This is good news for emergencies. But bad news when the emergency is over but the threat response cycle continues. The release of endorphins with resulting dissociation is meant to be temporary, as it is with mammals who live in the wild. Unfortunately, too often, shutting down and spacing out become the brain/body default mechanism for youngsters who are living with unresolved trauma.

When the energy is not fully released, it remains as a preset, implicit (unconscious body) memory that can be easily triggered. In this way, a lethargic, depressed student can be sitting quietly one minute, and suddenly lunge into a defensive reaction the next. A simple, innocent gesture, word, glance, or touch that hints of danger (real or not) sets off the same cascade of physiological reactions. What can be done to interrupt trauma-induced reactivity and replace it with self-awareness of the body/brain connection? And, how can this knowledge, so easy to do in a one-on-one situation, be adapted for classrooms and agencies so all students can become more conscious? Daniel Goleman (1995) brought the concept of *emotional intelligence* into public popularity. But cognitive/emotional approaches by themselves fall short with trauma. There is a need for experiencing *interoceptive intelligence* (awareness of physical sensations) to release toxic stress and reset the autonomic nervous system; thus, alleviating trauma symptoms. It also answers the question of how to simplify practices so they become part of school and community agency policy.

The Resilience Roadmap Model has two pathways:

- Develops internal resources: Teaching kids (and their adults) about their brain/body connection with guided practice in tracking their own arousal/settling cycles. This builds *interoceptive intelligence* (or sensation awareness) and a resilient autonomic nervous system that responds appropriately.
- Provides external resources: Rectifying relationship deficits through nurturance using the 'Eight Essentials of Healthy Attachment.' These tone the ventral vagal branch of the autonomic nervous system necessary for both co- and self-regulation and are the foundation for physiological and emotional regulation.

Putting the puzzle together: The evolution of the Resilience Roadmap Model

As a school psychologist and a family therapist in private practice, I began adapting art, movement, and play to reflect the skills I had learned from Dr. Peter A. Levine's Somatic Experiencing® (SE), a cutting-edge psychobiological approach to healing trauma. In particular, I applied the concepts of safety and containment, along with sensation awareness, tracking physiological and sensory-motor changes, releasing frozen survival responses, and restoring healthy self-protective mechanisms. All this needs to happen in a delicately titrated way to avoid inadvertently unleashing destructive aggression or disabling anxiety in the process. The idea is to release a flow of warmth and vital energy to restore equilibrium, confidence, and wholeness. SE skills are often sufficient to empower kids to rebound after a terrifying incident. Interoceptive intelligence, or sensation awareness, and the ability to track sensations from heightened arousal to calming and settling is the first of the two-fold Resilience Roadmap. It has proven time and again to be a magical antidote, despite the magnitude of the event(s). But this is if, and only if, the youngster had formed a secure attachment.

Unfortunately, not all youngsters have the 'attachment advantage' for a myriad of reasons. Those with the most challenging symptoms and behaviors at school, home, and in therapy, typically had traumatic interruptions during the vulnerable years from pre-natal to age five. Dr. Stephen Porges teaches that the process of myelination (or insulation) of a branch of the nervous system known as the ventral vagal complex develops within the safety and co-regulation of a secure caregiver(s). This stage with a regulated parent is critically important in making it possible for young children to eventually self-soothe, cooperate, make friends, have empathy, and regulate their emotions. Healthy function or 'tone' of the ventral vagus nerve puts us in touch with what makes us feel fully human; namely, to feel calm, grounded, present, joyful, and connected, rather than stuck in a traumatic past. When there are too many ACEs (adverse childhood experiences) and/ or too much unrepaired medical, surgical, or birth trauma during this delicate period, without early interventions, complex trauma will likely result. The second pathway in my two-fold model can be adopted by school staff to provide nurturance and ameliorate the deficits children with an insecure attachment have suffered.

The first pathway of the Resilience Roadmap – developing interoceptive intelligence to calm the threat response and reset the autonomic nervous system and body/brain connection

The first pathway to resilience is teaching kids the magic of their own *interoceptive intelligence* (sensation awareness) to downregulate overactive survival brain circuitry. This body wisdom is accomplished through SE skills using art activities, often together with organic movements inspired by the child's own drawings. These address the widespread issues traumatized children suffer: nightmares, anxiety, fear of being alone, inability to express distress in words, anger, depression, the inability to relax, and somatic symptoms like head and stomach aches. The activities in this chapter incorporate the SE skills of:

- creating safety
- tracking sensations
- using artwork as image in the SE SIBAM model (see below)
- pendulation between comfortable and uncomfortable images, sensations and/or emotions
- releasing activation
- integration of the triune brain and body.

Part 1 of the Resilience Roadmap promotes self-awareness. It answers the questions, 'Where do my anxiety, love, anger, or safety live inside me?' and 'How do I know that I know what I feel, need, and want?' Why is it important to guide youngsters to develop internal awareness of the various nuances of the peaks and valleys of their sensations? One reason is that traumatic and stressful events overwhelm the capacity to cope. Thwarted fight/flight/ freeze mechanisms are released via our sensory-motor and autonomic nervous systems. Moving into present time to leave past traumatic patterns behind is a physiological process. Completing incomplete, involuntary threat cycle responses happens within the oldest, deepest brain structures responsible for survival. Mastering the ability to notice and befriend physical sensations stemming from these subcortical instinctual circuits returns the brain and body to equilibrium. Rather than a temporary fix through coping mechanisms like 'reframing' or 'taking a deep breath,' the ability to sense and redirect arising nervous system activation transforms trauma into triumph through new experiences of feeling empowered, embodied, and connected.

To understand trauma-responsive strategies, it's important to understand the different functions and languages of our triune brain. Unlike the neocortex that communicates with words or the midbrain that feels emotions, the primitive brainstem and cerebellum, hardwired for survival, do not understand words. Their language is the language of sensations. And, it is through this awareness that we relieve stress, release traumatic activation, and develop a sense of self.

Table 15.1: The triune brain speaks three distinct languages

Neocortex or thinking brain	Speaks with words
Midbrain or mammalian brain	Speaks with emotional feelings
Instinctual/Survival brain	Speaks with physiological sensations

An excerpt from Brain-Changing Strategies to Trauma-Proof Our Schools (Kline, 2020)

Learning to name and navigate this inner landscape creates homoeostasis, which regulates our moods and emotions. It also improves physical well-being, such as our immune, cardiovascular, and respiratory health. Interoceptive intelligence (sensation awareness) can be learned in the classroom through guided practice. Teachers and other school staff can engage students in making sensation vocabulary lists and posters. They can be taught that thoughts come from the neocortex, while emotional feelings arise from our body and the limbic circuits in the midbrain. Interoception is the awareness of the sensations or physical feelings that arise quickly from the lower brain circuits wired instinctually to keep us alive. Interoceptive intelligence is developed through repeated practice of noticing physical sensations and how they change over time. Humans are familiar with the ups and downs of emotions – irritation, joy, dread, sadness, calm, annoyance, curiosity, disappointment, elation, relaxation, angst, pride, shame, surprise, grief, rage, terror, triumph, gratitude, grumpiness, elation, disgust, excitement, and helplessness to happiness, love, and affection. The list goes on. Yet, it is the rare few who make it a practice to go inward, awakening body consciousness by noticing the current of physical sensations running just beneath those waves of human emotion. And this is pivotal in trauma recovery.

With guidance, kids (and their adults) become self-observers of their sensations. Feeling, labeling, and locating sensations is key in breaking loose from habitual reactive patterns from past hurt. They can be taught to track the activation of their own threat arousal cycle and follow it as it deactivates, leaving them settled. This can be accomplished with simple grounding exercises and active games by 'taking a pause' that allows time for everyone to 'check-in' long enough to notice their present state of being. Learning a sensation vocabulary is important for everyone. Having interoceptive intelligence is a lifelong competency that can minimize the accumulation of stress, increase resiliency when traumatic events happen, and prevent long-term symptoms. The table below gives a small sampling of three types of sensations when working with a stressful situation: comfortable sensations indicate movement toward expansion into healing; uncomfortable sensations show how the body is reacting to stress or trauma; while sensations of letting go indicate that our autonomic nervous system is releasing the stress.

Table 15.2: Sensation vocabulary box

Comfortable	Uncomfortable	Releasing/Letting go
spacious	tense	trembling (without fear)
warm	numb	hot/sweaty (without fear)
heavy (grounded)	heavy (frozen)	shaky (without fear)
strong	weak	tears of relief
easy breathing	shallow breathing	spontaneous full deep breath

An excerpt from Brain-Changing Strategies to Trauma-Proof Our Schools (Kline, 2020)

When introducing sensations and teaching kids to track them, both comfortable and uncomfortable feelings will arise. To help build tolerance, encourage exploration with curiosity until sensations release. Typically, there might be a bit of shaking or tears followed by a spontaneous breath, yawning, or relaxation. Offer extra support to locate sensations that feel safe, strong, comfortable, and resourced. Learning to release stuck sensations is an SE skill. However, suffice it to know that befriending them and pausing long enough to notice what changes happen next, frequently lessens distress. If it does not, the adult will need to assist the child in finding internal or external resources that shift focus to a positive experience.

Gently orienting children to something fascinating, beautiful, or calming in the environment brings awareness of the present moment in time and place.

Educating children that shakiness, trembling, and other nervous sensations are extra energy to move arms and legs quickly to run, hide, and fight helps allay fears. To access the underlying physiology where trauma is held, invite an exploration. Noticing the color, shape, and size of the physical feeling focuses attention long enough to provoke a shift. For example, if the child feels scared, explore the sensations underneath. It might be trembling, jumpiness, shakiness, or butterflies. Next, have the child befriend those sensations by using a reassuring voice to explain that the 'scary' feelings are the fuel to escape from danger. As they feel their 'energy tank' getting ready, ask where the energy wants to go. The ANS is the engine, and the muscles and joints of the limbs provide the defense. Encourage the movement of the energy into the limbs and watch the fascinating (sometimes mysterious) automatic impulses release into arms for fight, legs for flight or kicking, and/or neck for orientating away from danger or toward safety. The body has a mind of its own! The following story of a girl named Jump illustrates the effective use of artwork, and the basic SE skills of tracking sensations as anxious energy from her ANS moves into her limbs as described above. This is how traumatic activation is released.

The story of Jump and the healing power of art with SE basics and movement

Helping children discover their underlying physical sensations is important, because their physiology may be either escalating or blunting strong emotions. Drawing is one of the easiest and most fruitful ways to help kids access and express what words cannot. The two most efficient and non-threatening strategies I have found to increase awareness, befriend sensations, and evoke movement are 'The Magic of Opposites' and 'The Gingerbread Person Body Map'. I first combined the principles of SE with 'Drawing the Opposite' while volunteering in Thailand after the Southeast Asian tsunami where I met 13-year-old Jump at her school. She was frozen in shock with vacant eyes and a collapsed, limp body from witnessing the devastating tsunami. After asking her class to draw anything they wanted, many, including Jump, drew their lifeless fishing village. Her first drawing was devoid of people and homes, showing stumps of dead palm trees with birds scattering in all directions. Even in a catastrophe where children have witnessed mass fatalities, leaving thousands homeless and, in many cases, orphaned, combining the principles of SE with art brought children out of shock and back into their bodies.

Despite the cloudy skies and the decimated empty landscape in Jump's drawing, the sun peeked out from behind the strong mountain she referred to as 'the high ground,' safe from the rushing tsunami waters. It is easy to see in her drawing what Peter Levine calls the trauma vortex, and also the beginning of its opposite, or counter-vortex, in the tiny nascent sun. When an individual is able to embody the opposites, the dynamic of both polarities creates the catalyst for transformation. Before having the children describe their first drawing, which, like Jump's picture, showed mostly destruction, they were asked to make a second drawing. To stimulate the counter-vortex, the instruction was simply to draw the opposite. For those who have studied SE, the drawings become the 'I' in the SIBAM model which stands for 'Image.' The opposite image brings along with it the internal resources that become the counter-vortex when the other elements of SIBAM are added: 'S' for Sensations, 'B' for Behavior, 'A' for Affect, and 'M' for Meaning.

Using both drawings in a brief SE session helps children identify sensations. This a process that can provoke a release of extremely high arousal, which was showing up in Jump's case as overwhelming depression and collapse, alternating with bouts of anxiety.

While looking at her first drawing, Jump described the sensation of heaviness in her chest. She said, 'I feel sad. All nature is being destroyed.' Next, her heart started to pound. She also described shakiness inside her belly. I explained how a fast heartbeat and shaky feelings ignite the fuel inside our bodies to move very quickly when there is danger. Next, I asked her to look at both drawings side-by-side. As we worked together with her two sketches, sensations and movements organically arose. The shaky feelings increased, moving into her legs. I asked her to notice how the shaky energy might help her move. She pointed to the stream flowing from the mountains and said, 'I would run to the high ground!' After gently guiding her to let her legs move, Jump began running in place slowly as she imagined moving alongside the stream to the safety of the solid mountains and radiant sun that she had drawn.

Jump ran for several minutes while imagining making it to the mountain until she felt safe. Then, she slowly came to a stop. She sensed her trembling legs stop shaking as they gradually became solid and strong, like the mountain. She sat down and examined her second drawing again. Jump described a warmth around her heart as she looked at the sun and the coconut palms that had grown back. She smiled and said, 'I feel glad in my heart. The natural environment is beautiful.'

Of course, there is much grief to be processed after such cataclysmic losses, including the breathtakingly beautiful landscape swept away with people and possessions. That goes without saying. But it's important to understand that the process of healing the emotional grief begins after the nervous system physiology is attended to in such a way that one releases the bound energy that was mobilized to escape. If the body is stuck in readiness, the mind believes that the disaster has not ended. Processing shock trauma using SE releases the body to begin grieving within the cultural and spiritual norms and rituals within one's community.

The second pathway of the Resilience Roadmap – rectifying relationship deficits using the 'Eight Essentials of Healthy Attachment'

The first pathway to resilience – supporting the development of interoceptive intelligence as a system-wide classroom practice – increases both self-awareness and awareness of others. It can increase compassion and kindness, and foster improved social relationships by stimulating the growth of the anterior insult. It aids in self-regulations and can be used to reset the nervous system after an overwhelming event. But, alone, it is not enough for children with complex developmental trauma. Episodic trauma, such as a natural disaster, fall, accident, medical procedure, death of a loved one, or witnessing violence can leave any child with anxiety, nightmares, numbness, stomach aches, and other experiences. A resilient youngster fortunate enough to have enjoyed a secure attachment can easily be guided to slow down and navigate sensations. Just like Jump's story earlier in this chapter, secure children can quickly be supported to release trauma's physiological grip. Gently coming out of traumatic shock after a traumatic episode can prevent, or greatly reduce, long-term post-traumatic psychological symptoms. Building sensation awareness as a curricular practice and using the case example of Jump as a model for resetting the nervous system can help children restore a sense of stability and wellness. If only it could be so easy for all children!

Unfortunately, not all children have had the advantage of a secure attachment. There is a huge difference between those with complex developmental trauma and those who experienced an episode of tragedy. This is where the second pathway enters the picture. The characteristics of familial and societal trauma require a longer-term two-pronged approach. Before a child shapes their physiological states, she requires the loving kindness and bond of trust that provides the security missed during their early years. For youngsters struggling with social, emotional, and behavioral issues arising from early separation, abuse, neglect, or other mitigating factors that rupture attachment and bonding, the 'Eight Essentials of Healthy Attachment' were designed to build the external environmental resources necessary to support an internal felt-sense of safety. The 'system,' whether it be community agency personnel or school district staff, requires a shift in policy for how traumatized youth are treated. A commitment needs to be made to replace punishment with nurture.

Descriptions, rationale, and sample activities for the 'Eight Essentials of Healthy Attachment'

Deficiencies of any or all of the eight essentials can be remedied at any age. Due to the hierarchical nature of brain development, cortical development will be arrested when the earliest needs have gone unmet (Perry, 2013). Stages of development cannot be skipped. The activities, attitudes, and social games outlined in the Eight Essentials below are designed to stimulate positive brain/body growth by strengthening connections at the preverbal, subcortical levels of development. Some can be used with the entire class, while others are for use in a one-on-one situation, such as with a counselor. Ordinary games that you may already be familiar with can be adapted into trauma healing and resiliency practices by adding one or more of the eight essentials and guiding students to pay attention to internal changes. As my social work friend, Nathan Swaringen, developer of 'It's About T.I.M.E.' to support classroom teachers and students, says: 'You don't have to be a therapist to be therapeutic.' This is about changing the culture and the climate of school to include social-emotional growth together with goals of academic success. It is not one or the other – it is both.

No matter their age, all humans heal in the context of pleasurable relationships. But with the little ones, co-regulation shapes the anatomy and physiology of their rapidly developing brains and bodies. For those deprived of a secure attachment, relationships that repair those deficits are critical for lifelong mental and physical health. The dire consequences of early relational breaches can be mitigated by providing the Eight Essentials at school. They are the bedrock that supports underlying relational health. Everyone needs a safe harbor, nurturing touch, and playfulness throughout life. However, when missed during the formative years, just like malnourishment needs extra aliment, mental health needs supplemental nurturance. With these essentials, there can be a felt-sense that it's okay to trust and make friends, feel protected, and even joyful. Close proximity to regulated adults and older cross-age mentors with a mega-dose of attachment play incorporating the Eight Essentials serve as robust remedies. Schools and community agencies have the opportunity to provide these in the classroom, office, and as out-reach to the families at home. Psychobiological approaches for healing both episodic and complex developmental trauma are demonstrated in Lance's story that can be found following a brief description of the Eight Essentials.

The Eight Essentials of Healthy Attachment

Combining as many of the following Eight Essentials within any activity is most potent for building secure attachments. They are necessities for infants to thrive but can be appropriately adapted for teen and adults. Some can be used with the entire class; others are more suitable for a counseling or home setting.

1. Safety, containment, and warmth. Transmitted nonverbally through an adult's co-regulating presence, a calm nervous system with relaxed muscles helps children's bodies settle down and feel protected; wrapping a blanket or shawl around the back and upper arms so boundaries can be felt; holding; rocking; using weighted blankets; bilateral tapping of upper arms; teaching butterfly self-hugs.

2. Soft mutual eye gazing for infants. Soft kind eyes for children and teens. Words are powerful, but nonverbal cues 'speak' louder. Mirror neurons automatically entrain children to those close to them. Adults can soothe children and help shape a relaxed nervous system by being aware of the quality of their presence. An adult's awareness of their own grounding and facial expression can relax a tense child. For example, offering help to a student struggling with an assignment by connecting through soft eye contact and friendly expression first rather than focusing on the student's mistakes.

3. Shared intention, attention, and focus. Awareness of body language is key. This intimate attunement is experienced as a desire to learn the wishes, intentions, and energetic rhythms of the other, and be in synchrony or somatic resonance. This skill of recognizing cues develops with interoceptive practice. This helps the adult to know when and how to offer support and when to back off.

4. Skin-to-skin molding for infants. Safe nurturing touch for children. Nurturing touch from a calm adult can transmit a sense of safety via the heart-to-heart electromagnetic field of a warm human connection. An adult in a ventral state can soothe a young child with the following ways of relaying connection: holding, rocking, hugging, cuddling; hair brushing, stroking or braiding; and gentle massage. With older children, supportive touch of the head, back, shoulders, or feet; high fives and contact games such as piggyback rides and hand-clapping. Notice what types of touch affect the child in a positive and age-appropriate way. Plush toys, burrowing into pets' soft fur, and comfy pillows can be used for those not ready to accept touch.

5. Sweet soothing sounds and rhythmic movement for all ages. Being rocked in someone's arms; soft, soothing voice; music; chanting; drumming; rattles and other percussive instruments; hammocks; dancing; swings; and rocking chairs help calm the nervous system. The tone, pace, and rhythm of the adult's voice is key. Singing and humming to or with children while moving, rocking, dancing, or

resting together can be a mighty healing force that stimulates the ventral vagal complex for resting, digesting, and while experiencing the joy of connection.

6. Synchronized movement and facial gestures for all ages. Spontaneous silly games and mirroring activities such as funny expressions or a surprising incident can trigger a synchronization where both participants simultaneously burst out laughing. This nonverbal play increases bonding.

7. Pleasure. Smiles + play + laughter = fun for all ages. Play can be structured or spontaneous – the key is that everyone is having fun; any variety of active and passive games from patty-cake to puppy piles; chase games and board games, silliness for no reason.

8. Alternating between stimulating and quiet activities. For young kids: 'itsy bitsy spider,' 'ten little piggies go to market,' and 'fox in a box'. For school-age kids: chase and hide-and-seek games such as 'wolf comes at midnight.' For older kids and teens: athletics and team sports such as ball play, relay races, rough-and-tumble, jumping jacks or jump rope, juggling sticks. These activities are followed with debriefing by sharing post-activity sensation and emotional changes. Follow-up quiet activities can include coloring; story time; reading or being read to; meditation; yoga; listening to calming music or nature sounds; the body map gingerbread person drawing of sensation/emotion; expressive arts; verbally sharing experiences, hopes, dreams, worries, and goals.

As you read 17-year-old Lance's story below you will see how the Eight Essentials of Healthy Attachment are woven into our time together to build a solid, trusting, relationship. These demonstrate the concepts, attitudes, and activities that guide me when working with students with complex developmental trauma. Lance suffered egregious neglect, plus physical and sexual abuse by both biological parents. This caused severe and pervasive symptoms and, because of the shock to his immature nervous system, resulted in a disorganized, insecure attachment. The ventral vagal system, which requires nurturing touch, feelings of safety, and pleasurable dyadic play, is fundamental to later emotional self-regulation and social relationships. Co-regulation precedes self-regulation. His story demonstrates how to provide pre-cortical nourishment, absent during infancy, to an adolescent.

LANCE'S STORY: A TEEN WITH COMPLEX PTSD DUE TO PARENTAL NEGLECT AND ABUSE FROM BIRTH

Lance was a high school junior returning to public school after expulsion due to aggressive acting out. His challenging behavior was the result of interrupted development due to a history of abuse and neglect from infancy, which ended when Lance was adopted at age five after social workers removed him from endangerment. He had a mild traumatic brain injury, presumably from being shaken as an infant. He was a slow learner, diagnosed with attention deficit disorder (ADD) and low average cognitive ability. Although he received special education support, his intense emotions were out of control. By the time we met, Lance was on a cocktail of three pharmaceutical drugs and had been hospitalized 11 times due to psychiatric problems, including both depression and violent aggression.

At our first meeting, Lance flopped lethargically onto my office couch. 'I know what you want,' he said. 'Oh?' I replied curiously. With his legs sprawled out in front of him and arms crossed tightly over his chest, he told me that he had 'been through this before,' that he had seen many therapists since elementary school and did not like counseling one bit. Lance wasted no time telling me he did not want to come and it would do no good. 'You're gonna want me to talk about my feelings' and, without skipping a beat he put me on notice... 'Well, I won't.' I loved his forthrightness from the beginning – it made me feel playful.

Lance's resistance was no deterrent. I was blessed to have studied with Peter A. Levine, one of the masters of trauma transformation. Dr. Levine, author of *In an Unspoken Voice: How the Body Releases Trauma and Restores Goodness* (2010), teaches that the body speaks louder than words through posture, gesture, expression, and the nuances of its physiology. The crippling effects of physical, sexual, and medical disaster, war, and social trauma, along with emotional abuse and neglect, leave an unmistakable imprint. Lance had endured at least four of these atrocities during his earliest years – way before narrative memory. Of course, he did not want to talk about his feelings! Why would he? How could he? Why should he? Before learning how to treat trauma, I most likely would have been stumped. Certainly, I would have done my best to establish rapport and, then, taken a long and winding trail with plenty of detours and roadblocks. Instead, I created the Resilience Roadmap Model by synergistically combining SE skills with attachment play essentials and embodied meditation to give Lance the nurturance he never received.

After a slightly slouched posture in synchronized solidarity with Lance, I sat upright, wiping pretend sweat off my forehead. Spontaneously, and with a relieved sigh, I responded, 'Well, thank goodness, Lance! People have been telling me their feelings all day long and I'm actually quite tired of listening. Let's have some fun instead. Okay?' He looked at me incredulously, as if thinking, 'Is this lady for real?' Lance looked confused. He was intrigued by my genuine interest in his likes and dislikes, what he found funny, and his favourite pastimes. My priority was to help him to feel comfortable, safe to be himself, and to have choices (missing for traumatized kids). Helping youngsters like Lance with complex symptoms, including bouts of depression that could quickly ignite into explosive, hurtful rage, requires precision in focused attention and attunement.

Lance had no problem sharing that he was a skateboarder and wanted to learn how to surf. I told him I had just the thing for him. He livened up with curiosity as I stood up and reached around behind the couch to pull out my wooden balance board. Its graded, angular blades (resembling ice skates) can be adjusted from easy to very challenging. We played and laughed, and we played and laughed some more. I stood next to him like a spotter in gymnastics. I communicated that his safety was important to me. We took turns. Lance challenged me to try the toughest blade. He performed better on the board than me. We laughed as his face glowed and his chest expanded with pride. We spent the hour with the 'back and forth' of dyadic relationship – what Harvard's Center on the Developing Child refers to as 'serve and return' in its podcast for caregivers as healthy brain architects. Just as with infants, there was no goal or expectation. My presence as an anchor and my genuine desire to share joyful moments was the beginning of his transformation. When time was up, Lance asked when he could come back.

By the third session, Lance and I took turns with juggling sticks. We sat close enough to catch each other's sticks when we had mishaps that sent them flying through the air. We had fun – every time we laughed, our playful eyes and warm smiles would meet. We took breaks to rest a bit, gently alternating between active play and quiet time to settle. The distance between us was less than a meter. Again, this was intentional, a bit like peek-a-boo that babies love. Playing in proximity makes co-regulation more possible.

A new kind of 'selfie' for building interoceptive sensation awareness

After several sessions of active back-and-forth, rhythmical dyadic play using the juggling sticks, I sensed that Lance had enough security within our relationship to build self-regulation and resilience skills using Part I of the Resilience Roadmap. Our bond was strong and the time seemed ripe to set up exercises for him to explore and pay attention to his own physical sensations. To help him build interoceptive intelligence, I asked him to draw a 'selfie' outline that resembled a gingerbread cookie with lots of open space. Felt-tip pens could then be used to fill in the shades, shapes, and colors of his internal landscape. Because Lance could shift from a depressed mood to aggressive violence within seconds, this next step was critical to his growth. His autonomic nervous system pattern, like many who had experienced early abuse, was to move from frozen parasympathetic lethargy to sympathetic fight activation without any awareness of the nuances of the emotions or moods inside that were triggered. Without interoceptive intelligence, it is easier to blame others, rather than experiencing the locus of control within ourselves.

Teaching kids to notice, locate, label, and track bodily sensations and pay attention to how they change moment-to-moment is the first step in building a capacity to sense nuances and subtle shifts in emotions before feelings become too intense to bear. Since Lance felt fatigued and numb most of the time, I invited him to draw his 'selfie' directly after the juggling stick activity that would provide sympathetic nervous system arousal in a pleasant, playful way. Lance, who just a few weeks before was not interested in 'feeling' anything, drew himself with spiked hair.

Lance's 'Gingerbread' body map
First, Lance used the red marker and drew his center with squiggly lines to represent 'tingling energy equals happy feelings,' with energy moving into both arms and arrows pointing downward into both legs. Next, I asked him to 'hang out' and notice what might happen next if he took a little time to explore his internal movements with curiosity. After a few minutes, he chose a yellow marker to show his energy slowing down and moving down into his feet and toes. Lastly, he noticed that his feet relaxed.

Once Lance became aware of his sensations, he opened up spontaneously. He felt safe to share how easily and quickly he became angry and lost control. Now that we had formed a trusting relationship and he had developed a bit of interoceptive capacity, I introduced him to a focused breathing meditation to deepen his interoceptive awareness and his attention span. This also became a tool for him to settle when he was mad. As trust built, Lance also allowed me to gently hold his shoulders (like swaddling an infant for containment), then cradle the occipital area of his head with soft, warm hands to help him settle when he felt upset at some incident at school. He asked me to teach his mom how to hold his head the same way to soothe him at home, which I gladly did!

Focused breathing exercise (embodied meditation)
The following exercise that I used with Lance is a simple breathing meditation I first developed to bring body awareness to 35 under-achieving, mostly delinquent teenagers, who were in a special class because they

had all failed eighth grade. In order to focus Lance (and others with attention challenges), I gave him a colorful Post-It. I asked Lance to number from 1 to 4 on the Post-It in preparation for a 'quiz' where he could record his observations like a scientist. This was to stimulate his reticular activating system (RAS) – the part of the brain that puts motivation on auto-pilot. I gave him the four simple questions beforehand to facilitate ease in sustained focused awareness and ensure his success:

- How did your breathing change over time?
- Did you notice a pause before your inhale and exhale?
- Were your inhalation and exhalation even or uneven?
- How are you feeling now?

Next, I softly invited Lance, with eyes open or closed, to get as comfortable as possible. I encouraged him to notice the minutest details of his breathing, such as the temperature of the air entering his nostrils, noticing if his nasal passages were congested or clear, and if he could feel the tiny hairs inside.

My voice became softer and slower and more rhythmical as I continued to guide him to notice the width and depth of his breath. I suggested that he place his hands on his rib cage to easily feel the expansion and contraction as air entered his chest and lower diaphragm, and to notice the rhythm of his breathing.

A resilient breath has four phases: inhale, pause, exhale, and pause. I invited him to notice if he had one pause, two pauses, or no pauses. Focusing on details such as comparing the length of each inhale and exhale brought acute focused concentration. After eight minutes, I invited Lance to open his eyes, allow them to explore the room, and notice how he was feeling. There is no agenda to change anything; only to notice what changes happen. This is an exercise that builds awareness and the capacity to feel without fear. Despite the fact that Lance felt tired, he liked the exercise. I gave him the Post-It pad as a transition object and reminder to practice daily. I suggested that when he was upset, he could excuse himself to take a 'time-in' using his Post-It pad to help him focus on the rhythm of his breath until he felt his heartbeat calming, his muscles relaxing, and his agitation settling. Lance began practicing this 'homework' activity and his angry outbursts subsided substantially. He needed no reminders because he thought the Post-It idea was 'pretty cool.'

As time went on, Lance became more and more regulated. Play, laughter, smiles, the back-and-forth dyadic face-to-face game playing, genuine relationship-building, touch, and fun alternating with quiet, meditative tracking of interoceptive sensations and focused breathing exercises made a huge difference. Much to the delight of Lance and his parents, he graduated with a diploma, passing all required state tests. He became more and more regulated. When I first met Lance, he had no friends. Before graduation, he enthusiastically asked me to teach him how to dance because he had asked a girl to senior prom and she had said 'yes'!

Conclusion

Schools and agency caregivers can become change-makers. With research on neuroplasticity, embodied meditation, interoception, the neuroscience of trauma, and Somatic Experiencing®, we know that trauma is not in the event; it resides in the nervous system. Symptoms are reversed physiologically. A movement is needed to facilitate systemic change so that more institutions adopt psychobiological interventions that reset the autonomic nervous system. These practices interrupt a maladaptive threat response cycle, preventing long-term post-traumatic stress symptoms. The Resilience Roadmap Model presented in this chapter offers hope for prevention and healing of episodic trauma through sensation-based activities that build interoceptive intelligence. These foster a sense of self, a robust ability to bounce back after a terrifying or stressful event. The chapter also offers solutions that schools can adopt to build secure relationships between school staff and students with complex developmental trauma using the attitudes, concepts and activities from the 'Eight Essentials of Healthy Attachment'.

KNOWLEDGE AND PRACTICE REFLECTION

Joe Tucci, Janise Mitchell, Ed Tronick and Stephen W. Porges

Maggie Kline offers a tangible example of how a coherent knowledge architecture underpinning a therapeutic and educational approach can extend traditional ways of doing and create novel solutions to challenging real-world problems.

The problem Kline is aiming to address is the mind-body dualism and its progeny – cognitive behavioural traditions in which talking about feelings has been likened to the experience of the bodily sensations of those feeling states. This is how the field has ended up with constructs such as emotional literacy, and posters with list of words that can help children and young people choose language that best represents the way they are feeling on the inside of their bodies.

Kline challenges this problem practically and conceptually. First, she replaces emotional literacy with the construct of *interoceptive intelligence* – building from Goleman's work on emotional intelligence (1995). It is both familiar and new at the same time. The term interoceptive draws on the writing of Steve Porges, as he summarized so eloquently in his chapter in this book. It is the emergent properties of a dynamic which attunes to the qualities of the body sensations that emanate from the physiological systems of human neurobiology. Using her deep understanding of somatic psychotherapy, attachment theory and her own joyful, open-hearted practice wisdom, Kline outlines an approach to supporting children to identify physiological sensations not for the purposes of naming and categorizing them but for the purposes of befriending them. Offering children the opportunity to get to know their own body in a guided way that incorporates the presence of collaborative and trusted adult relationship is a resource that Kline is now attempting to build into the competency of the school system. She is not teaching regulation skills for children. She is helping adults to know how to reconnect to children who are in desperate need of attachment relationships so that they can seek out comfort and support to the very draining costs of living with the ongoing effects of adversity and trauma.

For the purposes of this book, it is the way that Kline has marshalled her knowledge areas that is most important. She has used knowledge about neuroscience, trauma, attachment, and somatic experiencing and coupled all of that with her own insights from years of working with children and the implicit feedback that children have provided her with in the minutiae of their playful interactions in the therapeutic processes that she invites them into.

This active assembling is a quality that we are proposing be included as part of the way that *trauma-transformative practice* is conceptualized and realized. It is the effort of articulating the knowledge domains that are being used (e.g. research evidence, theory, cultural knowledge, voices of those with lived experience, practice insights) and the way they are deliberately connected into a coherent whole – a framework for practice that has its ambition to make a difference to the lives of victims and survivors of violence.

The use of *trauma transformative* is discussed in more detail in the concluding chapter. But it is important to recognize that the use of the word *transformative* is not meant to be a bold claim to effectiveness in healing the effects of past trauma. It is used in the way to support practitioners, organizations and systems to be more than informed about trauma. It is encouraging them to organize themselves around purposefully achieving change, not hoping that practice change will occur because the people working in the service have a better awareness of trauma and its effects.

The theme of holding complexity needs to be operationalized in reality.

This is one of the steps in its implementation – articulate and make explicit knowledge frames, test them rigorously to ensure that the values underpinning each domain are compatible, develop a coherent framework for their integration, and never lose sight of the needs of the individuals, families and communities that are being served.

Trauma-transformative practice is not an incremental evolution in the trauma-informed movement started by Harris and Fallot over 20 years ago. It does not aim to be a revolution either. It is an act of heart to try and lift its influence to a more significant level.

References
References for chapter

Goleman, D. (1995). *Emotional Intelligence: Why It Can Matter More than IQ*. New York, NY: Penguin Random House.

Kline, M. (2020). *Brain-Changing Strategies to Trauma-Proof Our Schools: A Heart-Centered Movement for Wiring Well-Being*. Berkeley, CA: North Atlantic Books.

Levine, P.A. (1997). *Waking the Tiger: Healing Trauma: The Innate Capacity to Transform Overwhelming Experiences*. Berkeley, CA: North Atlantic Books.

Levine, P.A. (2010). *In an Unspoken Voice: How the Body Releases Trauma and Restores Goodness*. Berkeley, CA: North Atlantic Books.

Perry, B. (2013). Bonding and attachment in maltreated children: Consequences of emotional neglect. Adapted in part from *Maltreated Children: Experience, Brain Development and the Next Generation*. New York, NY: W.W. Norton and Company.

References for Knowledge and Practice Reflection

Goleman, D. (1995). *Emotional Intelligence: Why It Can Matter More than IQ*. New York, NY: Penguin Random House.

CHAPTER 16

Complexity, Uncertainty and Therapeutic Intent: Trauma-Transformative Care for Children and Young People

Janise Mitchell and Noel Macnamara

Introduction

The complex needs of children living in out of home care arising from abuse, neglect and violation are widely recognized (Mitchell *et al.*, 2020a; de Wilde *et al.*, 2019; Murray *et al.*, 2011; McLean *et al.*, 2011; Oosterman *et al.*, 2007). These children have generally been exposed to multiple traumas in the form of family violence, exposure to alcohol and drug abuse, or sexual, physical, and emotional abuse. They are usually known to child protection authorities at an early age. Children who enter out-of-home care are more likely to have been exposed to multi-type abuse, poly-victimization, and multiple adverse childhood experiences (ACEs) (Finkelhor *et al.*, 2007). Sadly, their journeys in care can be no less problematic for them. Many experience histories of placement instability as foster carers, kinship carers, and residential carers struggle to attune and respond to their trauma (Mitchell *et al.*, 2020a) in the context of the systems around these children finding it difficult to galvanize to meet their needs. Blythe *et al.* (2014) found that carers' difficulties in sustaining placements are impacted by experiences of managing children's challenging behaviors, and often compounded by difficult relationships with professional support services.

Attachment is the secure base from which a child moves out into the world. Having a safe haven promotes self-reliance and instils a sense of sympathy and helpfulness to others. From the intimate give-and-take of the attachment bond, children learn that other people have feelings and thoughts that are both similar to and different from theirs. In other words, they get 'in sync' with their environment and with the people around them. They come to develop self-awareness, empathy, impulse control, and self-motivation, and build an internal locus of control, the key factor in healthy coping throughout life. Forming a secure base with a carer can be a challenging experience for a traumatized child who has been unable to experience this in their early attachment relationships (Taylor, 2012).

Children in out-of-home care have commonly developed deep survival-based attachment strategies owing to their necessity to adapt to the threatening environments within which they lived prior to coming into care (Meadows *et al.*, 2011) These behaviors, which served them well in a threatening environment, can become problematic by impeding their capacity to form trusting relationships in their new family, at school, and in relationships in general. These trauma-based behaviors may appear alarming, uncontrollable, unpredictable, and even inexplicable to carers. Hobday (2001) aptly used the metaphor of falling into a 'time hole' that captures children's sudden mood changes accompanied by extreme behavioral difficulties. These behaviors may be externalized (aggressive/controlling) and/or internalized (dissociative/rejecting) (Cecil *et al.*, 2014). They are more likely to hold negative views about the self and have difficulties sustaining relationships. So much trust has been broken.

There are many ways in which the care system can unintentionally exacerbate, rather than heal, adverse childhood experiences, trauma, and loss. Even in a safe setting where an overactive alarm response is no longer adaptive, traumatized children may continue reacting in an extreme way to neutral and even apparently positive cues (Streeck-Fischer and van der Kolk, 2000). These difficulties can be long-lasting and may even grow more challenging while in out-of-home care (Octoman and McLean, 2014).

The complexity of the task of foster, kinship, and residential carers (carers) is 'inescapable' (de Wilde *et al.*, 2019; Day *et al.*, 2018). The complex needs of the children in their care can leave carers feeling overwhelmed, ill-equipped and unsupported. There may be additional complicating factors depending on the nature of contact with birth families and on-going statutory involvement and decision making. For many years it has been argued that out-of-home care has been in a state of crisis (Mitchell, 2008; Geiger *et al.*, 2013; Leloux-Opmeer *et al.*, 2017; Randle *et al.*, 2016; Riggs *et al.*, 2009), with carer retention a critical challenge as the demands of meeting the complex needs of children are mismatched with the level of support and training carers receive. Murray and colleagues (2011) noted:

> The challenges of providing sensitive and structured care for children in foster care go well beyond normative experiences of parenting. The developmental status of children in foster care is characterised by high levels of impairment across multiple domains, largely as a consequence of early maltreatment and deprivation… (p.149)

Although out-of-home care systems, for the most part, keep children and young people physically safe, it often neglects their need for emotional and psychological safety. As Browning (2020) says:

> Foster carers may attempt to create a nurturing environment for the children. However, the way the children behave can evoke powerful and unwelcome feelings in carers, such as rage and hatred towards those they look after... (p.185)

Caring for these children is full of paradoxes, complexity, and uncertainty. Good intentions alone will not help these children.

Children feel safe when they have stable, secure, nurturing, and enduring connections to aware and attuned adults (NICE, 2015). With a map of the world based on trauma, abuse, and neglect, these children often anticipate rejection, ridicule, and deprivation, and are reluctant to try new options, certain that they will fail. This lack of experimentation traps them in a world of fear, isolation, and scarcity, where it is impossible to welcome the very experiences that might change this basic perspective. Much has been written about understanding and managing the challenging pain-based behaviors of children who have experienced trauma and live in therapeutic or out-of-home care. Anglin (2003) coined the phrase 'pain-based behavior' to denote behaviors arising from traumatized reactions of children in out-of-home care. Carers are confronted with the need to offer children transformative healing on a daily basis.

> The importance of clear and consistent structure, along with a need for flexibility, patience, and empathy demonstrates the complex nature of successful fostering. Caring successfully for teens placed in out-of-home care requires a myriad of characteristics, knowledge, skills and abilities that blend together to meet the challenges... (Anglin, 2003, p.165)

It is within this context and the rise of the trauma-informed movement that the practice of 'therapeutic care' has evolved. Trauma-sensitive, compassionate care is underpinned by a biopsychosocial theoretical framework of trauma-informed care (Bath and Seita, 2018) based on an integration of neurobiology, trauma, attachment and compassion research (Blaustein and Kinniburgh, 2010).

This chapter will explore therapeutic care as a vehicle for transforming trauma in the lives of children in out-of-home care. The care environment is no longer considered the place where children live while healing and recovery are achieved through traditional approaches to psychotherapeutic one-on-one counselling. Rather, it is imbued as an active agent of change in the healing process. The case study is offered by way of example to highlight the critical dimensions of building safety and meaning making within therapeutic care.

Therapeutic care as trauma transformation: The role of therapeutic intent

Therapeutic care is an intentional approach to the care and support of children who have experienced developmental trauma and is concerned with their needs, their entitlements, and their voice (Tucci *et al.*, 2020).

> It is informed by the consilience of knowledge (Siegel, 2016) distilled from a range of disciplines and practice areas encompassing interpersonal neurobiology, trauma, therapeutic intervention, child protection and children's rights... (Tucci *et al.*, 2020, p.55)

We (Tucci *et al.*, 2020) have previously suggested that therapeutic care is underpinned by the following principles:

- Therapeutic care recognizes that trauma related to abuse and violence has a differential impact on each child and young person, leading to a unique configuration of impact and downstream consequences.
- Therapeutic care practice privileges children's needs as the basis of all of its decisions.
- Therapeutic care understands that children's behavior communicates the efforts made by their internal systems to protect them from the traumatic experiences of violation.
- Therapeutic care adopts a lifespan approach to planning for children and young people as they grow and change.
- Therapeutic care honours the strengths of cultural heritage as resources for children and their relationship networks.
- Therapeutic care adopts the view that children's experiences of deep visceral safety are both an outcome and a form of intervention.
- Therapeutic care is active in ensuring that children and young people who have experienced abuse and neglect are not further disempowered by the way practice is implemented.
- Therapeutic care fosters the authentic participation of children and young people in decision-making processes that are about them.
- Therapeutic care empowers relationships to be therapeutic.
- Therapeutic care conceptualizes the physical and sensory environments that children inhabit as therapeutic.
- Therapeutic care expands the role of therapists to become relational

brokers, network enablers and system advocates for children in out-of-home care.
- Therapeutic care is resourced by coordinated collective decision-making that serves the needs and interests of children.

Therapeutic care is, at its heart, trauma-transformative relationship-based practice across multiple dimensions. Relationships offer the opportunity for hurt to be understood, shared and ultimately, as Bonnie Badenoch suggests, 'digested' (2018). This approach:

> ...considers the needs of the child, the needs of the carer and others in a relationship with the child and the space between them, each influenced by the other individual, their unique life experiences and knowledge, as well as the shared interactions between them... (Mitchell *et al.*, 2020b, p.114)

It works from the premise that the relationships closest to children have the most capacity to contribute therapeutic effort toward change for children (Tucci and Mitchell, 2019). It empowers all relationships to be therapeutic or hold 'therapeutic intent,' particularly carers and other significant relationships in the lives of children (e.g. teachers). It posits that all relationships have the therapeutic potential to be reparative and corrective. It achieves this through sequenced strategies that promote the ability of carers and others to know, understand and engage with the mind of the child in relationship with them. Based in the mentalizing work of Peter Fonagy and colleagues (Allen *et al.*, 2008; Fearon *et al.*, 2006; Fonagy and Adshead, 2012; Fonagy *et al.*, 2002), it makes reference to the emotions, feelings, thoughts, intentions, and desires of another, and creates an understanding of each other in the lived experiences of relationships.

Therapeutic care holds a commitment to meaning making, viewing behavior as a form of communication and seeking to understand the meaning behind all forms of communication. The program supports the carers and others to bring into conscious awareness the meaning behind both what is said and what is done on the part of both the child and themselves (Mitchell *et al.*, 2020b).

Therapeutic care integrates therapeutic intent into the daily practices of care and support for children, offering the healing properties of safety, attunement, trust, predictability, and stability. Drawing on the milieu-based 'life-space' work of Smith (2005), Taylor (2005) and Torrenon (2006), and Ward's (2006) 'opportunity-led' approach, all interactions between children and carers and others are conceptualized holding therapeutic capacity. The therapeutic intent unifies expectations about the care and support of the child within the care environment and other environments (such as school) and how it can work to provide the basis for growth and transformation to occur. Therapeutic intent underpins everyday moments that carers and others can use to assist children to increase their flexibility and adaptability in the face of their locked-down trauma-based feelings, thoughts and behaviors, and in the process building new understanding of themselves and how to relate to others. In doing so, the child is offered compensatory experiences that serve to counteract the negative effects of earlier traumatic experiences as well as complementary experiences that build resilience (Mitchell *et al.*, 2020b).

A relational environment holding therapeutic intent enables growth and transformation to occur in the form of the children developing a strong sense of safety; developing and/or practicing empathy; regulating emotions; processing traumatic memories; changing or managing their behavior consistent with the context; experiencing congruence between their thoughts, emotions, and behaviors; experiencing a sense of acceptance, comfort, or positivity about themselves 'in their own skin'; developing a strong sense of identity; mastering new skills that they may not have had an opportunity to engage with previously; developing resilience to difficult experiences; developing a capacity for calmness; and having fun (Mitchell *et al.*, 2020a).

To be effective, therapeutic care must also 'focus on the complex and collaborative relations demanded of stakeholders in the provision of...care' (de Wilde *et al.*, 2019, p.296).

Therapeutic care programs perform optimally when embedded within trauma-informed organizations and systems, including child protection, education, policing, health, and justice. The needs of children are rarely met by one agency alone, rather requiring the coordinated and collaborative efforts of many. The capacity to develop a 'shared lens' within the system about a child's needs and how to best meet them is a key challenge, but nonetheless critical to the goals and intent of therapeutic care (Mitchell *et al.*, 2020a). Having the processes for active and constructive engagement with interfacing agencies and organizations in relation to creating a consistently therapeutic environment for children is fundamental to the achievement of good outcomes. One vehicle for the achievement of this in therapeutic care are care teams.

Care teams

Care team members (carers, support workers, case managers, teachers, clinicians, family members, and the children themselves) work cooperatively and share responsibility to jointly develop, implement, monitor, and evaluate an integrated, collaborative therapeutic plan that sets goals and defines therapeutic intent. The care team is more likely to be successful when care team members approach decisions in an open-minded manner (Tullberg *et al.*, 2019). Members must be willing to provide their own perspectives, with a commitment to focus on strengths and opportunities in addressing needs, and work to ensure that others have opportunity to provide input and feel safe doing so. Each care team member must be committed to the care team goals and the integrated therapeutic plan for the child. Interactions between care team members are governed by the goals in the plan. This includes the use of resources controlled by individual members of the team. When legal mandates or other requirements constrain decisions, care team members must be willing to work creatively and flexibly to find ways to satisfy mandates while also working toward the child's goals.

The care team does not give up on, blame, or reject children, their carers, or family members. When faced with challenges or setbacks, the care team continues working toward meeting the needs of the child and carer and toward achieving the therapeutic goals. Undesired behavior, events, or outcomes are not seen as evidence of child or carer 'failure' but, rather, are interpreted as an indication that the plan should be revised to be more successful in achieving the positive outcomes. At times, this requires care team commitment to revise and implement a therapeutic plan, even in the face of limited system capacity or resources (Macnamara, 2020).

A care team approach provides a systems framework to drive a whole-of-practice approach to understanding, supporting, and working through the needs of children in a way that is child-centred, holistic, and connected.

Therapeutic leadership

Therapeutic specialists provide therapeutic leadership across all the critical relationships around the child in order to develop a shared understanding of the needs of children and deliver congruent and collaborative trauma-informed responses which are consistent across the settings in which children live, learn, and play. They broker these relationships, moulding them into a collective that works to keep the whole child in perspective.

As we have previously noted, therapeutic specialists:

> ...offer carers the intersubjective resource (Hughes, 2007, 2015, 2017; Hughes and Baylin, 2012) that enables them to stay open to the relationships with children, which can in themselves be stressful if not traumatising to the carer. Therapeutic Specialists provide the neurobiological brace that carers can rely on in the face of the activated states of the children and their implications back into the implicit memory systems of the carer, who may be carrying reverberating experiences of loss, disruption and even direct experiences of violence and abuse... (Tucci et al., 2020, p.54)

The reflective practice offered by therapeutic specialists to support carers and care team members aims to review the relational space between themselves and the child, to seek to understand what the child is experiencing and needs in the context of each interaction, in addition to supporting self-reflection. Such a process builds the capacity of carers and others to engage with a higher form of understanding of their 'relational mind' and remain present in their relationship with the child. Carers are assisted to reframe trauma-based behavior in terms of its function or the unmet need it is communicating. This reframing supports different perspective-taking and enables compassionate and attuned ways of making meaning of the behavior, replacing traditional approaches to responding to behaviors.

Trauma sensitive, compassionate care in action: A case study

No child chooses to be angry, afraid, or immersed in deep shame. Certainly, there are lots of behaviors that have big negative consequences for children in out-of-home care and those around them. But understanding, knowledge, support, and compassion can provide a framework for transformative change. The following case vignette illustrates the need for and application of trauma sensitive, compassionate care.

JOHN'S STORY: PART 1

John (not the child's real name), who was seven years old when he entered our therapeutic foster care program:

- had experienced multiple placement breakdowns
- had had his needs met with dismissive or aggressive reactions rather than a nurturing response from his primary carer and other carers from whom he sought comfort
- struggled to regulate, regularly attacking adults
- showed emotions and feelings through aggressive, violent outbursts
- was unable to trust others
- engaged in self-rejection – he had a negative regard for himself, and believed he was unworthy and unlovable
- lacked compassion for others
- held a deep-rooted belief that adults were unable to keep him safe
- had a diagnosis of ADHD and took regular medication to aid regulation and support his sleep routine
- hoarded food
- had poor standards of personal hygiene.

John's emotional presentation included negative self-evaluations, low self-esteem, and guilt, perhaps due to a belief that he was responsible for the failure of his family to care for him. He appeared to fight against feelings of being thrown away, of being disposable, unwanted, and needing to go into a stranger's homes, and these emotional struggles led to feelings of shame. Perhaps due to the multiple placement moves, John had developed an unstable sense of self-identity as well as a tenuous belief system.

John was boisterous, confused, and dysregulated. He felt let down by the world and the adults who should have cared for and protected him and made him feel safe and loved. He was predisposed to expressing his emotions through aggressive, violent outbursts and would regularly attack his carers to get what he wanted or when he felt a disruption in their relationship. John would throw things at his carers. He showed limited understanding of his actions, believing that hurting others showed strength and power and would ultimately achieve the results he wanted. John had been removed from his family when he was five years old. In the last two years he'd had three foster care placements and a number of short-term care arrangements.

John struggled with routines and boundaries, had no sleep pattern to speak of, and was afraid to have his bedroom door closed or the light turned off. This meant he slept intermittently, waking several times throughout the night when he would leave his room, frequently running about the house.

John felt unable to trust others, feeling the need to control everything and everyone around him to feel safe – this impacted his ability to form relationships with adults and other children. His need for control often manifested in aggression, threats, or violence.

John's previous foster carers did not have a deep understanding of, or a tolerance for, his fear and pain-based behaviors. As he began to display his pain, it become too intolerable or risky for them. John was punished, shamed, and blamed by his past carers and ultimately the placements ended, reinforcing to John that he was unlovable and could be tossed away.

John could not accept responsibility for his decisions or actions, firmly believing that others were to blame and deserved the things he did. He refused to acknowledge incidents once they were over.

During his introduction to his new foster carers, he told them that they had better be careful and that they should not attempt to hurt him because he had friends who protected him. He went on to say: 'I have a friend called Buster and he is good at fighting, and he will bash you up if you do anything to me. I also have a friend called Simo and he has a knife.' Finally, he said, 'I also know a dog and he bites really bad, so you better watch it.'

While at times during the first months of the placement John could accept the carers' offer of nurture, this could become too much for him. To accept it, he needed to be open to their warmth and tolerate an emotional space that required an inner vulnerability. Vulnerability was not a space John could afford in his prior placements.

Over the course of the first months of the placement, John's difficult behavior persisted, abating and escalating at regular intervals. The carers provided a very consistent, sensitive, warm, and empathic environment for him where John could feel safe, contained, and held – literally and emotionally. To do this required an ability to be adaptive to the spontaneous experiences of John.

At the same time, they attempted to place boundaries by creating routines and structure in an effort to contain John's feelings of being overwhelmed and out of control. This type of therapeutic parenting required the carers to be sensitive and responsive and gradually allow John to experience and tolerate frustration.

Bedtime was often a contested space for John, as it can be for many children in care, in that it recalled experiences of separation and abandonment, accompanied by difficulties in feeling safe enough to relinquish himself to the empty space of his room and go to sleep.

John had not developed the capacity to be alone. As an integral part of this developmental process, the capacity to be alone is founded on reliability, since the child's expectation of care is reinforced by the caregiver. The seminal author Winnicott (1974) writes that the child is able to 'build up belief in a benign environment' as a result of being in the presence of a consistent, attuned other.

Without the presence of a reliable primary carer to facilitate in John the capacity to be alone he was unable to build up a belief in a benign environment and to learn self-soothing techniques – there was no one who initially soothed him.

John's trauma was ongoing. Every new encounter and event were contaminated by the past in an endless loop. His carers were sufficiently attuned to John to know when he could tolerate them maintaining firm boundaries around the bedtime routine and when he needed flexibility. In the latter case, they often accommodated his needs by placing a mattress alongside their own bed in their room so as to soothe his distress, while keeping other aspects of the bedtime routine in place.

Building a support system for John

The complex needs of children like John need to be matched with similarly complex solutions to their care and support needs, which requires multiple stakeholders and systems. In this case, the care team approach provided a 'shared lens' that could be systematically applied to better connect and integrate the array of service providers and points of service delivery capable of matching flexibly to John's needs and preferences over time and at various stages of his care. The core function of John's care team was the establishment of holistic arrangements that were explicitly geared to his needs, inclusive of his wishes and goals and those of the carer family. Shared meaning making was built within the care team about John's needs and the drivers of his behavior. The care team gathered information and built a coherent narrative about John and his care history and shared this with his carers.

The care team supported the development and implementation of John's therapeutic care plan, comprising interventions or strategies that could be replicated or at least congruent across environments.

The care team approach promoted horizontal rather than hierarchical relationships so that people treated each other on equal terms, developing share ownership for the success of their common purpose – John's best interests. In the first months, the care team met on a weekly basis. There were also individual sessions with the carers and John began therapy and work with his occupational therapist.

The therapeutic specialist worked with the carers on a weekly basis, established a trusting relationship that provided a crucial foundation for the work surrounding John's difficulties. The consistency of this input played an important role in the carers feeling supported through their own experience, holding an emotional space whereby they could articulate their feelings and have them acknowledged and understood within a compassionate frame of reference. Gilbert (2014) defines compassion as 'the sensitivity to suffering in self and others, with a commitment to try to alleviate and prevent it' (p.19).

Compassion has been found to have a number of benefits for physiological health, mental health, and emotion regulation (Keltner et al., 2014; Seppälä et al., 2012), and in improving interpersonal and social relationships (Crocker and Canevello, 2012).

Much of the work with John's carers focused on helping them to develop and maintain self-compassion. Neff (2003) defined self-compassion as having three components:

- being mindful, rather than over-identifying with problems
- connecting with others, rather than isolating oneself
- adopting an attitude of self-kindness, rather than being judgmental.

All three elements are essential for the effective care of children like John if the emotional impact of caring for a highly traumatized child is to avoid creating shifts in the internal world of the carer, undermining their sense of identity and confidence as facilitators of children's well-being.

Creating a sense of safety for John

Research has shown that trauma exposure affects both the perception of environmental threat (i.e. lack of safety) and an individual's response to per-ceived threats. Specifically, a history of trauma can alter brain development and cause detrimental changes to children's neurobiological reactions to stress (Teicher *et al.*, 2016; Shonkoff *et al.*, 2012). These changes can interfere with a child's ability to understand and regulate emotion and prime them to detect threats in typically benign circumstances – leading them to respond in ways that may seem extreme and 'out of the blue' to others (Sweeney *et al.*, 2016). Porges' (1995, 2004) pioneering work in Polyvagal Theory and the neuroception of safety is fundamental to therapeutic care practice.

The Polyvagal system is a brain-body science (or neuroscience) of con-nection, trust, and safety. As Porges (2015) says: 'Polyvagal Theory helps us understand how cues of risk and safety, which are continuously monitored by our nervous system, influence our physiological and behavioral states… (p.144).

It explains how feeling safe optimizes spontaneous social interactions by turning off defensive states and increasing social behaviors through our social engagement system. Starting from birth, babies learn to regu-late their physiological and behavioral state through engagement with their caregivers. The building blocks of connectedness typically start with a mother nursing her baby, a two-way interaction system which is both receptive and expressive. This ability to mutually (synchronously and recip-rocally) regulate each other's physiological state (through soothing and stimulation) forms the core of the development of this social engagement system (Porges, 2011), thus helping us navigate relationships by promoting connectedness, trust, play, and intimacy. The ability of a child to be socially successful in adolescence and then adulthood is largely based on the devel-opment of the social engagement system in earlier years.

Because of its role in making contact between different people reward-ing, the social engagement system is a way of achieving personal safety. But there is a catch. The social engagement system requires a sense of safety to develop or stay employed. When we experience our environment as safe, we operate from our social engagement system. Prolonged stress or threat or stress early in life tends to weaken or impair the development of the social engagement system.

Dana (2018) summarized all of this thinking with her reflection:

Neuroception results in the gut feelings, the heart-informed feelings, the implicit feelings that move us along the continuum between safety and survival response. Neuroception might be thought of as somatic signals that influence decision making and behavioral responses without explicit awareness of the provoking cues... (p.144)

Dana goes on to suggest that when Polyvagal state shifts occur we create a story to explain why – a concept she called 'Story Follows State.' Stories may sound something like this:

- 'There's no point in trying.'
- 'I deserved it.'
- 'No one can be trusted.'
- 'I'm worthless and unlovable.'
- 'It's my fault.'

These 'stories' are there to explain the world and attempt to make sense of what caused the autonomic state shift. However, these stories do not necessarily reflect reality – they serve the function of creating an explanation.

Children in out-of-home care are constantly scanning their relational environment for cues of safety or danger. It is said to be constantly ticking below our subconscious, although humans are likely to be aware of the physiological responses it causes. They are sent to the brain, which is then tasked with making sense of it – in other words, a story. The problem is that the children like John may be telling themselves the wrong story, or at least very unhelpful ones. In John's case, his story was built on the belief that no adults were safe and he needed to take care of himself.

Unfortunately, for many children like John this function of the nervous system is shut down and underdeveloped. Conditions of relational and physical safety and repeated positive nurturing experiences are essential for it to develop and come back online.

In our work with children like John we know that we have to help our carers to support children in experiencing 'felt safety.' It is essential that the carers understand that being safe does not equal feeling safe. As Porges (2017) explains:

...safety is not the removal of threat and that feeling safe is dependent on unique cues in the environment and our relationships that have an active inhibition on defence circuits and promote health and feelings of love and trust... (p.43)

We have all had that feeling where we say to ourselves: *'I know it is true, but I don't feel like it is true.'* The conscious brain can know it is safe, but the unconscious brain and heart do not feel that it is safe.

To recover from traumatic events and adverse histories, children like

John need to experience felt safety. Felt safety is probably the most important part of the therapeutic caring process. With an impaired ability to access the logical thinking brain, the lower unconscious parts of their brain are asking 'Am I safe?' four times every second (Rock, 2008).

'Safe?' 'Not safe?' 'Safe' 'Not safe' 'Safe' 'Not safe.' This constant questioning/fear-based response is the basis of the John's ongoing behaviors and why at times his carers asked themselves, 'Why does he keep doing that? We are safe people, and our home is a safe place.'

In the case of John, we conceptualized this super-fast safety detector as looking in three different places.

- *Inside* (e.g. heart rate, hunger, genetics, biology, inflammation, neuroimmune systems):
  - For John who has a history of intense deprivation including hunger in the past, then even very mild symptoms of hunger can create a full-blown fight/flight response.
  - For John who has a history of having a fast-beating heart only when something was dangerous (as opposed to when playing or having fun), then a fast-beating heart at recess when nothing is truly dangerous may trigger a full-blown fight/flight response.
- *Outside* (e.g. consistency, predictability, structure, and routine):
  - The first Christmas John was in his therapeutic foster care placement, the carers had relatives come to stay unexpectedly. John found the changes in structure and routine within the home intolerable and he was triggered into rages and destructive behaviors.
  - On one occasion, the carers got a call from school telling them that John had been extremely upset and very disruptive for no reason. When they collected John, he told them that he had had a substitute teacher that day.
- *Between:*
  - One of the places John's brain looks to decide if he is safe is whether his carer is feeling safe or not.
  - If his carer is outside their window of tolerance and in their own fight/flight or fear-based state – regardless of how well they are trying to hide it – John will experience them as 'not safe.'

Three places, four times every second. Safe – Not safe – Safe – Not safe. It is actually hard to wrap our brains around! In order to address the issue of felt safety, the caring environment must support all three aspects of safety.

In John's case, this involved high levels of environmental and relational predictability, consistency and routine, minimizing unexpected changes, and planning for expected changes (such as substitute teachers, family contact, visitors to the house, weekends and school holidays, and school excursions). It also involved repeated messages, communicated through what the carers said and how they were with John, that he was safe, lovable, and valuable, and that they could tolerate 'the worst that he could throw at them' because he was more than the sum of what he did. It involved healthy food being made accessible to John at all times, and him having a say in family meals. It involved spending time together doing things that John enjoyed, experiencing mutual play and fun together. It involved validating his big feelings and helping him to make sense of them. It involved active steps to repair relational disruption between John and the carers at times when things got difficult for him.

John had many unmet developmental needs from his early life that the carers were supported to understand, adjusting their expectations of him so that he experienced success rather than failure. The care team was supported to use the same or similar strategies across the environments he moved between. In doing so, a high level of congruence was built in how John's needs were understood and responded to, regardless of which member of his care team he was engaging with. Frequent communication between care team members was critical, as a challenge at school was very likely to lead to a difficult evening at home, and a bad night at home was likely to lead to a difficult day at school the following day. John's ability to feel safe was contingent on the capacity of the care team to work together. The therapeutic specialist became an interpreter of John's world with the carers and care team as they made meaning of his behaviors and needs, and an enabler of the adults in John's life to maintain a reflective stance and remain present to John's needs while understanding and developing strategies for meeting their own needs.

JOHN'S STORY: PART 2

Approximately nine months into his placement, John began to see and feel changes in his experience of safety with his carers and others. One evening when he was having a bath, he spoke to his carer about the fact that the [imaginary] friends he had told her about when they first met were gone now. He did not need them anymore. When the carer asked why, John responded by saying, 'It's because I feel safe now.'

With the support of the care team, the carers were able to:

- implement consistent routines and predictability
- follow the principles of trauma-informed care, ensuring John experienced a felt sense of security and safety
- provide a safe, secure home with adults John could trust to care for him

- work with the school to enable them to better meet John's needs
- ensure that John was supported to attend weekly therapy sessions.

During this period, it was becoming evident that there had been a palpable shift in John. While he continued to have outbursts, they became less frequent and when they did occur, they did not seem to last as long or have the same intensity. He was sleeping in his own bed, albeit with the lights on and the door open. There was a sense that he had unconsciously stepped back from the extreme of his attacks on the carers and the environment. This shift was accompanied by a significant change in the atmosphere of the placement over time, with a greater sense of calm and containment. The carers demonstrated more confidence and appeared less tired.

Prior to John coming into his therapeutic foster care placement, his experience of school was turbulent and conflictual and resulted in many school exclusions. He spent his time in school in isolation from other children, sitting outside the principal's office. The care team supported a move of school for John and a fresh start.

Members of the care team held educational sessions for all school staff about the impact of trauma on learning. This provided essential knowledge and built relationships between the care team and the school. The therapeutic specialist met with John's class teacher and the deputy principal on a regular basis. John was fully aware of the connections between home, the care team, and school.

Due to the carers and the new school's immense efforts to emotionally 'hold' John, the pattern of escalations declined at school. Initially, John went to school for only a few hours a day, for a few days a week and through this gradual introduction, after nine months he was attending full time. John had a full-time support worker to help him to integrate into the school environment and support his classroom experience. He began to develop friendships and a positive relationship with his classroom teacher.

Lost in time and place – the process of meaning making

Memories are the stories of our lives and offer interpretive frames for meaning making. They tell us who we are, where we belong, what is possible and what the future might be. As Siegel (1999) puts it, 'Memory is the way past events affect future function' (p.24).

The consequences of trauma impinge on children's lives in various ways, including their capacity to make sense of their experience. For many, traumatic memories invade their lives and intrude on their sense of self in a myriad of ways. Memories become fragmented – they are not time-stamped or well organized with the 'who,' 'what,' 'when,' 'where,' and 'why' of experience. They lose the story of their life – the past and present are intertwined. It's confusing and disorienting. It's hard for children to separate safe events happening now from dangerous events that happened in the past. A consideration of memory is primary in the understanding of the consequences of trauma and the development of healing and recovery practices (Seigel, 2012; van der Kolk *et al.*, 2015).

Safety is the brain's core organizing principle. Most other functions are subservient to this need (Perry, 2004). To assist this our brain blends the information that it is processing right now with all the information it has stored in our memory networks. That is a lot of information! Those two streams of information (then and now) merge together to create our conscious experience of now.

It is important for carers to remember that children like John experience safety or the perceived lack of it not only on objective information that is happening right now. *'These are safe people; where I live is a safe place.'* There is a lot of the 'past' that is influencing that perception. Integrated memories allow the past to flow gently into the present (Levine, 2015). However, trauma does not tell time. When an unintegrated implicit memory gets triggered, it does not have access to information that tells John, *'Hey! That happened a long time ago! You are safe now!'* Trauma seizes John's body in the moment and thrusts him back into those terrifying times when the trauma was happening. Trauma is largely remembered as physical sensations, automatic responses, and involuntary movements (Ogden *et al.*, 2006), as well as unconscious 'acting out' behaviors (Levine, 2015). This happens in milliseconds. It is fast and furious and John has no brakes on his system.

If this understanding of trauma memory is applied to a traumatized child, it starts to become clear why their behavior is very difficult for them to consciously understand and explain in terms of their past traumas. All of the child's abuse and/or neglect experiences will have been remembered but not necessarily in a way that they can access consciously or give language to. Memories that are not integrated, often due to overwhelming emotion at the time of the experience (Siegel, 2012; van der Kolk, 2015), do not flow gently into the stream of now. They are fast and furious and crash into the stream as if a dam has been released, overflowing and overtaking. Past experiences dominate children's experience of the now, shaping their behavior.

For example, John was severely neglected when he was an infant. He was left alone for hours at a time. He has no conscious memories of being left alone but his body remembered the terror and helplessness. This terror and helplessness were connected to other everyday things, including the sound of the television and the house phone. He would react very badly at times. As the brain that 'wires together fires together,' Barfield *et al.* (2012)

would argue that terror and the telephone or television may have been wired together. This can be extremely confusing for carers, teachers, other significant adults, and the children themselves.

When carers and others understand this confusion we can support children to slow the tsunami of input their brains are trying to deal with. To put brakes into the system. To help the rivers of then and now meet gently, connecting in harmony to create something that has never been created before. This can all happen in seconds.

And while there are lots of ways to support this gentle connection of then and now, in our view the best way is compassion. Compassion is the combination of empathy and action. Compassion is the energy that is needed to slow the tsunami. And eventually when a struggling child receives enough compassion (with boundaries) they begin to develop self-compassion. Self-compassion is exactly the energy that is needed to bring the then and the now together more slowly – allowing the then to inform the now but without knocking it on its backside and destroying everything in its path.

By helping children learn to practice self-compassion (*I am worthy*) you help dislodge shame-based beliefs, such as you are worthless, defective, bad, unlovable. You will also increase their capacity to accept compassion from others, helping to build stronger social connections.

Rapidly flowing water has the power to destroy everything in its path, but all it is trying to do is be water. Seeing behaviors as what they are – the result of two rivers, their past and present, coming together in the best way the child knows how – is a central tenet of therapeutic care. Compassion will help the river slow down and enable children to experience felt safety.

Using this frame of understanding, it starts to become clear why John's behavior is very difficult for him to consciously understand and change. Recognizing the relationship between repetitive, problematic behavior and unresolved trauma allows carers to make sense of emotional outbursts that can seem to come without warning and explain why reward-punishment and logical consequences approaches to child rearing are unhelpful in bringing about change in the child's behavior.

In John's case compassion, calmness and closeness was key. John's carers and teachers helped build his memory capacity by helping him to tell the story of his experience over the course of his day, locating the who, what, where, when, why, and how of experience in a story that was coherent, made sense, and could be recalled. They helped him connect his feelings to these stories and make meaning of his experience. Time was spent in counseling and with his carers, locating what had happened in the past, who had been there, and why things had happened, working through the good memories and bad. His growing capacity to feel safe and develop shared meaning and narrative about his life was a turning point for him.

JOHN'S STORY: PART 3

Four months later and the carers and the care team program have continued to provide John with a consistent and predictable environment within which he has been offered repeated experiences where adults can be trusted and relied on. He has developed a sense of security and belonging and is beginning to understand family life and what being a part of something really means.

He has started to form friendships with other children and is more able to enjoy time playing together with others. He can now think of others and recognize their needs, as well as his own, and is able to show his natural, loving, and affectionate nature.

The routines, boundaries, and compassion the carers have offered John have allowed him to be a child again. John no longer requires night-time medication and he sleeps soundly through the night with the door closed. John is able to form friendships. and he is more self-aware and able to identify a range of feelings.

John attends school full time and is highly engaged in the school community. He is liked and supported by his teachers and the deputy and principal of the school.

Although John's journey is not yet complete, his life has been transformed from a little boy who lived a life of fear and uncertainty to a little boy who feels safe and can connect with and show compassion for himself and others.

John was helped to experience felt safety by his carers offering him attuned and responsive care. They paid attention to his nonverbal cues suggesting he felt unsafe. Over time, they were able to name and tame John's big feelings. By naming John's emotions, it helped him to create some distance between the emotion and the intense feelings that accompany it. John began to feel seen, heard, respected, and calmed.

Irrespective of what they already knew, the carers always allowed John to voice his point of view. They validated his emotions. This helped John to feel held and not alone. The carers allowed John to experience control by giving choices. This reduced the power battles that he had been used to having with his previous carers and that were the basis of much conflict.

The carers remained curious and open to why John might be behaving the way he was. This not only reduced conflict but also allowed John to begin to be curious about his own thinking and behavior. They were also playful in their interaction with John. John had not experienced a 'playful parent.' John started to see himself as someone who could be experienced as a joy.

Conclusion

The Beatles sang that all you need is love and love is all you need. The children in the out-of-home care system certainly need love but it is not all they need. For these children, the creating of felt safety is probably the single most important aspect of their therapeutic care. As van der Kolk (1996) says: 'Safe connections are fundamental to meaningful and satisfying lives' (p.124).

Through this chapter and the case study of John we have attempted to paint a picture about how therapeutic care can be transformative in the lives of the children living in out-of-home care. It is a complex task that requires carers and other significant adults in the life of a child to share an understanding of the way in which the internal brains and bodies of children have been changed and continue to be changed in the present by past experiences of harm and violation. It requires carers to understand their own brains and bodies and the relational space between themselves and the child. The therapeutic intent of relationships that are resourced to withstand the maelstrom of trauma-based behaviors and infused with the capacity to remain present, compassionate, consistent, non-judgmental, and congruent are the magic healing properties of therapeutic care (Caw and Sebba, 2014). It requires an investment of time and energy on the part of all the important adults in a child's life (the care team) to provide reparative and compensatory experiences, through the vehicles of their relationships that serve to counter the messages of abuse and violation, and give children hope. The care team must hold the complex needs of children in their care, provide for their feelings, and allow distress to be borne healthily. It must hold hope for their future, with the intent and aspiration for them to find a way toward a happy, productive adult life.

Transformational change is slow and can be painful. It requires dedicated and sustained support for all those who surround the child in care. This is a challenge for our carers, as well as the organizations and systems around them. The children living in out-of-home care are some of the most vulnerable in our communities. The literature is replete with the failings out-of-home care systems to meet this vulnerability and resource children's complex needs. Children need adults to not give up on them. The clarion call is clear. The experiences we offer children in care, and the enduring relationships we scaffold around them, are the architecture of changed trajectories and hopeful futures for them. We can do better. Therapeutic care is a critical step in the right direction.

KNOWLEDGE AND PRACTICE REFLECTION

Joe Tucci, Janise Mitchell, Ed Tronick and Stephen W. Porges

This chapter by Mitchell and Macnamara illustrates how a trauma-transformative frame can resource the practice of those in important roles supporting children and carers in out-of-home care. As powerfully described, the practice of therapeutic care moves well beyond a trauma-informed paradigm.

With concepts such as therapeutic intent, it actively deconstructs the delineation between trauma informed and trauma specific (SAMHSA, 2014), viewing the relationships closest to the child as active agents of therapeutic change and healing. It appreciates that all the relationships around the child can influence and reshape their inner neurosomatic states and external capacities. Cozolino, Drulis and Samuelson, in their chapter, refer to this as the 'social synapse' – the space between us.

Therapeutic care respects the developmental context of childhood and the dependency of children on the relational environments that adults offer them to shape and interpret experience, to grow, learn, and change. In doing so, healing and transformation are found in the minutiae of day-to-day, moment-by-moment exchanges between children and their significant adults. It does not exclude traditional approaches to one-to-one therapy but views them as an adjunct to what a therapeutically oriented care and support environment can achieve – the 'other 23 hours' (Trieschman *et al.*, 2002).

It holds central to its work the need for children to have a deep, visceral feeling of safety and meaning making. As Tucci, Weller and Mitchell (2018) have previously noted:

> ...children learn to tolerate the boundary of activation so that their physiology can be coaxed back into the safe zone of proximity and relational connectedness. Children come to feel themselves as being safe through their experience in relationship with a caring and protective adult. They become more open and less fixed. They use their own social engagement system to approach the adult and seek mutually satisfying interactions. They play and experience curiosity. They test the reliability of the safety being offered. They reach out and begin to hold on to safety for what it offers them. They change. They begin slowly to shed the habitual patterns of activation that have defined by their trauma-based responses to the world. Their heart opens itself to the adult's affection... (p.102)

This story was so beautifully told in the case study of John, which highlighted what Porges refers to in his chapter as the 'resilience' that John came to embody as a product of his feelings of connectedness and safety.

Similarly, this chapter elucidated the importance of meaning making with children. In his chapter, Tronick referred to meaning making – a dynamic and continuous process of making sense of 'one's self in relation to the world of people and things, and to one's own self' as a core organizing concept in therapeutic approaches. Within a therapeutic care approach, this is embraced in the slow and considered ways in which we disentangle the past from the present and thicken the coherent narratives about our lives.

Therapeutic care integrates different knowledge domains into a complex approach. Together with the science of interpersonal neurobiology, trauma, and attachment, this approach privileges the lived and living experience of children, carers, and family members as credible knowledge holders, engaging them in participatory processes that deconstruct professional authority and expertise in true collaboration. It brings to bear knowledge about compassion in the ways in which children and carers are responded to. Compassionate thinking filters into the ways that children are attended to.

Finally, it exemplifies how therapeutic intent across the system is able to create opportunities for change. It maintains the multiple needs of children, carers, practitioners, and the system, in view all the time. This approach has ways of interpreting the complexity so that it can be understood and enacted easily. It also creates different kinds of roles that have not been in existence before to support the system in implementing a trauma-transformative role. The role of therapeutic specialists and care teams highlights the importance of introducing translator/meaning-makers into a system of care so that understanding of trauma, child development, family systems, and therapeutic responses is held in view when considering how the needs of child and carer are identified and then responded to over time.

A hallmark of trauma-transformative practice is its capacity to bring together, in meaningful ways, relevant knowledge frames that can more effectively address the needs of a specific cohort, in this case children in out-of-home care. The art and science of translating and synthesizing knowledge, in all its forms and from different domains, into a process of meaning making and conceptualizing is the richness of this approach. It is relevant to acknowledge that the practice wisdom of Mitchell and Macnamara over many years is seamlessly integrated into the fabric of the conceptualization of therapeutic care. It is critical to recognize that multiple voices are necessary in the development of approaches that resource victims and survivors. Practitioner experience is important, as is implementing strategies that involve seeking input from service users. This commitment to power sharing is to be found in the trauma-informed literature. Trauma-transformative practice gives weight to how such knowledge frames are assembled, with the value base of the practitioner/researcher being uncovered for analysis if required.

References

References for chapter

Allen, J.G., Fonagy, P. and Bateman, A.W. (2008). *Mentalising in Clinical Practice*. Arlington, VA: American Psychiatric Publishing.

Anglin, J. (2003). *Pain, Normality, and the Struggle for Congruence: Reinterpreting Residential Care for Children and Youth*. London: Routledge.

Badenoch, B. (2018). *The Heart of Trauma: Healing the Embodied Brain in the Context of Relationships*. New York, NY: W.W. Norton.

Barfield, S., Dobson, C., Gaskill, R. and Perry, B.D. (2012). Neurosequential model of therapeutics in a therapeutic preschool: Implications for work with children with complex neuropsychiatric problems. *Journal of Play Therapy*, 21(1), 30–44.

Bath, H. and Seita, J. (2018). *The Three Pillars of Transforming Care: Trauma and Resilience in the Other 23hours* (Kindle ed.). The University of Winnipeg, Faculty of Education Publishing.

Blaustein, M. and Kinniburgh, K. (2010). *Treating Traumatic Stress in Children and Adolescents: How to Foster Resilience Through Attachment, Self-Regulation, and Competency*. New York, NY: Guilford Press.

Blythe, S.L., Wilkes, L. and Halcomb, E.J. (2014). The foster carer's experience: An integrative review. *Collegian*, 21(1), 21–32.

Browning, A.S. (2020). The impact of complex and unwanted feelings evoked in foster carers by traumatised children in long-term placements. *Adoption and Fostering*, 44(2), 185–196.

Caw, J. and Sebba, J. (2014). *Team Parenting for Children in Foster Care. A Model for Integrated Therapeutic Care*. London: Jessica Kingsley Publishers.

Cecil, C.A.M., Viding, E., Edward, D., Barker, E.E., Guiney, J. and McCrory, E.J. (2014). Double disadvantage: The influence of childhood maltreatment and community violence exposure on adolescent mental health. *Journal of Child Psychology and Psychiatry*, 55(7), 839–848.

Crocker, J. and Canevello, A. (2012). Consequences of self-image and compassionate goals. In P.G. Devine and A. Plant (eds), *Advances in Experimental Social Psychology* (pp.229–277). New York, NY: Elsevier.

Dana, D. (2018). *The Polyvagal Theory in Therapy Engaging the Rhythm of Regulation*. New York, NY: W.W. Norton.

Day, A., Willis, T., Vanderwill, L., Resko, S. *et al.* (2018). Key factors and characteristics of successful resource parents who care for older youth: A systematic review of research. *Children and Youth Services Review*, 84, 152–158.

de Wilde, L., Devlieghere, J., Vandenbroeck, M. and Vanobbergen, B. (2019). Foster parents between voluntarism and professionalisation: Unpacking the backpack. *Children and Youth Services Review*, 98, 290–296.

Fearon, P., Target, M., Sargent, J., Williams, L.L., *et al.* (2006). Short-Term Mentalisation and Relational Therapy (SMART): An Integrative Family Therapy for Children and Adolescents. In J.G. Allen and P. Fonagy (eds), *Handbook of Mentalisation-Based Treatment* (pp.201–222). Chichester: John Wiley and Sons.

Finkelhor, D., Ormrod, R.K. and Turner, H.A. (2007). Poly-victimisation: A neglected component in child victimisation. *Child Abuse Neglect*, 31(1), 7–26.

Fonagy, P. and Adshead, G. (2012). How mentalisation changes the mind. *Advances in Psychiatric Treatment*, 18(5), 353–362.

Fonagy, P., Gergeley, G., Jurist, E. and Target, M. (2002). *Affect Regulation, Mentalisation, and the Development of the Self*. New York, NY: Other Press.

Geiger, J.M., Hayes, M.J. and Lietz, C.A. (2013). Should I stay or should I go? A mixed methods study examining the factors influencing foster parents' decisions to continue or discontinue providing foster care. *Children and Youth Services Review*, 35, 1356–1365.

Gilbert, P. (2014). The origins and nature of compassion focused therapy. *British Journal of Clinical Psychology*, 53, 6–41.

Hobday, A (2001). Timeholes: A useful metaphor when explaining unusual or bizarre behaviour in children who have moved families. *Clinical Child Psychology and Psychiatry*, 6(1), 41–47.

Hughes, D.A. (2007). *Attachment Focused Family Therapy*. New York, NY: W.W. Norton.

Hughes, D.A. (2015). The complex journey of traumatised children: Discovering safety in order to experience comfort, joy and self-discovery. *Children Australia*, 40(2), 147–151.

Hughes, D.A. (2017). Dyadic Developmental Psychotherapy (DDP): An attachment-focused family treatment for developmental trauma. *Australian and New Zealand Journal of Family Therapy*, 38, 595–605.

Hughes, D.A. and Baylin, J. (2012). *Brain-based Parenting: The Neuroscience of Caregiving for Healthy Attachment*. New York, NY: W.W. Norton.

Keltner, D., Kogan, A., Piff, P.K. and Saturn, S.R. (2014). The sociocultural appraisals, values, and emotions (SAVE) framework of prosociality: Core processes from gene to meme. *Annual Review of Psychology*, 65, 425–460.

Leloux-Opmeer, H., Kuiper, C., Swaab, H. and Scholte, E. (2017). Children referred to foster care, family-style group care, and residential care: (how) do they differ? *Children and Youth Services Review*, 77, 1–9.

Levine, P. (2015). *Trauma and Memory. Brain and Body in a Search for the Living Past*. London: Penguin Books.

Macnamara. N. (2020). Therapeutic Care Teams: Horizontal Teams in a Virtual World. In J. Mitchell, J. Tucci and E. Tronick (eds), *The Handbook of Therapeutic Care for Children: Evidence Informed Approaches to Working with Traumatised Children and Adolescents in Foster, Kinship and Adoptive Care* (pp.219–240). London: Jessica Kingsley Publishers.

McLean, S., Kettler, L., Delfabbro, P. and Riggs, D. (2012). Frameworks for understanding challenging behaviour in out-of-home care. *Clinical Psychologist*, 16(2), 72–81.

Meadows, P., Tunstill, J., George, A., Dhudwar, A. and Kurtz, Z. (2011). *The Costs and Consequences of Child Maltreatment: Literature Review for the NSPCC*. London: NSPCC.

Mitchell, J. (2008). A case study in attempted reform in out of home care: A preliminary examination of the introduction of the Circle Therapeutic Foster Care Program in Victoria. (Unpublished Master's Thesis.) Monash University, Victoria.

Mitchell, J., Royds, K., Macnamara, N. and Bristow, G. (2020a). *Practice Guide: Client Mix and Client Matching in Therapeutic Care*. Sydney, NSW: Centre for Excellence in Therapeutic Care.

Mitchell, J., McPherson, L. and Gatwiri, K. (2020b). 'Support and Love and All That Stuff': Evidence of Impact in the Treatment and Care for Kids Program. In J. Mitchell, J. Tucci and E. Tronick (eds), *The Handbook of Therapeutic Care for Children: Evidence-Informed Approaches to Working with Traumatised Children and Adolescents in Foster, Kinship and Adoptive Care* (pp.109–134). London: Jessica Kingsley Publishers.

Murray, L., Tarren-Sweeney, M. and France, K. (2011). Foster carer perceptions of support and training in the context of high burden of care. *Child and Family Social Work*, 16, 149–158.

Neff, K. (2003). The development and validation of a scale to measure self-compassion. *Self and Identity*, 2, 223–250.

NICE (2015). *Children's Attachment: Attachment in Children and Young People Who Are Adopted from Care, in Care or at High Risk of Going into Care*. NICE Guideline, No. 26. National Collaborating Centre for Mental Health (UK). London: National Institute for Health and Care Excellence (NICE).

Octoman, O. and McLean, S. (2014). Challenging behaviour in foster care: What supports do foster carers want? *Adoption and Fostering*, 38, 149–158.

Ogden, P., Pain, C. and Fisher, J. (2006). A sensorimotor approach to the treatment of trauma and dissociation. *The Psychiatric Clinics of North America*, 29, 263–279.

Oosterman, M., Schuengel, C., Wim Slot, N., Bullens, R.A.R. and Doreleijers, T.A.H. (2007). Disruptions in foster care: A review and meta-analysis. *Children and Youth Services Review*, 29(1), 53–76.

Perry, B.D. (2004) *Understanding Traumatised and Maltreated Children*. The Child Trauma Academy. www.childtrauma.org.

Porges S.W. (1995). Orienting in a defensive world: Mammalian modifications of our evolutionary heritage. A Polyvagal Theory. *Psychophysiology*, 32, 301–318.

Porges, S.W. (2004). Neuroception: A subconscious system for detecting threats and safety. *Zero to Three*, 24, 5, 19–24.

Porges, S.W. (2011). *The Polyvagal Theory: Neurophysiological Foundations of Emotions, Attachment, Communication, and Self-Regulation*. New York, NY: W.W. Norton and Company.

Porges, S.W. (2015). Making the world safe for our children: Down-regulating defence and up-regulating social engagement to 'optimise' the human experience. *Children Australia*, 40(2), 114–123.

Porges, S.W. (2017). Vagal Pathways: Portals to Compassion. In E.M. Seppala, E. Simon-Thomas, S.L. Brown, M.C. Worline, C.D. Cameron and J.R. Doty (eds), *Oxford Handbook of Compassion Science* (pp.189–202). New York, NY: Oxford University Press.

Randle, M., Ernst, D., Leisch, F. and Dolnicar, S. (2016). What makes foster carers think about quitting? Recommendations for improved retention of foster carers. *Child and Family Social Work*, 22, 1175–1186.

Riggs, D., Delfabbro, P. and Augoustinos, M. (2009). Negotiating foster families: Identification and desire. *British Journal of Social Work*, 39, 789–806.

Rock, D. (2008). SCARF: A brain-based model for collaborating with and influencing others. *NeuroLeadership Journal*, 1(1), 44–52.

Siegel, D.J. (1999). *The Developing Mind: Toward a Neurobiology of Interpersonal Experience*. New York, NY: Guilford Press.

Siegel, D.J. (2012). *The Developing Mind: How Relationships and the Brain Interact to Shape Who We Are* (second edition). New York, NY: Guilford Press.

Siegel, D.J. (2016). *Mind: A Journey to the Heart of Being Human*. New York, NY: WW Norton & Company.

Seppälä, E., Rossomando, T. and Doty, J.R. (2012). Social connection and compassion: Important predictors of health and well-being. *Social Research*, 80, 411–430.

Shonkoff, J.P., Garner, A.S., Committee on Psychosocial Aspects of Child and Family Health, Committee on Early Childhood, Adoption, and Dependent Care *et al.* (2012). The lifelong effects of early childhood adversity and toxic stress. *Pediatrics*, 129(1), 232–246.

Smith, M. (2005). *Working in the 'Lifespace'*. In Residence, 2. Glasgow: Scottish Institute for Residential Child Care.

Streeck-Fischer, A. and van der Kolk, B. (2000). Down will come baby, cradle and all: Diagnostic and therapeutic implications of chronic trauma on child development. *Australian and New Zealand Journal of Psychiatry*, 34, 903–918.

Sweeney, A. Clement, S. and Filson, K.A. (2016). Trauma-informed mental healthcare in the UK: What is it and how can we further its development? *Mental Health Review Journal*, 21(3), 174–192.

Taylor, C. (2012). *Empathic Care for Children with Disorganized Attachments. A Model for Mentalising, Attachment and Trauma-informed Care*. London: Jessica Kingsley Publishers.

Taylor, L. (2005). Theoretical Perspectives. In M. Smith, B. Forrest, P. Garland and L. Hunter (eds), *Secure in the Knowledge: Perspectives on Practice in Secure Accommodation*. Glasgow: CELCIS.

Teicher, M.H., Samson, C.J., Anderson, C.M. and Ohashi, B. (2016). The effects of childhood maltreatment on brain structure, function and connectivity. *Nature Reviews Neuroscience*, 17(10), 652–666.

Torrenon, M. (2006). Community in a children's home. *Child and Family Social Work*, 11(2), 129–137.

Tucci, J. and Mitchell, J. (2019). Therapeutic Services for Traumatised Children and Young People Healing. In R. Benjamin, J. Haliburn and S. King (eds), *Humanising Mental Health Care in Australia: A Guide to Trauma-informed Approaches* (pp.319–320). London: Routledge.

Tucci, J., Mitchell, J. and Macnamara, N. (2020). What are the Key Elements of Therapeutic Care? In J. Mitchell, J. Tucci and E. Tronick (eds), *The Handbook of Therapeutic Care for Children: Evidence-Informed Approaches to Working with Traumatised Children and Adolescents in Foster, Kinship and Adoptive Care* (pp.35–58). London: Jessica Kingsley Publishers.

Tullberg, E., Vaughon, W., Muradwij, N. and Kerkera, B. (2019). Unpacking 'support': Understanding the complex needs of therapeutic foster parents. *Child and Youth Services Review*, 105, 104420.

van der Kolk, B.A., McFarlane, A.C. and Weisaeth, L. (2015). *Traumatic Stress – The Effects of Overwhelming Experience on Mind, Body and Society*. New York, NY: Guilford Press.

Ward, A. (2006). *Working in Group Care: Social Work and Social Care in Residential and Day Care Settings*. Bristol: Policy Press.

Winnicott, D.W. (1974). Primitive Emotional Development. In D.W. Winnicott (ed.), *Through Paediatrics to Psychoanalysis* (pp.145–156). London: Karnac Books.

References for Knowledge and Practice Reflection

Substance Abuse and Mental Health Services Administration (SAMHSA) (2014). *Trauma-informed Care in Behavioural Health Services – Treatment Improvement Protocol (TIP) Series 57* (HHS Publication no. (SMA 13-4801).

Trieschman, A., Whittaker, J. and Brendtro, L. (2002). *The Other 23 Hours: Child-care Work with Emotionally Disturbed Children in a Therapeutic Milieu*. New York, NY: Transaction Publishers.

Tucci, J., Weller, A. and Mitchell, J. (2018). Realising 'Deep' Safety for Children Who Have Experienced Abuse: Application of Polyvagal Theory in Therapeutic Work with Traumatised Children and Young People. In S.W. Porges and D. Dana (eds), *Clinical Applications of the Polyvagal Theory: The Emergence of Polyvagal-Informed Therapies* (pp.89–105). New York, NY: W.W. Norton and Company.

CHAPTER 17

Strengthening Community Capacity to End Interpersonal Violence: A Trauma-Transformative Application

Joe Tucci and Janise Mitchell

Introduction

For more than a decade now, there has been increasing awareness of the scale and nature of family violence in Australia. It is estimated that one in six women have experienced physical or sexual violence by a current or former partner, while for men it is one in 16. Seventy five percent of victims of domestic violence reported the perpetrator as male, while 25 per cent reported the perpetrator as female. On average, one woman every nine days and one man every month is killed by a current or former partner (Australian Institute of Health and Welfare, 2019).

Family and domestic violence is the main reason women and children are being forced to leave their homes in Australia (Australian Institute of Health and Welfare, 2022). Almost half of those received support from Specialist Homelessness Services were women and children escaping family violence (Australian Institute of Health and Welfare, 2022). A child or children were present at 29.8 per cent or 26,284 family violence incidents occurring in the state of Victoria alone between July 2019 and June 2020 (Crime Statistics Agency Victoria, 2022). Approximately 2.5 million Australian adults (13%) experienced abuse during their childhood; the majority knew the perpetrator and experienced multiple incidents of abuse (Australian Bureau of Statistics, 2017).

In the opening to her 2002 book, *Trauma Trails, Recreating Song Lines: The Intergenerational Effects of Trauma in Indigenous Australia*, Professor Judy Atkinson defines violence as:

> ...unjust force, actions or words used, without informed consent, to intimidate or harm; actions that are irreverent or disrespectful of another or others, and that are used, consciously or unconsciously, to obtain power

over another or others, causing pain to the whole person (body/mind/soul/ spirit)... (p.ii)

She argues that violence is both an activity and an experience. Atkinson uses the word experience to:

...acknowledge that a person (including a child) who is violated in an act of violence experiences violence; that a person who commits an act of violence experiences violence; and that a person who sees or hears violence experiences violence... (p.11)

Using these definitions, acts of violence are experienced by many individuals. The impacts of violence are also experienced by many individuals.

While violence occurs between people who are not in any form of prior relationships, family violence is specific to that which is experienced within families, intimate relationships, extended families, kinship networks and communities. Applying this understanding in smaller communities, violence and family violence is often one and the same set of experiences. The impact of such violence not only affects the individuals, but it serves to destabilize, harm and destroy the relationships that exist between people in that community.

The trauma of violence is remembered with pain and loss. For many people, it is not only the violence of the present, but there is an inextricable connection to the violation of the past. This is particularly the case for First Nations peoples who carry with them the deep hurt of historical and ongoing colonization. Violence interrupts the future as well. Parents and grandparents worry for their children who are exposed to violence early in their lives. The hopes of a community can become diluted as they face the day-to-day moments in which disrespect, abuse and violation are present.

Trust, compassion and belonging are undermined by violence. Relationships become in themselves the sites of tension and distress. In the face of violence, it appears that there is little strength and comfort to be found. The resources available in individuals and in relationships with which violence can be resisted become increasingly difficult to locate. This is how violence takes hold in the community and stays. It replicates itself by rendering invisible and inaudible the actions and words of those in the community who challenge its presence, its arguments and its persuasiveness.

This does not mean that such opposition evaporates. It remains but becomes less available. It requires unearthing, amplifying and collectivizing.

However, just as acts of violence are experienced by many individuals in the community, acts of resistance come to be experienced by many individuals in the community (White and Epston, 1990; Epston and White, 1992; White, 2006; Reynolds, 2010).

The key to strengthening community capacity to end violence is the respectful and patient engagement of those living and working in that community in dialogue that seeks to understand the tactics of violence, names its effects in the lives of the individuals who live in the community, and validates the acts of resistance already being enacted in the community.

The aim of this chapter is to highlight how a trauma-transformative model can operate as a framework for action. It draws on our work as child abuse and violence prevention practitioner/researchers over the last 30 years. We have worked alongside over a hundred organizations and communities to evolve a way of approaching the task of enhancing individual, community and systemic capability to end interpersonal violence, with a specific focus on reducing the prevalence of child abuse. We have named it *trauma-transformative practice* because it brings together our knowledge of trauma, community development and narrative and justice-based models of practice. In this sense, it has always been a step beyond trauma informed, seeking to integrate a range of knowledge sources so that it is applicable to local contexts and local needs.

As we head into the text in more detail, we would like to acknowledge and express our appreciation to all of our service and community partners over this period who have helped us to refine our thinking and given us the support to pursue what seems to be an unattainable ambition. They have offered the realization that violence does not arrive overnight into a community. It builds over time, standing on the foundations built by racism, gender inequality, discrimination, and violation of basic human rights. In response, it takes time to uncover how all of these dynamics have eroded the qualities of love, care and respect in a community. As we find those again and connect to the significance of their presence, we find the ways that violence has been resisted and its effects challenged. This is the core of efforts to prevent violence. Understanding trauma so that it is blended into models of community resilience makes the process transformative.

This chapter traces the knowledge analyses that rest behind the evolution of the model, then gives a description of it and a tentative example of how it can be applied in reality.

How have we understood how violence occurs in communities and how is it challenged?

It is essential that we listen to the people who live and work in communities, and hear their experiences of violence. Over the years, we have heard a number of significant themes that we have summarized below:

- Violence is an expression of power from those who are privileged by it over those who are subjugated by it.

- Ongoing acts of racism, sexism, subjugation, discrimination and colonization have served to undermine ways of knowing and showing respect, trust and mutual care. It has damaged, but not totally destroyed, people's experience of interdependence and the importance of connections that individuals have to family, community, culture and place or country.
- It is critical to develop and hold complex frameworks of understanding that acknowledge the intersection between acts of oppression and gendered acts of violence which continue to shape the experiences of all people in communities.
- Violence can take over families and communities to the point that it feels so overwhelming for individuals that ways to challenge it or address it seem non-existent.
- There are individuals and groups in the community who oppose the violence and want it to end.
- There is a great deal of agreement that violence affects children and young people significantly. This unanimous view has led to an increasing degree of concern and worry for children and young people. There is a strong desire to end violence in the community, particularly for the sake of children and young people.
- The power to name violence, its causes and its effects is important in supporting a community's commitment and capacity to address violence. Communities will come together around words and ideas that hold meanings about safety and protection when they are relevant to them.
- Acknowledging and tracing the lines of trauma, past and present, is a significant consideration for understanding the ways in which violence emerges, continues and affects the lives of individuals, families and communities. There is always the need to appreciate how much trauma and loss shapes the everyday experience of people.
- Meaningful actions to address violence in the community will come as individuals realize the ways in which they are already prioritizing safety in the face of violence. This knowledge will give them hope that change is already occurring. It will also open the possibility to enlist others into their own efforts. This will lead to collective action that will influence individual behaviour.
- Every community has leaders who are able to demonstrate that violence can be stopped.
- Symbolism is important to help communities see that attitudes and behaviour which condone violence can and are changing.
- The voices of women, men, children and young people are all important in addressing violence.
- Violence in the community is a problem that can be changed.

Strategies to end violence will not work if they are imposed in the community. The most effective strategies are those which can amplify, extend and resource acts of resistance to violence that are already being enacted by individuals in the community. Working alongside the community will facilitate dialogue which unearths the changes that communities are already making and indeed wanting to make more of. Such acts of resistance are sourced in the experiences of community action, community rituals and community narratives. It is the strength of connection to these community aspects and often, cultural qualities that are pivotal to ending violence in the community.

How have we understood how to work with a community's own efforts to resist and challenge violence?

There are a number of models of practice that reflect a commitment to working with individuals, families and communities in ways that support their own efforts to resist and challenge the pervasiveness of violence itself and its effects. At the forefront of contemporary approaches are those that find their traditions in the postmodern constructs of power and oppression, such as narrative therapy (White and Epston, 1990; Epston and White, 1992) and justice-based community work (Reynolds, 2010, 2013).

> No-one is a passive recipient of trauma. People always take steps in endeavouring to prevent the trauma they are subject to, and, when preventing this trauma is clearly impossible, they take steps to try and modify it in some way or modify its effects on their lives. These steps contribute to the preservation of, and are founded upon, what people hold precious. Even in the face of overwhelming trauma, people take steps to try to protect and preserve what they give value to... (White, 2006, p.28)

Drawing on his collaborative work with David Epston, Michael White articulated an approach to working therapeutically with individuals, families and communities that sought to honour even the smallest actions that people take to keep themselves and others safe in the face of violence. White sought to deeply listen for the two stories of people's experiences of violence – the story of trauma and the story of struggle to hold onto conviction, belief, hope and value. As people reconnect with the story that preserved them, their family and their community, they come to see themselves with intent and power, rather than at the mercy of violence (White, 2006).

This is an approach that is also mirrored in the works of Vikki Reynolds (2010, 2013), Johnella Bird (2002) and the Just Therapy Centre (Waldegrave et al., 2003; Waldegrave, 2012) and sourced in the early writings of Freire

(1972), Foucault (1972, 1977), Gergen (1985, 1991) and Laing (1967), among others.

For example, Freire (1972) argued that the oppressed cannot be liberated by education because education has been used as an instrument of oppression as 'an act of depositing knowledge, in which the students are the depositories and the teacher is the depositor' (p.45).

Education in this sense is not as much of an act of empowerment as it is purported to be. Instead, it serves to change the consciousness of the oppressed so that they come to accept their position as deviant, incompetent and a source of difficulty for the rest of society who are defined as good, organized and just. The helper cannot dominate the helped according to Freire (1972). Authentic help occurs when 'all who are involved help each other mutually, growing together in the common effort to understand the reality which they seek to transform' (p.8).

At its core, this narrative and justice-based pedagogical way of working with individuals, families and communities adopts a critical lens for understanding the genesis of individually experienced problems. It locates the experiences of individuals in the histories and continued practices of oppression that construct identities which perpetuate the use and abuse of power by those who have it over those who do not. The focus of this approach is to uncover the layers of language and entrenched beliefs that normalize pathology, victimhood and blaming.

Practitioners using this approach work alongside those they seek to support. They do not seek to empower them, as empowerment itself mirrors the actions of the privileged in their self-defined efforts to help those in need. In contrast, practitioners work to engage individuals, groups and communities in critical and sensitive dialogue which makes visible the pervasive social and historical discourses that limit the definitions of what is deemed as true and untrue, real and not real, worthy and not worthy. Freire defines such processes as a form of praxis – liberating through reflective conversations and consideration.

These are the practice elements which emanate from a narrative approach:

- *Externalizing conversations:* These are conversations that involve talking about problems as problems rather than people as problems. It decouples the pathology from the person and relocates the source of the problem to the social and historical contexts that have led to the problem being experienced. The outcomes of such externalizing processes, according to White (1988):
  - decrease conflict between people over who is responsible for the problem

- reduce the sense of failure people have in response to not having solved the problem
- unite people against the problem rather than against each other
- open the way for people to reclaim their lives from problems
- liberate people to view the problem in new ways.

- *Deconstructing dominant narratives to co-develop alternative stories:* As individuals engage in externalizing conversations, they become more aware of the strategies used by discourses of power to align their identities with the problems they experience. These dominant narratives hide the actions and intentions that individuals take to not succumb to the totalizing effects of the social conditions which led to the problems in the first place. They gradually access this differentiated story about themselves, which opens them up to experience themselves as separate to those practices of oppression. An alternative story, one that has always been there, takes over as the preferred way of living.

- *Outside witnessing:* White (1999) used outsider witnessing processes in the form of reflecting teams to underscore the significance of an individual's emerging alternative narrative. The reflecting team or groups of community members supported and inquired about the ways in which an individual was able to maintain a commitment to their ambitions for their life in the face of their experiences of the problem. This enabled acts of resistance to be amplified and experienced as more resonant and congruent in the life of the individual.

The work of Vikki Reynolds (2010) represents a contemporary re-imagining of these concepts into a framework that moves community work from identifying and connecting to acts of personal resistance to working with communities in practices of collective solidarity. For Reynolds, her 'Doing Justice' framework revolves around engaging in dialogue as a transformative practice with communities. It involves the following six guiding principles:

1. *Centering ethics:* It is important for community workers to actively adopt ethical positions that are consistent with their own lived experiences and connect with the lived experiences of the people they work with. As part of this ethical stance, workers accept the task to actively change the real conditions of people's lives created by the historical and current discourses of power rather than helping them to adjust to oppression.

2. *Doing solidarity:* Solidarity is part of and derived from the interconnectedness of the struggles towards achieving social justice and the outcomes that are possible from the collective experiences of strength, hope and sustainability. It is based on finding and engaging

with moments of affinity or interpersonal experiences of connection that transform the lives of people in the community and the workers themselves. It recognizes that different forms of oppression exist in the lives of people and that such difference creates opportunities for people to be united in collective practices of resistance. Solidarity arises from experiences of community-making dialogue resourced by workers and the community together.

3. *Addressing power:* There are multiple practices with which Reynolds addresses power, including witnessing resistance, examining the influence of discourses, and addressing identities made possible by power. They all recognize that acts of resistance are spontaneous and occur in the moment that oppression occurs. They require complex analysis of the themes associated with abuse and violation.

4. *Fostering collective sustainability:* This involves practices that connect workers, maintaining a commitment to hope and change. It avoids cynicism and builds sustainability of efforts among community workers within an organization and between workers from a range of organizations. It also connects workers with the optimism in their communities, which is often diminished because of experiences of violence and oppression.

5. *Critically engaging with language:* This principle highlights the centrality of language in shaping and reshaping the scope of the dialogue. Change leaders listen deeply to the language of their community, highlighting phrases, specific constructs and metaphors as the basis of transformative dialogue. It also recognizes that language includes the many forms that communities find to communicate what is important to them, including song, music, art, dance and other forms of performances. It is the symbolism of the relatedness that is the vehicle through which change is resourced and experienced.

6. *Structuring safety:* Safety is co-created in relationships. It is a prerequisite for community work based on practices of solidarity. It includes co-creating collaborative agreements, creating opportunities to maintain dignity, being prepared to learn from the people in the community, and building coalitions of allies that are sustained over time.

Why is it important to understand how to enhance community resilience?

There has been growing interest in re-conceptualizing resilience. Instead of it being understood as how easily an individual can bounce back from adversity, resilience is now seen as a dynamic process of adjustment, adaptation and transformation of communities in response to challenges and demands.

In particular, research points to the influence on the level of community resilience of:

> ...stories of identity and transformation at a personal and collective level. The idea that resilience might reside in the ways we have of narrating our lives...making sense of their own predicaments and mapping possibilities for adaptation and a positive vision of the identity and future prospects by drawing on collective history, myths and sacred teachings. At the same time, these collective forms of narratives serve not only to help people make sense of their experience and construct a valued identity but also ensure the continuity and vitality of a community or a people... (Kirmayer *et al.*, 2011, p.86)

In other words, strategies which aim to strengthen resilience focus on finding shared meaning across different members of a community about what has helped that community to survive and attempt to hold on to its values, beliefs, rituals and relationships, often in the face of overwhelming forces that have sought to destroy them. The modality used is collective dialogue. Its purpose is to unearth symbolic and historical practices that have maintained people's connection to their cultural heritage. It is this common quality that is viewed as being the most significant factor in moving a community along a continuum from oppression to resistance to resilience. In the past five years, there has been growing interest in re-conceptualizing resilience so that it can be applied relevantly to First Nations communities.

The capacity of stories to act as feedback speak to the *transformability* of a community which:

> ...refers to collective capacities to create a fundamentally new system when ecological, economic, or social conditions make the existing system untenable. In other words, external forces of change can provide windows of opportunity to transform systems... the notion of social memory, as a crucial transitional element, is significant here. It may lead to a learning and adjustment phase based on past experiences... (Vaneeckhaute *et al.*, 2017, p.74)

This shared and communal construct of resilience offers an antidote to the collective experience of trauma that occurs as a result of violence which ripples through a community. The honouring of social narratives of resistance engages specifically with the ways that communities can find interdependent qualities of courage to use against violence and abuse.

Why is it important to understand trauma and its consequences?

Trauma knowledge is critical because it highlights the ways in which the ongoing reverberations of violence affect the lives of those living in communities, both individually and collectively. Trauma keeps memories of pain and hurt alive. It promotes postures of defensiveness. It keeps individuals and networks of individuals tuned into and constantly vigilant for possible signs of danger. It supports reactivity and degrades ways of solution building. Trauma is the long tail of violation that keeps snaking through the community, silently affecting it.

It is an experience in the here and now, often taking the form of patterns of behaviour that aim to protect individuals from threat that are present in real time or emerge from memories of their past.

Trauma shapes the belief systems of individuals and groups affected by it. It forces them to be vigilant and constantly scan their environment for any small indicator that they will be hurt again. It reinforces that risk is at every turn in life. It stops them from being able to settle and engage in safety. And time is needed to make sure that perceptions of unpredictability and change do not increase their ongoing sense of unease and peril.

For many who experienced trauma in childhood, it leaves behind a set of developmental needs that stay unmet and tend to act as self-organizing themes in their lives as they grow. If they felt pain at the time of the trauma, they will need comfort, seeking it out in relationships around them. If their violation was invisible, they need validation, seeking it in all areas of their life. If they felt responsible for the violence, their shame separates and isolates them from the support and care that they need. If they were separated from loved ones, the fear of it happening again will haunt them in ways that they do not even understand.

Trauma affects the approaches that individuals use to adapt to their context. They are often reactive to small changes which they perceive may lead to an increase in risk of further terror and fear. They are not able to easily problem solve or apply strategies that have been helpful in the past into new situations. They run on instinctive behavioural routines that serve to keep them stuck following ineffective practices of care and self-care. Often, individuals can isolate themselves from others as a way of making themselves feel less frightened and more in control. While this may work in the short term, in the long term, it reduces the network of support that is needed by everyone at some point.

Where trauma is left unresolved, people can begin to internalize a toxic sense of responsibility for causing their own pain and, in more severe and sustained cases, whole communities can begin to think that suffering and chaos are normal.

Trauma is healed through the experience of relationships which are nurturing, predictable and safe over time. It is important to have a deep appreciation for the impact of trauma in the lives of the individuals, families and communities that practitioners work alongside and with. Trauma requires a specific kind of understanding that is sensitive not only to the current needs of people, but also to the needs they bring with them from their past. It is an orientation to the way that relationships are formed, oriented and maintained.

In our trauma-transformative model, practitioners not only understand trauma themselves, but they also work to ensure that this knowledge base is used by other workers and community members in the ways they interact with each other over time.

What are the principles underlying the model?

We work alongside communities to identify and amplify individual and collective efforts to end violence.

Strategies to end violence will not work if they are imposed in the community. The most effective strategies are those which can amplify, extend and resource acts of resistance to violence that are already being enacted by individuals in the community. Working alongside the community will facilitate dialogue which reveals the changes that communities are already making and indeed wanting to make more of. Such acts of resistance can be sourced in experiences of culture and its expression in forms of ceremony, origin stories, healing practices, spiritual beliefs and values. It is the strength of connection to these community and cultural qualities that has been identified as pivotal in consolidating community resilience.

We believe that efforts to end violence in a community will be led by individuals or groups who hold a strong intent to galvanize a collective focus.

Ending violence in the community will occur when it is supported and championed by an individual and/or group who will act to lead the change. These are community advocates who are interspersed in the community itself. They are from the community and are positioned as leaders. There must be specific strategies aimed at building their capacity, confidence and skills to influence the hearts and minds of the community. These individuals and/or groups should receive direct support from services so that they can galvanize the community to take stands against the tactics of violence.

We believe that violence adds toxic levels of stress to the lives of children, young people and adults.

Stress is the common feature of all experiences of interpersonal violence. Toxic and high impact levels of stress have significant effects on the functioning of individuals, families and the community as a whole. Such stress can make it increasingly difficult for individuals to learn and adapt to new environments and challenges. Its experience is pervasive and cumulative. It limits the capacity of children, young people and adults to form and maintain positive networks of relationships that are based on trust and understanding. The longer that children, young people and adults are exposed to high impact and toxic levels of stress, the more entrenched are their behavioural routines aiming to avoid its effects. These patterns of interacting and being can become increasingly difficult to change with time.

We believe that the effects of trauma must be recognized in order for communities to be able to engage in strategies which aim to end violence.

It is clear that often even engaging in the topic of violence will activate arousal systems in individuals, families and communities who have experienced violence previously. In these states, it is less likely for individuals to be able to examine the topic, consider its impact and seek to implement changes aimed at addressing violence. As such, the explicit creation of emotional, physical and cultural comfort and security is a prerequisite prior to any form of collective dialogue.

We believe in the importance of creating emotional, physical and culturally strong and secure places and relationships in all our work.

Safety is critical to transformation. Culturally, relationally and personally safe spaces are paramount during the difficult process of healing and change. These are places to reclaim history, find fragmented and lost stories, and talk about a painful past. It must be devoid of physical harm to property, oneself and others. When in a safe place, a person can commit to and participate in the making of behavioural rules. In this state, they are more likely to be able to identify elements of their culture or worldview that can act as resources to resisting forms of violation.

We understand that safety is also co-created in relationships. We help establish safety with community by letting people know that we are committed to:

- keeping everyone safe from violence. We will always act to stop violence if it is occurring or at risk of occurring
- being respectful in our interactions at all times
- being informed about and abiding by their cultural norms and expectations
- conveying a sense of collaborative effort

- supporting them to keep their environment predictable and consistent
- spending consistent time in the community.

We understand enough about the effects of toxic and high-impact stress that we can tailor our communication with people in the community in ways that acknowledge and consider how their experiences of violence influence their responses to our work.

We will always work towards co-creating collaborative agreements, creating opportunities to maintain dignity, being prepared to learn from the people in the community, and building coalitions of allies that are sustained over time.

We believe that active collective dialogue with and by the community is the way to work to end violence.

A community has a range of pre-existing sets of naturally forming groups with shared interests. Effective strategies to end violence will identify and work with each of these groups methodically. The process of engaging these groups starts with being invited. The practitioner or change champion must learn the norms and rules of each group. They will need to be prepared to offer some form of resource to that group as a symbol for acknowledging its willingness to open itself up to someone external to it. Beginning with a need in the group, the practitioner engages in dialogue about community resilience, the impact of violence, and actions which have been taken to end violence. This collective process of sharing stories of understanding leads to potential meanings that can be used as starting points for further conversations with other groups in the community, each following a similar protocol. As concurrent dialogues occur, collaborative meanings about ways to resist violence can be shared, with permission, across the community.

We believe that focusing on the impact of violence on children and young people is likely to be the best point to start dialogue about ending violence in the community.

Coming to realize the extent to which violence can affect the development and functioning of children and young people is often a powerful motivator for adults to want to take action to end violence. Children come to hold an important position in families and communities. They offer a sense of continuity. They reflect conditions of love and care – qualities that everyone in a community needs. They provide the basis on which the community can think about itself into the future. For these reasons, their importance in the life of a family and community is critical. The narratives about childhood in culture and community communicate the need to protect and keep children safe.

We believe in using strengths-based models that aim to enhance individual capability and community resilience.

Strengths-based models of intervention have been shown to be replicable and effective in supporting adults experiencing disadvantage to change. A strengths-based approach enables people to take control of their lives in meaningful and sustainable ways. Its aims are to:

- empower people to take a lead in their own care process
- work in collaborative ways on mutually agreed on goals
- draw on the personal resources of motivation and hope
- create sustainable change through learning and experiential growth.

A strengths approach is a specific method of working with and resolving areas of concern experienced by individuals. It does not attempt to ignore the problems and difficulties. Rather, it attempts to identify the positive resources available to individuals (or what may need to be added) as the basis for addressing the challenges resulting from the problems. Specifically, a strengths-based model:

- seeks to understand and support the important variables contributing to individual and family/community capability
- provides a common language that does not further disadvantage people by ascribing them as causes to the problems they experience
- works to ensure that strategies are driven by the community
- engages distressed people with respect and understanding
- perceives capacity building as a dynamic process that evolves over a lifetime
- affirms the reparative potential in people
- aims to enhance strengths as opposed to deficits.

We believe that all of our work should strengthen family relationships and/or build networks of sustainable support.

Family relationships represent a significant source of support for children, young people and adults. In the formative years, families provide young people with experiences of interdependence as the precursor to independence. They allow young people the opportunity to adapt to increasingly challenging tasks associated with caring for themselves and engaging in their community with greater responsibilities. Interventions are effective when they include a component aimed at strengthening family relationships, helping them to be sources of comfort and understanding and templates for interpersonal resolution.

We believe in the importance of collaboration with each other and other services.

The most effective responses occur when practitioners take responsibility to sustainably build coalitions of mutual respect with others who live and work in communities. We invest in establishing trust, transparency and accountability as important qualities of networks of practitioners who are working together to support community. We coordinate our effort so resources are applied efficiently and effectively. We work with others by respecting differences in approach to enable networks to hold their unique relationships in the community but not jeopardize the overall outcomes being achieved collectively.

We believe that cycles of violence will end when they are replaced by cycles of mutual care, respect and resilience.

We understand that violence is likely to come to an end when people in the community feel valued by each other, their needs understood and met and they feel trusting and trustworthy. The interdependence of family and community life is respected and celebrated. Relationships are experienced as harmonious. Conflict can be addressed without it escalating to violence. Stress is experienced positively and is tolerable. In these circumstances, individuals and the community as a whole are more adaptive and hopeful. There is a sense of the future that it is building. Its sense of humour is available and actively experienced.

What is our model?

Our model aims to strengthen community capacity to end violence and consists of 11 stages of actions and strategies. It is presented as sequential in nature. But in reality, it is not. In real life in the community, the path to transformation is far from linear. It is more likely to double back on itself and be repeated as different forms of challenge and stress are experienced at times. However, it is important to note that momentum towards trans-formation cannot skip a step or fast forward. Sustained change occurs when those who live and work in the community keep going – striving towards resolution.

The 11 stages are presented in Figure 17.1. Each of the stages is explained in more detail in the content that follows it.

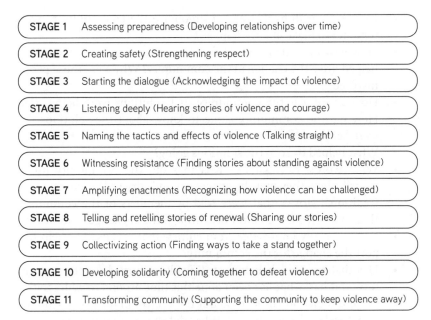

STAGE 1	Assessing preparedness (Developing relationships over time)
STAGE 2	Creating safety (Strengthening respect)
STAGE 3	Starting the dialogue (Acknowledging the impact of violence)
STAGE 4	Listening deeply (Hearing stories of violence and courage)
STAGE 5	Naming the tactics and effects of violence (Talking straight)
STAGE 6	Witnessing resistance (Finding stories about standing against violence)
STAGE 7	Amplifying enactments (Recognizing how violence can be challenged)
STAGE 8	Telling and retelling stories of renewal (Sharing our stories)
STAGE 9	Collectivizing action (Finding ways to take a stand together)
STAGE 10	Developing solidarity (Coming together to defeat violence)
STAGE 11	Transforming community (Supporting the community to keep violence away)

Figure 17.1: Strengthening community capacity to end violence.

Stage 1. Assessing preparedness

The first stage is to evaluate the community's preparedness to end violence. It is based on practitioners creating positive sets of relationships with people across a community over time. A partnership approach reflects a respect for collective self-determination and being responsive to community needs and aspirations. Developing an effective partnership takes time, trust and personal relationships.

Assessing preparedness is an informal process of consultation and gathering stories, which starts broadly and becomes more specific with time. Using a strengths-based approach, workers focus their interest on talking to different members of the community about what has helped them individually, as families and as a community to face and withstand challenges or difficulties in a broad sense.

In these discussions, practitioners help to identify challenges which were resolved positively and adopted by the community as a whole. Specifically, practitioners are seeking to understand the following:

- How was the challenge first identified by the community? Who was involved? How did the conversations first start?
- What attempts to address the challenge have been made?
- How were the solutions to the challenges generated? Were any of the solutions already occurring even before the challenge was identified as requiring action?

- How easy or difficult was it to mobilize the community to work together to make change happen?
- How easy or difficult was it for the solutions to be applied? Who helped drive the change in the community? Why were those people involved?
- How aware was the community that solutions were being tried? How did the community come to know about the solutions that were being tried?
- What helped to keep the solutions going?
- What words, expressions or sayings did the community use to describe how they met the challenges and survived? Were there any traditional stories that were told by members of the community that supported the community through the challenge or difficulty?
- Was there any knowledge from culture that was used to help support the change for the community?
- Has that specific challenge or difficulty returned for the community? If it has, what has been done this time around to address it?
- What did individuals learn about themselves in relation to the way they tackled that challenge? What did the community learn about itself in the way it addressed the challenge? What part of the solution could be used again for a different type of problem?
- What part of the solution was connected to the community's culture? Were there any rituals, ceremonies, traditional practices that helped to formulate and implement the solutions to this challenge? If there were, how important were these elements to the effectiveness of the solutions?

The answers to these questions help the practitioner understand the strengths inherent in the community to identify and design solutions, work together and be effective in achieving and maintaining change. As far as possible, strategies that have worked in the past from the community's perspective for other challenges or difficulties should form the basis for developing strategies that address violence specifically.

Importantly, practitioners should also inform themselves about the level of violence that is experienced in the community. This includes identifying:

- the frequency of the different types of violence that are committed
- who is committing the violence
- who are the targets of the violence
- the conditions in which the violence emerges.

Information should also be gathered about the quality of the service response to violence from police and other services in the community. This is critical in understanding the extent to which safety in the community can be assumed at the initial stage of this work.

This is all intelligence that can be used by practitioners to plan the next stage strategies aimed at ending violence.

Stage 2. Creating safety

Creating safety is an essential platform to forms of practice which have at their core the prevention of interpersonal violence in the community.

Ending violence in the community starts with practices that take into account how such violence, over time from multiple sources, has affected the capacity of the relationships within communities to address its consequences. This is an important consideration as it acknowledges the following concerns that will need to be addressed through the implementation of careful and planned activity in the subsequent stages of this process:

- The patterns of behaviour associated with the trauma of past violence will be triggered again in individuals in response to cues in relationships which have led to the violence occurring in the first place. These are cycles of helplessness that individuals and/or the community will not feel can easily be interrupted.
- While many topics can be raised in the community for discussion, those related to violence have in themselves references of loss, pain and tension which are likely to be re-experienced by individuals in their relationships in an ongoing way. Their ability to remain cognitively capable to logically work though these issues will be limited.
- Discussion about violence will activate arousal systems in children, adults and the whole of the community. These heightened states may in themselves trigger subsequent rounds of violent behaviour.
- Different people in the community will have different reactions to past effects of violence related trauma. Those who are able to tolerate their reactions will need to be supported to engage others in relationships that help mediate the emotional and psychological impacts of discussing strategies to end violence. Establishing or supporting groups with ways of understanding the impact of trauma will provide a sustainable base for the additional layered strategies that will be required to end violence.
- Practitioners who work across communities in different roles will need ongoing opportunities to learn about and use frameworks that use continuums of stress to understand the needs of children, young people, families and the community as a whole.
- The signs of the impact of trauma on children and young people are highly visible, in particular in small communities. Ending violence

and attending to the needs of those young people affected by violence forms a natural starting point for beginning dialogue about resisting and challenging the potency of violence in the lives of the community as a whole.

Safety is negotiated in the relationship between practitioners and individuals and groups in the community. The orientation of the practitioner to the conversations they have and the questions they ask should preface permission on minute-by-minute basis. There should be an onus on working with the different ways of understanding and learning styles of individuals. It should take into account that experiences of past violence or other stressors (e.g. exposure to drug, alcohol and other substance abuse) can affect the ways that individuals are able to consider new information and engage in reflection. Practitioners are responsible for not asking questions that seek detail about the violence. In general, practitioners will use the following guidelines to create safety for all future stages:

- Introduce yourself and where you are from, if you are not already known within the community.
- Introduce conversations and their purpose and seek input into which topics can be included and excluded.
- Be prepared to discuss your own experiences of topics to facilitate the experience of the conversation being a shared activity.
- Leave space for silence.
- Ask permission of the individual again before a topic is explored.
- Be mindful of your gender and the gender of the individuals/group with whom you are engaging.
- Allow time for conversations to be led by the individual or group.
- Think about stories and metaphors that the individual or group is used to using and explore these in the way you frame questions and hold curiosity.

Finally, it is important to consider the physical setting in which dialogue is to occur. Engage individuals and the community to identify places in which a dialogue about violence will not contaminate the primary use of the space. The place itself should be culturally safe, and available for individuals or specific groups to talk about violence without the threat of repercussion.

Stage 3. Starting the dialogue
Children and young people hold a special position in the heart of a community. There is general agreement that their well-being and protection are critical for people in the community. For this reason, a good place to start

the dialogue about violence in the community is to gradually focus on the developmental needs of children.

The first part of this dialogue aims to mobilize the focus and motivation of individuals or groups in the community to consider the consequences for children and the community as a whole if violence is not addressed.

The dialogue can take the form of conversations about the development of the brains of children, how they grow and learn, and how they react to stress. There are simple yet powerful metaphors about the brain that can be used to explore the needs of children. One example is to talk about the brain as a tree which requires solid roots in order for it to be healthy. The roots are the early experiences that children are exposed to. If children are exposed to high-impact or toxic levels of stress, the roots of the tree will be shallow and not strong. Then the whole of the tree is unsteady.

These conversations in the first instance should target people with responsibility to care for children in the community. These are the individuals who are heavily invested in the children's development and often express concern for their care.

The metaphor of the brain and the tree can be extended to adults and the community as a whole. Over time, through ongoing conversations, the community can be supported to find its own metaphors that make sense and resonate with community members.

This opening dialogue does not have an educational aim. Its primary purpose is to make dialogues about violence accessible to the community. The aim of the practitioner is to minimize reactions of shame and promote the strengths associated with a collective commitment to caring for the community's children.

In this dialogue, opportunities will open up to hear about what individuals and the community as a whole do already to protect children and young people from violence. These are critical acts of resistance, which are relationally focused on the needs of children. In this stage, these small stories of challenging violence should be noted for future acknowledgement. The language used by individuals to describe their experiences is essential to note.

Stage 4. Listening deeply
This is the process whereby the practitioner attends to both the story of the violence and its impact in the lives of the community and to the stories of courage, challenge, defiance and opposition to violence that are inevitably present during the course of violence.

Practitioners sensitively hear and validate the experiences that individuals want to share about their experience. They also attend to the steps that people engage in to modify, reduce, or protect themselves and their loved ones from the violence or the effects of that violence. This process of deep listening by the practitioner offers their attuned interpersonal resources to the individual or group with whom they are in dialogue to support their arousal regulation. It acknowledges their pain and provides the individual or group in the community with the experience that they are not alone in wanting to put a stop to violence. This joining is the first step in building coalitions of commitment to work together towards a common goal.

Stage 5. Naming the tactics and effects of violence

Throughout this process, individuals and groups will describe their experiences of violence. They may not do this directly as it may be too painful. They may talk about stories of other people, other communities rather than their own. They may elicit descriptions about past experiences of abuse and violation in their community committed by outsiders to that community. These are conversations that practitioners will hear and participate in.

The practitioner's orientation in this phase is to listen and explore the effects of violence in the lives of the community. The sorts of questions in which a practitioner would be interested include:

- Who has been most affected by violence in the community?
- Who in the community has used violence? How has being violent changed them?
- How did violence shape trust in the community?
- How did violence influence the way that people are cared for?
- How did violence affect who people could talk to or not talk to?
- What do people think was lost in the community because of violence?

Simultaneously, practitioners are also interested in conversations that identify the strategies used by violence to take hold in the community and the extent to which such violence has come to be viewed as normal. It should be clearly noted that this conversation is not aimed at diffusing responsibility for violence. Those who commit violence should be held accountable in law and by the community. Accountability is a significant element of the next stage of this process in relation to witnessing resistance. In this phase, drawing out the way that violence is accounted for by the community has as its purpose the development of understanding about the causes of violence at a local level. It is an attempt at holding dialogue that reduces the shame inherent in families when violence is attributed to their own failures. It connects violence with historical and present forms of oppression that contribute to other problems that can escalate to violence; for example, consuming excessive alcohol as a means, unconsciously or consciously, of responding to the internal pain of having lost connection to family and friendship circles.

Questions that practitioners can pursue in naming the tactics of violence include:

- How has violence achieved its goals?
- How does violence stay once it has arrived in the community? Does it use secrecy? Or threats?
- How does violence convince people to use it?
- When are people in the community most susceptible to violence?
- How does violence react when it is challenged? Is there any kind of payback if violence feels threatened?
- How have the resources to be found in culture been overlooked for violence to be allowed to take hold in the community?

Stage 6. Witnessing resistance

By naming the tactics of violence in the community, the opportunity is opened up to consider how individuals and groups have stood up to it. This dialogue enables the community to start to be aware of its own power to change attitudes and behaviour that support violence. The focus is on finding examples of actions that the community has already implemented – regardless of whether they have worked or not. It is the meaning that the community attributes to the effort in resisting violence which is the outcome of this phase.

The orientation of practitioners in this stage is not celebratory or overly positive as acts of resistance are identified by individuals and groups. This is a temptation which needs to be resisted. Instead, practitioners focus on creating rich descriptions of these acts of resistance, slowly and patiently – never overtaking or over-emphasizing the value that is placed on them by the individual or group. In this way, the individual or group is able to explore how the resistance was organized, resourced and experienced. The richer the detail, the more likely the individual or group will feel that they own their actions and experience them as part of their intentions and ambitions they hold for their families and community.

An important component of this stage is to identify if and how those who have used violence were held accountable for their actions.

Questions that practitioners can pursue in witnessing resistance include:

- Were there any times when someone in the community acted to oppose violence? What actions did they take? How did they know that it was the right way to go about it?
- Were there times when a group of people in the community stood up against violence? How did they come together in the first place to do that? What did they do together that they could not have done on their own as individuals?

- What did anyone do to make sure that the person who had used violence knew they had hurt someone else in the community? What was it like for them if someone called in the police? What was it like for the family if someone called in the police? What was it like for the rest of the community if the police had to charge a person for using violence in the community?
- What does the culture say about standing up to violence? What stories have been told in the community about how violence was not allowed to win?
- When people were standing up against violence, what were they standing up for? What did they notice they were promoting about the way that people should treat each other?
- What was found in the community again that had been lost as a result of violence taking over?
- How did respect become part of the community again? How did trust become part of the community again?
- How have people been able to ensure that they have been protected from a person who has hurt someone by using violence? How has safety been present in the face of violence?
- What did you learn about yourself when you stood up to oppose violence? What did the community learn about itself when it stood up against violence?

Stage 7. Amplifying enactments

In this stage, the rich descriptions of actions that people in the community have taken to resist violence are amplified to support others in the community to find out about the opposition to violence that has already begun to take hold and how it had originated in the community. This is a sensitive process that must take into account family and community dynamics to ensure that conflict between people is not inadvertently promoted.

The practitioner in this stage is oriented towards an active dialogue that supports the individual or group in considering the views of others they know in the community. This is not yet an exercise in engaging those others in a real conversation. It is a rehearsal for what will happen in later stages. It is also a conversation that seeks to extend recognition of the acts of resistance in a way that the individual or group feels the effects of the acknowledgement without exposing them yet to the potential for criticism or negative attention.

In this stage, practitioners are interested in the following kinds of questions:

- Who else in the community may have noticed the steps you took to stand up to violence? How might they have come to know about it?

- If I asked them to tell me what they thought about the actions you took, what would they say? What would they say were the qualities in you that enable you to act in the way you did? What would they know about you that would have left them not being surprised that you took this action?
- Who might have predicted that you would have taken the sort of action that you did to oppose violence? Who would have known that you were capable of doing that ever since you were a child? What would they have seen in you back then that would have made them think that way?
- Who do you think would join you in the community in taking action like you did? What do you have in common that would tell you that they would support you in what you did?
- Who might change their mind about what you are capable of achieving if they knew you had acted in the way that you have against violence?
- Who would be the most proud of what you did?

Stage 8. Telling and retelling stories of renewal

In this phase, the practitioner continues the dialogue with the individual and/or group by retelling them the story that has come to be told about the way violence came to the community, how it affected people and how it was opposed and challenged. This retelling provides the opportunity for the individual and/or group who have participated in the process so far to hear the story in its entirety from the position of the audience. This change in perspective allows another layer of dialogue aimed at reflecting on themselves as actors in their own narrative of resistance. This process helps to consolidate the narrative as purposeful and valid.

As they retell the story, practitioners can also check to see if there are other elements that have been omitted or need to be strengthened. The act of participation from multiple perspectives facilitates the take up of the story in an embodied and meaningful way. Practitioners can ask the following questions to support this level of reflection:

- What was the experience of hearing the story from start to end like for you?
- What are the things you like about yourself when you hear that story?
- Where in your body did you feel any reactions to what was happening in the story? How do those qualities that were identified in the story about you feel like when you hear them being described?
- Did the person that was you in the story feel as if it was you? How do you know that?

- If other people in the community heard that story, what do you think their reaction would be? What would they say to you? Would they be more likely or less likely to join you in standing up to violence if you asked them after they heard that story?
- What parts of that story are still going?
- How much of that story was similar to stories that you have heard told in the community?
- What parts of that story are connected to the way that culture influences your way of living?
- How important were relationships to you in that story? What do these relationships mean to you still?

Stage 9. Collectivizing action

It is at this point the practitioner needs to assess whether the individual or group feels safe to extend their dialogue to others in the community. This is the period in which the practitioner supports the development of coalitions of support in the community who may take the lead from individual or small-group resistance and allow its effects to spread across the community. Coalitions of support form in concentric circles of relationships around the individual or group who has already been engaging in the dialogue of change to this point. The safest starting point is those with whom the individual or group has an affinity or a pre-existing relationship of support. Practitioners need to consider how information is communicated so as to map out the people who may be resourced to join a collective movement aimed at implementing community-wide actions of resistance to violence. At this point, practitioners and the individual/group that have been in dialogue together initiate processes to recruit others in the community into their plans. Informal and formal leaders of a community should be considered as possible sources of support and direct engagement.

This is a process of small-group discussion, with an effort being made to connect the stories of the original individual or group with other stories of opposition to violence that others in the community can tell. The practitioner does not lead these conversations or try to push an agenda. Instead, the individuals or groups in the community engage with each other through shared opportunities to meet informally or informally. These processes lead to the momentum for change driven by the community itself, taking with it its own lessons about what has been effective in its history and in recent times in convincing violence to leave.

Practitioners should consider at this stage how shared meaning is generated between members of the community by asking the following questions:

- What stories are common among people in the community about how violence has been challenged or opposed?
- What do the people who have stood up to violence share in relation to their qualities or relationships?
- What common goals have been used by people in the community to oppose violence?
- How do people know that their actions have worked?
- What are the qualities of relationships that have emerged as violence has started to leave the community?
- What has entered the community in a positive way to take the place of violence as it left?

Combining stories of individual resistance into a collection of stories of community defiance and resilience is the outcome of this stage.

Stage 10. Developing solidarity

In this stage, the community is mobilized to take collective action against violence. Here the practitioner seeks out community symbols or metaphors that can be enacted and highlight the solidarity of the community in its shared intention to end violence. It can take the form of a community project that depicts a celebration of safety or a community activity that engages in cultural stories about respect and care. This symbolic action serves as reminder about the story of community coming together to prioritize the protection of all of its members from violence. If the symbolism is powerful enough, it can also be shared with other communities as a sign of hope that violence can be defeated when people act in concerted and collaborative ways with a shared commitment.

Stage 11. Transforming community

In this final phase, practitioners continue to support the community's ongoing transformation. The process of deep listening continues in order to source stories that contribute to community resilience. The focus should be in particular on qualities of trust, hope, respect and care across the whole community. Telling and retelling these stories at an individual, group and community level resources the transformation of community in a sustained way. It is also important that these narratives are integrated where appropriate with traditional cultural stories of healing.

Conclusion

Trauma-transformative practice for ending violence offers important resources to the field of violence prevention. It recognizes that one of the implications of trauma is that it supports violence in keeping hold of a community once it has found its way there. Trauma makes it hard for people to come together to talk about their efforts to challenge the effects of violence. It makes living in a community feel frightening and overwhelming. Every time that violence is mentioned, the neurophysiological patterns of the past re-engage in overdrive, keeping people apart, making them feel isolated and disempowered. Once this tactic of violence and trauma has been unmasked, people have a chance to understand it and look into their relationships to find the resources that they have used to stand up to them both.

They do this by holding vigils, calling community meetings, enlisting the support of other communities that are struggling with the same problems. They listen to those with lived and living experience of violence and trauma as experts in what may help. They form committees. They call for resources. They advocate to take charge of the rules and laws that make sense to them.

They act compassionately towards victims and survivors and declare their intent that violence does not have the right to undermine trust, care and love in their community. Compassion is the collective act of resistance to violence and it is an antidote to trauma. It engages systems of cooperation and regulation – sharing the mutuality of life, its responsibilities and its joyfulness.

Art, sport, culture and music become the valued qualities of a community that has violence on the retreat. Engaging in the capacity to play again and to experience relationships with safety are powerful indicators that healing is emerging and that the experience of trauma itself is starting to shift.

KNOWLEDGE AND PRACTICE REFLECTION

Janise Mitchell, Joe Tucci, Ed Tronick and Stephen W. Porges

In this example of trauma-transformative practice, a number of the emerging principles that have been forming as part of the reflections of each chapter are identifiable.

The model integrates trauma knowledge with complementary approaches of working so that there is coherence to the ways in which it is conceptualized, described and implemented. Trauma knowledge is interspersed relevantly throughout. The model holds the complexity of the task of ending violence alongside the complexity of explanatory frames for how violence is perpetrated and how it can be challenged. Language is used deliberately as a deconstructive system to open up possibilities for individual and collective action.

The model recognizes that trauma will manifest challenges to the strategies that the model seeks to employ. Members of the community who have experienced violence may react to the processes of even the most respectful and sensitive dialogue. Understanding the nature of safety in communities and being prepared offers interactions with victims and survivors as possible resources to their own past, instead of magnifying the likelihood of activating defensive postures and physiological responses to threat.

It is oriented to listening deeply for stories of shame and loss. Compassion is at the heart of the approach.

Throughout the model, collaboration between community members and between community and services is promoted and relied on. The collectivizing of action coupled with acts of solidarity, so eloquently described by Vikki Reynolds (2013), reflects the power of joint purpose, relationship-based forms of knowing and doing. Without partnership, individuals remain isolated, families remain stymied by the control of violence. The community holds no visibility into how it is already challenging and resisting violence.

The meaning of violence is pitted against the value of safety, respect and appreciation. In this context, trauma-transformative practice uses the insights from resisting violence in the past to form the basis on which future responses are configured and put into play. Discourses of power and oppression are questioned through subtle forms of inquiry that serve not to overwhelm but to encourage community members to consider how violence benefits perpetrators, their ways of thinking and the values they surreptitiously plant as seedlings. When these truths emerge, they do so strongly with the inherent belief that they feel unassailable. It is why trauma-transformative practice actively considered how to engage in ways that do not perpetuate, either deliberately or unintentionally, the worldviews that normalize violence and its aftermath.

This approach offers hope. It draws on practices of cooperative play to connect people through symbols and rituals which in themselves offer transformed forms of meaning that are used in looping effect to change the community even further.

It is by no means a perfect example of trauma-transformative practice. It could speak more about the ways that trauma can hold back progress. It could consider more deeply the impacts of poverty and the gendered nature of violence, especially family violence. There is always more to understand, more to know about trauma and the experience of violence from which it is derived. The integration with community-based approaches could be stronger and more aligned. It could be more specific and outline more detailed examples.

It does begin to take a step beyond a trauma-informed framework. It offers a glimpse into the next possible phase of the paradigm shift in the trauma movement. Trauma-transformative practice dimensions reflect the intention of more complex outcomes. They aim to deliver transformative opportunities at a relational level, which, once embedded, can make change more sustained for those with lived and living experiences of violation, their families and their communities.

References
References for chapter

Atkinson, J. (2002). *Trauma Trails: The Transgenerational Effects of Trauma in Indigenous Australia*. Melbourne: Spinifex Press.

Australian Bureau of Statistics (2017). *Characteristics and Outcomes of Childhood Abuse*. Canberra: ABS.

Australian Institute of Health and Welfare (2019). *Family, Domestic and Sexual Violence in Australia: Continuing the National Story 2019*. Canberra: AIHW.

Australian Institute of Health and Welfare (2022). *Specialist Homelessness Services Annual Report 2021–22*. Canberra: AIHW.

Bird, J. (2002). *The Heart's Narrative: Therapy and Navigating Life's Contradictions*. Auckland: Edge Press.

Crime Statistics Agency Victoria (2022). *Victoria Police Law Enforcement Assistance Program, July 2022*. Melbourne: Crime Statistics Agency Victoria.

Epston, D. and White, M. (1992). *Experience, Contradiction, Narrative and Imagination*. Adelaide: Dulwich Centre.

Foucault, M. (1972). *The Archaeology of Knowledge*. London: Tavistock Publications.

Foucault, M. (1977). *Discipline and Punish: The Birth of the Prison*. London: Penguin Books.

Friere, P. (1972). *Pedagogy of the Oppressed*. London: Penguin Books.

Gergen, K.R. (1985). The social constructionist movement in modern psychology. *American Psychologist*, 40, 266–273.

Gergen, K.R. (1991). *The Saturated Self*. New York, NY: Basic Books.

Kirmayer, L., Dandeneau, S., Marshall, E., Phillips, M. and Williamson K. (2011). Rethinking resilience from indigenous perspectives. *Canadian Journal of Psychiatry*, 56, 84–91.

Laing, R.D. (1967). *The Politics of Experience*. London: Penguin Books.

Reynolds, V. (2010). *Doing Justice as a Path to Sustainability in Community Work*. www.taosinstitute.net/files/Content/5693763/ReynoldsPhDDissertationFeb2210.pdf.

Reynolds, V. (2013). *Justice-Doing at The Intersections of Power: Community Work, Therapy and Supervision*. Adelaide: Dulwich Centre Publications.

Vaneeckhaute, L.E., Vanwing, T., Jacquet, W., Abelshausen, B. and Meurs, P. (2017). Community resilience 2.0: Toward a comprehensive conception of community-level resilience. *Community Development*, 48, 5, 735–751.

Waldegrave, C., Tamasese, K., Tuhaka, F. and Campbell, W. (2003). *Just Therapy – a Journey: A Collection of Papers from the Just Therapy Team New Zealand*. Adelaide: Dulwich Centre Publications.

Waldegrave, C. (2012). Developing a 'Just Therapy': Context and the Ascription of Meaning. In A. Lock and T. Strong (eds), *Discursive Perspectives in Therapeutic Practice*. Oxford: Oxford University Press.

White, M. and Epston, D. (1990). *Narrative Means to Therapeutic Ends*. New York, NY: W.W. Norton.

White, M. (1999). Reflecting team work as definitional ceremony revisited. *Gecko – A Journal of Deconstruction and Narrative Ideas in Therapeutic Practice*, 2, 55–82.

White, M. (2006). Working with People who are Suffering the Consequences of Multiple Trauma: A Narrative Perspective. In D. Denborough (ed.), *Trauma: Narrative Responses to Traumatic Experience* (pp.25–86). Adelaide: Dulwich Centre Publications.

References for Knowledge and Practice Reflection

Reynolds, V. (2013). *Justice-Doing at The Intersections of Power: Community Work, Therapy and Supervision*. Adelaide: Dulwich Centre Publications.

CHAPTER 18

From Trauma Informed to Trauma Transformative: Core Dimensions for Practice, Organization and Community Change

Janise Mitchell and Joe Tucci

Introduction

Over two decades on from the original article by Harris and Fallot (2001), the interest in trauma-informed practice has not waned. In fact, it can be argued that it is growing. As we have already noted, there has been a proliferation of models and applications of the construct across a diverse range of human service organizations and systems. The hope remains that it will deliver improvements to the experiences of all service users, but in particular victims and survivors of interpersonal violence.

We share this view. Given the prevalence of such violation across the lifespan, there is an absolute need for practitioners, organizations and systems to better appreciate the pervasive influence of trauma in the lives of victims and survivors and make wholesale changes in the way that programmes and services are designed to support them.

Our sense is that trauma-informed practice as it is currently conceptualized is unlikely to produce all the benefits that were expected without further evolution. For us, that progression is a move to what we have called *trauma-transformative practice*. It is a set of coordinating principles and interpretive constructs that aim to transform the ways that practitioners, organizations and systems operate with *collective therapeutic intent* to make the continuing effects of trauma become less influential in the lives of victims and survivors and reduce the pain and suffering they experience over time. It collapses previous constructs such as trauma-sensitive, trauma-aware, trauma-informed and trauma-specific interventions into one compelling metaphor that can integrate the nuances of each term so that the impact of the construct itself is in keeping with the language used to describe it. Trauma-transformative practice is defining both of its ambition and its name.

This book has set out a framework for the development of the paradigm that is required to incorporate important knowledge domains that are missing or should be further amplified. The first chapter traced the origins of trauma-informed practice as a paradigm. It also mapped out its benefits and its current status as it is being reported in the literature. We then used the knowledge and practice reflections after each chapter to underscore our argument for a shift to trauma-transformative practice and to point to the aspects that should comprise it. In Chapters 16 and 17, we have also offered two examples of how trauma-transformative practice is already being implemented.

In this final chapter, we bring together all of these parts to more fully describe the construct of trauma-transformative practice and its core constitutive dimensions.

Why is there a need to evolve the current paradigm?

From the very first chapter, we have laid out the limitations of the trauma-informed paradigm. In summary, we made the following points:

- The language of the trauma-informed construct has become confused and risks losing its potency due to a lack of differentiation between what constitutes 'good practice' in general and trauma-informed practice more specifically; a lack of shared understanding of what trauma-informed practice is and is not; and a lack of agreed ways to measure its impact.
- Differentiations between concepts such as trauma informed, trauma aware and trauma specific to name a few are at odds with contemporary conceptualizations of trauma knowledge and other critical knowledges (cultural, lived experience and practitioner) that argue a more inclusive theory of change that deconstructs the central power of one-to-one therapy in favour of an approach that acknowledges the therapeutic capacity of all interactions.
- There is a focus on the individual to the exclusion of collective experiences of interpersonal violence that can be experienced by groups of individuals and communities such that there is inadequate attention paid to the critical sociocultural context within which interpersonal violence occurs and is perpetuated.

The chapters contained in this book are testimony to the need to resist reductionist ways of thinking and conceptualizing interpersonal violence, complex trauma and its remedies. Each chapter, in its own way, has made an important contribution to the complexity that is inherent in conceptualizing trauma, its consequences and the steps to its amelioration.

The richness of ways of knowing, thinking and doing is highlighted by all the authors, who support the need to evolve the current conceptualization away from trauma-informed practice to one built around the construct of trauma-transformative practice. After each chapter, we have reflected on the knowledge and practice frames made available by each author, noting at times where the trauma-informed construct was somewhat limited conceptually and pragmatically.

Knowledge is not static, but rather dynamic and thus must constantly challenge our meaning-making processes. This book marks another point in time, mapping available knowledges about interpersonal violence and complex trauma and how to translate these evolving understandings into a framework for healing and recovery. The following is a distillation of what we believe are some of the key messages from the chapters contained in this book, acknowledging that the book is by no means an exhaustive exploration of all available knowledge on the topic.

We need to expand our understanding beyond the individual. Trauma was, and largely continues to be, conceived of as an individualized experience of a harmful event. A traumatic injury was conceived first as being held in the mind and then reconceptualized as being also stored in and by the body. In this frame, trauma may be viewed as a deficit pathologizing construct where the individual's state before the harmful event is perceived to be the healthy state that the individual must be supported through treatment to regain. Multiple authors in this book have questioned the validity of this way of thinking. In his chapter, Tronick identified that the meaning of a harmful event, such as the physical abuse of a child, does not start with the event and its aftermath. It should also include what was happening before. It must be oriented to the relational environment in which the child was living and the saliency of experiences in that environment. He maintained that:

> ...adults and children live in a world where an hour of any kind of therapy is lost in the welter of all the other hours. If the people in a child's life are not part of the process of change, then change will not occur; the same is likely true for adults ... they need immersion with therapeutic others...

Mitchell and Macnamara similarly argued this point, suggesting that all significant relationships in a child's life, when resourced with therapeutic intent, enable change to occur. This is the core of the work described by Baylin and Hughes. Kestly introduced the concept of the power of playful interactions between children and between children and adults as being the agent of change for those who have experienced trauma. As noted in our first chapter, the trauma-informed paradigm as it is currently conceptualized, '...denies the potential for *therapeutic intent* that can arise in environments, networks of relationships and communities.'

Trauma-informed practice approaches are also shaped by a historical view that locates the consequences of violation in the individual and not in the context of broader sociocultural discourses. In so doing, it replicates social norms that have reduced accountability for the violence. However, Becker-Blease (2017) rightly noted that complex trauma is inextricably linked to systems of power and oppression. In the first chapter, we argued that the reframe of the question 'What is wrong with you?' to 'What happened to you?' still does not go far enough because:

> ...the neutral tone of the second question reflects an undervaluing of the inherent dynamics of power on which abuse and violence are facilitated, including the gendered structure of society which privileges male world-views, racism that discriminates in favour of social groups with histories of colonizing and enslavement, the ways in which children and young people are rendered powerless through adult-centric perspectives and belief systems, and the wrongful perception that abled body frames of reference are more legitimate over those with disabilities.

This critique was explored further in the chapter by Atkinson *et al.*, which served to highlight the fallacy of trauma as emerging as the result of a harmful event. Atkinson has fought all her life for greater understanding of transgenerational trauma arising from the persistent and ongoing colonizing effects of white settler practices that dispossessed First Nations people from their inherent rights and agency. In their chapter, Courtois and Ford proposed a taxonomy for defining complex trauma that encompasses the trauma arising from colonization and from the oppression of women through gendered-based violence. For them, trauma that results from the systematic violation of individuals based on group or cohort characteristics related to perceptions of age, ability, socio-economic status, geography, gender and culture brings into question the adequacy of definitions of trauma contained in the trauma-informed paradigm. The reflections from many of the chapters highlighted the need for decolonizing and anti-oppressive practices to be included in the evolution of the trauma-informed paradigm (e.g. Cozolino, Kestly). Importantly, there is acknowledgement of the healing properties of strong connections to culture (Atkinson *et al.*) and specific cultural practices such as storytelling, somatosensory cultural experiences and social bonding (Atkinson *et al.*, Cozolino *et al.*).

It is acknowledged here that the framework developed by SAMHSA includes in its six key principles the need to integrate the wisdom and knowledge that address racist, gender and socio-economic biases in the ways that services are delivered. However, this element of the SAHMSA framework leaves out the experiences of discrimination based on age, ability and cultural identity. Critically, this core SAMHSA principle is not always found in other frameworks that purport to be trauma informed, such as the approaches described by the National Child Traumatic Stress Network (Pynoos *et al.*, 2008), the Office for Health Improvement and Disparities in the UK (2022) and the Welsh Government (2022).

We need to incorporate recent developments in trauma and related theory into how we conceptualize the critical needs of people who have experienced complex trauma including safety, shame, compassion and loss. Since the introduction of the trauma-informed paradigm, the science of safety has developed significantly, led by the work of Stephen Porges. From this work, we now understand the need to 'be safe' (the focus of the trauma-informed approach) and 'feel safe'. 'Felt safety' is experienced as an internal quality of an individual's neurophysiological states shaped by the experience of relationship to others' internal states and intentions. It has not been effectively integrated into the trauma-informed practice paradigm. The trauma-informed paradigm is also silent about the evolving knowledge base focusing on shame. The chapter by Ginot serves to highlight how shame accompanies trauma and, in most instances, amplifies its effects. Similarly, the chapter by Gilbert, Lee and Matos illustrates the significance of the study of compassion to the trauma field. However, it too is missing as a core element of trauma-informed practice. Finally, our reflection on the themes contained in the chapter about love by Carter has demonstrated the need for the love and its loss arising from violation to be more centrally configured into the next evolution of trauma-informed practice. Arguably, attention to an individual's need for safety in all its forms, and compassion, with sensitivity to experiences of shame and loss, will go a long way towards the ambitious goal of preventing re-traumatization described in the trauma-informed approach.

We need to more fully articulate the multisystemic dimension of practice that is required to achieve change. Throughout this book, there is a repeated reference to the need to work on a coherent and congruent way within and between the individual, family/group, community, organizations and systems. Cozolino talked about our need for supportive and cohesive communities to provide us with a sense of structure, security and meaning. Tronick referred to the need to move to a 'multiple competence approach, and/or a team approach to therapy and/or one that considers the whole range of experience and functioning of the individual.' Courtois and Ford described the need for multi-modal and multi-dimensional treatment. Atkinson and colleagues noted the need for both communities of care – groups of people who live together in small communities and who care for each other – and communities of practice – groups of people coming together in a common endeavour and shared practice.

Creeden reminded us of the need to work collaboratively with the child, their family, and any other members of the child's service system 'in a manner that promotes respect, safety, trust, competency, and optimism for change and growth.' Such collaboration is essential in ensuring that service systems are not fractured into silos which only respond to a specific compartmentalized problem or issue of concern. As pointed out by Mitchell and Macnamara in their chapter, it is also through such collaboration that collective commitment of therapeutic intent can be shared across the system. This enables the multiple needs of victims, survivors, their families, practitioners and the systems to be held in view all the time, helping to influence how relationships shape experience of change and transformation. Sharing of decision-making power about the nature of and approach to the support that is offered with victims and survivors and those in their network is critical in the evolution of the trauma-informed construct.

We need to have an increased focus on meaning making within and between individuals, families and communities. A number of chapters focused on meaning making as fundamental to understanding and responding to experiences of trauma. According to Tronick in his chapter, meaning making is a neurosomatic process that connects internal states with the inner states of others in mutually coordinated patterns of communication and through which micro-disruptions of the relationships occur all the time. Kearney and Lanius examined the bodily processes through which trauma comes to be known, experienced and ultimately processed. Baylin and Hughes showed through their work that intersubjective experience of another gives rise to changes in meaning about experience through compassion and careful attention to the way that a child's needs from the past come into the present. The two chapters by Kestly and Kline both illustrated how playful connections that are hopeful can serve to strengthen the ways that meanings are generated, held and understood by children. Their work can also easily be applied to adults.

Creeden emphasized that the final stage of intervention for children and young people who have engaged in harmful sexual behaviour is narrative meaning making. Given how much it features in the writing of our authors, it is clear that it is a core element of the evolution of the trauma-informed paradigm. Meaning making can be used to understand how trauma shapes the ongoing experiences of victims and survivors. But it is also a broader cultural dimension of organizations and systems which can use it as a metaphorical resource to support changes in practice, policy and culture. Critical to meaning making is the need for deep listening. Atkinson and colleagues extend the notion of deep listening (*Dadirri*) to the need for truth-telling in an effort to render transparent the colonizing practices and their impact. Tucci and Mitchell similarly talked about deep listening, allowing for the slow and detailed telling of stories in search of alternative narratives that spoke less of hurt and trauma and more of courage, strength and collective empowerment. Kestly's notion of relational presence similarly uses the underlying principles of deep listening and witnessing. Kline's openness to the adaptability expressed through the behaviour of young people in their interaction with her is a critical source of meaning making. Narrative and storytelling have been suggested by numerous authors as central to meaning making for individuals, families, groups and communities. Such processes can render transparent hidden assumptions and begin to privilege and honour values, beliefs and behaviours that foster belonging, connection, trust, respect, identity and rights. Tucci and Mitchell's chapter provided a clear example of the power of storying and re-storying in meaning making and empowering the community to take a stand against the influence of violence within it.

We need to more clearly articulate the centrality of the relational basis of healing and change. The foundation of human relationships to provide resources to individuals in pain arising from interpersonal violence reflects a deep and enduring connection between trauma knowledge and attachment knowledge. There are at least four chapters which directly reference attachment and trauma (Carter, McIntosh *et al.*, Mitchell and Macnamara, Baylin and Hughes). There are other chapters which describe and use it as well. However, while the trauma-informed paradigm alludes to the importance of relationships in some of its messaging, it is absent in many ways. Cozolino refers to is as the social synapse – the space between us that we can use to heal each other. Baylin and Hughes point to good care being able to rewire brain circuitry, while Atkinson and colleagues provide numerous examples of the power of relationships between a school principal and her students. McIntosh *et al.* point to the importance of understanding disorganized attachment as a property of relationships in which children have experienced violation and/or neglect. Kearney and Lanius note how the body's relationships to a range of internal and external experiences (posture, physiological cues, people, nature) contain the resources to healing.

The therapeutic potential of networks of relationships around children and adults has been referred to earlier in this chapter and adds weight to the need for greater articulation of relationships, and networks of significant relationships as vehicles through which healing and change be achieved. Importantly, there is also a need to expand the concept of relationships beyond the interpersonal to be inclusive of significant relationships which shape the sense of belonging and identity that forms through connection to country, land, nature, culture, spirituality and ancestors.

We need to be able to hold the complexity of views about trauma, interpersonal violence and oppression that is historical and current. There is a need, identified throughout the book, to resist simplistic and reductionist explanations of experience and encourage the acceptance of pluralist positions that can embrace multiple perspectives at the same time. In addition, the current trauma-informed paradigm has insufficient conceptual resources to integrate with other policy, service delivery applications and organizational values of agencies in their effort to support victims and survivors. In the first chapter, we maintained that:

> It is not as if organizations which attend to disadvantage and poverty should take up trauma-informed approaches to the exclusion of theories about how capitalist structures create social conditions in which the working class are exploited by those with greater financial resources. Or that domestic and family violence services would suddenly jettison their beliefs about the gendered nature of society as it contributes to violence against women and children solely in favour of trauma-informed perspectives. It is not meant to be an 'either/or' but more an 'and.'

The evolution of the trauma-informed construct needs to be more integrative in its design from the outset, to allow it to merge with and support practitioners, organizations and systems with approaches that are in the best interests of service users.

The lessons described above provide the pointers to a new navigational framework for the integration of a trauma lens into everyday practice. We need a *post-trauma-informed construct* which is delivered by the paradigm shift to trauma-transformative practice. The conceptual resources and frames of reference for what we proposed for trauma-transformative practice are explored in the next two sections.

What is trauma-transformative practice?

Our definition of trauma-transformative practice is:

> An inclusive set of coordinating constructs that aim to transform the ways that practitioners, organizations and systems function collectively with therapeutic intent to address the complex and reverberating effects of trauma so that it becomes less influential in the lives of victims and survivors of interpersonal violence, which will reduce the pain and suffering they experience over time.

The word *transformative* is used in two different respects. It is used to describe changes that are aimed at the ways that services and programmes are delivered so they hold the complexity of knowledge and experience required to address the needs of victims and survivors who seek out support. *Transformative* is also used to refer to the continuing adaptations that victims and survivors are supported to make as the impact of trauma is given meaning to, neurosomatically reshaped and relationally validated. Within our construct of trauma-transformative practice, we have sought to move from the notion of 'informed' to the more active intentionality ascribed in the term 'transformed.' We have also sought through the articulation of the construct to allow for greater clarity with regard to expected outcomes inherent in the component parts of trauma-transformative practice, thus lending itself to easier impact measurement. That is our hope.

We also believe that trauma should not be reduced to a definition that is confined to one sentence. Instead, we express our appreciation to Christine Courtois and Julian Ford for delivering a conceptually complex but clear taxonomy for defining and understanding the nature of trauma. We cannot think of a definitional framework that is more comprehensive and immediately applicable. For this reason, we replicate our summary of it again with the examples.

Table 18.1: Defining and understanding trauma

Category	Form	Example
Type I	Impersonal trauma	Sudden, unexpected, accidental, and unintentional events, such as a weather disaster or car accident.
Type II	Trauma experienced as a result of interpersonal violation and abuse	Child physical abuse, child sexual abuse, family and domestic violence, kidnapping.
Type IIA	Trauma from interpersonal violence perpetrated by strangers	Child sexual abuse perpetrated by an adult who physically traps the child at a public place, such as a shopping centre bathroom.
Type IIB	Trauma from interpersonal violence perpetrated by related or familiar individuals	Grooming of a child by someone in a position of authority such as teacher, sporting coach or religious leader. Bullying by a peer online. Child sexual, physical and emotional abuse perpetrated by parent. Physical and sexual assault by an intimate partner.
Type III	Individual and group identity-based trauma experienced as a result of discrimination and oppression	Based on major characteristics of the individual or group identity (e.g. gender, especially female, race, skin color, hair, facial and other body features, age, socio-economic status, ethnicity, sexual orientation and sexual identity, geography and educational attainment). These characteristics form the basis of or provide the rationale for prejudiced-based violation. Abuse and violence towards people with disabilities. Physical and financial abuse of the elderly.

Type IV	Group identity-based trauma experienced as a result of persecution, war, genocide	Ethnic cleansing and genocide. Combatants, prisoners of war, civilians exposed to warfare. Captives and hostages held for ransom, political prisoners, asylum-seekers, refugees and other displaced populations living in detention camps.
Type V	Group identity-based trauma experienced as a result of colonization and enslavement	Sale/trafficking of family members. Forced separation of First Nations children from families as a result of assimilationist government policies. Failure to recognize traditional ownership of land. Ongoing impact of historical massacres of First Nations people.
Type VI	Cumulative, continuous, and insidious trauma that encompasses multiple forms across all the different types	Exploitation of children and young people who are living in foster and residential care. Poly-victimization of children due to concurrent and ongoing experiences of physical, sexual and psychological abuse within the family.

In our reflection on their chapter, we noted that:

> Courtois and Ford offer an insight into the very nature of the damaging and ongoing impact of trauma when it arises from violation by another person or group of people. There are dynamics associated with interpersonal violence which in and of themselves cause hurt and pain. The betrayal of trust and care, the use of power, the historical reverberations of colonizing violence are all elements which compel the use of trauma, not in reductionist and simplified ways, but as experiences which intensely affect the very integrity of victims and survivors. Importantly...it is a salient reminder of how naming and clearly demarcating the effects of such violation can bring the needs of victims and survivors into much sharper focus for practitioners and organizations.

The construct of trauma-transformative practice demands a definition of trauma that is multi-layered. Courtois and Ford achieve this not through a definition but through a taxonomy. It illustrates how the trauma of interpersonal violence is so categorically different from impersonal trauma. It also delineates the impact of trauma on the individual as a result of violation that occurs by people known and not known to the victim and survivor, introducing Freyd's construct of betrayal trauma (Freyd, 1996; Birrell and Freyd, 2006; Foynes, Freyd and DePrince, 2009; Kaehler et al., 2013). It lays bare the need to understand the fundamental difference between identity-based trauma arising from persecution, war and genocide and the trauma that arises from the practices of colonization and enslavement which continue in the present time through acts of racism and other forms of discrimination that are built into societal structures of power. It finally attends to the different impacts of trauma that arise through cumulative, continuous and insidious experiences of violation, neglect and adversity across all the types of trauma described in Courtois and Ford's taxonomy.

Trauma-transformative practice uses these two foundational aspects (a definition that offers purpose and intent, and a taxonomy reflecting different types of trauma) to provide the conceptual resources that are needed to further encourage practitioners, organizations and systems towards more effectively responding to the needs of victims and survivors.

What are the core dimensions of trauma-transformative practice?

When a programme or practice lacks specificity, it is challenging for those delivering services to know what they should be saying or doing to achieve expected outcomes. This has been both the critique and challenge of the trauma-informed approach, leading to a lack of clarity and intent as to what the ambition is that was trying to be achieved. Practice principles should be articulated so that they are clearly defined, learnable, doable and measurable. In our conceptualization of trauma-transformative practice, we have attempted to articulate the core dimensions or practice domains on which it is based. We are intentional in our use of the term *trauma-transformative practice* rather than *trauma-transformative approach* to emphasize the active nature of what is required to achieve its goals. Practice is the actual application of an idea, belief or method, performed habitually or regularly, so that individuals, organizations and systems become proficient in its use.

Trauma-transformative practice is based on 12 core dimensions that, while described discreetly, inherently integrate with each other to best support victims and survivors to meet their needs and achieve the ambitions they hold for their life and their relationships.

1. *Safety dedicated:* Safety, to be safe and feel safe, is a commitment that all practitioners, organizations and systems must uphold. It includes ensuring that all service users are not physically or sexually abused in their interaction with practitioners, programmes or services. It relies on a value base which understands the impact of further violation of the physical and psychological integrity of victims and survivors. It is based on an understanding that felt safety is signalled in deep neurosomatic states where the intent of the cues offered to victims and survivors needs to be coherent with the actions that fulfil the commitment to being safe. Safety is negotiated in micro-exchanges between service users and service providers. As

such, safety and well-being are qualities that emerge when there is due consideration given to *context* (ensuring coherence between articulated positions/policies and behaviour), *choice* (a dimension of interactions that enable victims and survivors to determine how they will engage, if at all, with practitioners and other service personnel) and *connection* (the interdependence between experiences of self, others, nature, spirit and culture) (Dana, 2021).

2. *Trauma and healing resourced:* The knowledge from neuroscience has forever transformed our understanding of how healing from trauma is achieved. The potential for all relationships to hold therapeutic intent, the inclusion of body-based somatic interventions, along with sequenced and phased approaches that create safety, process experiences over time, support narrative meaning making and rebuild the relational capability of victims and survivors, have been significant in creating opportunities for healing and recovery to occur. In addition, embracing traditional, cultural practices that evoke healing has been critical in expanding Western methodologies of intervention and support. The integration of lived and living experience wisdom is an essential contributor to what is needed and what is helpful in achieving change. A commitment to a pluralist synthesis of relevant knowledge is thus a key dimension of trauma-transformative practice. It requires a deep understanding of how these integrated knowledges influence meaning making and an understanding of what change and healing can be, shaped by the goals, hopes and ambitions of the individuals, families and communities themselves. An understanding of the impact of trauma on the brain, body, mind, spirit and relationships of the individual and the group informs a theory of change, signals what the impact of change might look like and enables evaluation and measurement to occur.

3. *Shame responsive:* Shame often sits at the heart of trauma. It extends the social pain that interpersonal violation afflicts. As such, trauma-transformative practice must be responsive to the experience of shame that victims and survivors carry with them. A shame-responsive orientation recognizes the interwoven subjectivity of trauma and shame and responds to it directly. Practitioners, organizations and systems must design their interventions, programmes and services in ways that analyze beforehand how each element may risk amplifying the experience of shame and what can be done to directly reduce it. Strategies which communicate who is responsible for the violence, validate the impact that is experienced by victims and survivors, and act to erode the messages about identity built on humiliation, embarrassment and guilt are critical in trauma-transformative practice.

4. *Decolonizing and anti-oppressive committed:* Trauma-transformative practice commits itself to decolonizing and anti-oppressive ways of working. This includes an obligation to facilitate deep listening, 'truth-telling' and acknowledgement of past and current societal and systemic abuses. It includes, as Atkinson and her colleagues have argued, the need to promote and use First Nations peoples' ways of knowing, doing and healing. It compels acts which challenge the ongoing effects of colonization and oppression through practices which are led and determined by First Nations peoples. Similarly, anti-oppressive practice acknowledges and addresses the biases and ongoing forms of discrimination which lead to the systematic violation of individuals based on group or cohort characteristics related to social constructions of gender, age, ability, socio-economic status, geography and culture. Trauma-transformative practice cannot be realized without a commitment to engaging and integrating knowledge frames about the abuse and misuse of power and the way this is interwoven into social structures, relationships and institutions.

5. *Collaborative and participatory driven:* Collaboration between practitioners, organizations, systems and victims and survivors themselves, is a fundamental aspect of trauma-transformative practice. It recognizes that the needs of people who have experienced trauma are rarely offered within one organization, most often requiring a multi-dimensional and multi-systemic response. Service fragmentation does not serve the interests of victims and survivors of interpersonal violence. Collaborative and participatory processes ensure that individuals are responded to holistically, that there is a shared lens through which their needs are understood and congruence is held in the planning approach to meeting these needs. They deconstruct power and expert knowledge to develop ways of meaning making and solution generation that are inclusive of all knowledge holders and key stakeholders. Collaboration ensures that often scarce resources are used wisely and in the interests of victims and survivors. It also recognizes that victims and survivors and the key relationships around them, both formal and informal, can work in a coordinated way to promote change in the ways that violence is perpetrated. There is power in joint purpose, relationally driven forms of knowledge sharing and experiences of collective solidarity. This requires intentional effort and an investment of time to develop processes which support collective practice and collaboration that is inclusive of the voices of victims and survivors, their families, carers and communities.

6. *Meaning focused:* Trauma is acknowledged as the recalibration of meaning-making systems of victims and survivors and between

themselves and their network of relationships – both their informal social support networks and formal support offered by practitioners, organizations and systems. Trauma-based behaviour is understood as an expression of adaptation by victims and survivors to the experience of interpersonal violence. As such, meaning making is always strengths based. It attempts to hold both the possible impact of the behaviour with the positive adaptation that victims and survivors were forced to use in order to create the conditions conducive to their protection. Trauma-transformative practice respects the meaning-making efforts of individuals as endogenous and continuously operating. Meanings generated in turn affect the subsequent meanings that are made possible. It takes place at deep neurosomatic levels and shapes the brain and body's behavioural patterns, activation preferences, thresholds and arousal states. Meaning making also occurs at the level of families and communities as a dynamic and continuous process of making sense of relationships, truths and experience.

Practitioners, organizations and systems must organize themselves to build their own capability to be reflective so that meaning about practice is traced and recorded as forms of feedback that can help to encourage changes to practice and organizational culture. Meaning making is a resource that needs investment and has the effect of keeping organizations and systems more open and adaptive to new contextual information, feedback from service users and insights from their own personnel. Reflective practice, action research, supervision and mentoring are all practices that encourage reflective capability. Trauma-transformative practice actively considers how to engage in ways that do not perpetuate, either deliberately or unintentionally, the worldviews and biases that normalize violence, promote shame and fail to ensure accountability of perpetrators.

7. *Compassion oriented:* Compassion is an essential quality for responding to the pain and suffering of humans, its drivers sitting within our neurobiology. Compassion is the antidote to danger and fear. It acts to dampen internal neurosomatic cues of threat. It creates safety within relationships. Knowledge about compassion recognizes that the frames of reference held by those who use violence leave victims and survivors with experiences of shame and self-criticism which can spiral into cycles of self-blame and self-hatred. The integration of compassion into responses to victims and survivors cultivates kindness and self-care. It also orients the behaviour and attitudes of service providers towards greater empathy and understanding of the unique experiences of individual victims and survivors. It introduces

a less clinical frame of reference that acknowledges the therapeutic intent of all relationships and that tenderness and understanding are important qualities of practice and organizational culture to nurture. It renders important the concept of 'compassion fatigue' and the critical need to take due care of the 'helpers'.

8. *Complexity considered:* At the core of trauma-transformative practice is an embedded acknowledgement of broader 'therapeutic intent'. The therapeutic intent of every activity or strategy or interaction should be carefully considered because of the broader impact that relationships can serve for victims and survivors. A hallmark of trauma-transformative practice is its capacity to bring together, in meaningful ways, relevant knowledge frames that have the capacity to address the needs of specific cohorts with their own unique lived and living experience of trauma within their relevant context.

9. *Relationally integrative:* The power of relationships to support healing for victims and survivors of interpersonal violence is essential in trauma-transformative practice. Relationships support, encourage, process, anchor, soothe and meet the needs of individuals for whom the pain of trauma feels as if it is located within them. Relationships, when they are purposeful and are resourced to realize therapeutic intent, serve the interests of victims and survivors. Close relationships for victims and survivors act as agents of change and healing, influencing and reshaping their inner neurosomatic states and externally visible and available capacities. Through relationships, victims and survivors learn to tolerate the boundary of activation so that their physiology can be coaxed and supported back into safe zones of proximity and relational connectedness. Through safe and intentionally organized relationships, victims and survivors become more open and less fixed. They use their own self engagement systems to approach others and seek mutually satisfying interactions. The benefits of such experience form the basis of their future health and well-being. The critical task thus is the practice of resourcing of these relationships to hold therapeutic intent.

10. *Grief receptive:* Loss is a significant dimension of trauma. Trauma-transformative practice underscores the importance of supporting victims and survivors to grieve and process their experience of loss. Time and a receptive orientation gives significance to the ways in which compounding, and sometimes chronic, grief is experienced and held by individuals, families and communities. It is a specific kind of meaning-making activity that permeates the internal states of individuals as well as their own sense of identity. Grief must be witnessed, acknowledged and validated by an important other. Collective forms of bereavement can become part of the way that

trauma-transformative practitioners, organizations and systems enable the meaning making of victims and survivors, including ceremonies, vigils and memorials.

11. *Lived experience valued:* Power sharing with victims and survivors as lived experience knowledge holders positions relationships to respect the authority and insights that they bring with them in service relationships and processes of service co-design. It communicates that the practitioner, organization and system is committed to understanding the unique experience of each individual victim and survivor, not grouping their experiences into categories of common meaning. It respects the interpretations victims and survivors ascribe to experience, and perhaps for the first time, their own capability to shape the nature and limits of relationships they find themselves in.

12. *Hope inspiring:* Hope is a form of knowledge that results from the integration of neuroscience, practice wisdom and embodied experience. Hope emerges when victims and survivors are attuned to the acts of resistance they are engaged in against the violence and the ongoing effects of trauma in their lives. Hope is important because it motivates victims and survivors and practitioners, organizations and systems to stay the course in the face of the pervasiveness and brutality of violence and its ongoing effects. Hope is a resource for healing. It evolves in the moment-by-moment exchanges between victims and survivors and those who seek to support them. These exchanges communicate messages that trauma can be transformed, that the pain they carry will subside with support and that the intentions they have for their lives can be realized in some shape or form. It is the continuity of a promise that the impact of trauma can end. Hope often emerges when these exchanges involve playful qualities that are liberating of deeply held meanings which keep victims and survivors in states of protection and defensiveness. With hope, and through the energy that comes with it, victims and survivors are supported to keep going and not give up. Trauma-transformative practice privileges hope over despair and implements strategies that engender it across networks of practitioners, organizations and systems.

What are the considerations for the implementation of trauma-transformative practice?

Bloom (2016) reflected on the critical lessons learned in attempting to realize the potential of a trauma-informed approach when she likened the required paradigm shift to an 'internal earthquake' – a major change in the worldview, concepts and practices of how something works or is accomplished – and suggested that its achievement 'is no small feat and demands a new integration of mind, heart and spirit' (p.386).

It is a complex task that requires attention to both the affective and technical dimensions of implementing change.

Creating practice and systems change is a non-linear, interconnected process (Metz and Bartley, 2012). It engages the hearts and minds of all stakeholders. It addresses the critical dimensions of the capacity of practitioners, organizations and systems to implement and deliver on the desired change. It identifies barriers to change and develops strategies to address change and measure their impact. Failure to do so can result in misalignment of values and beliefs, absence of a collective vision for, or shared ownership of, the change, lack of motivation to sustain the effort, diversion of necessary resources to ensure success, distraction by competing priorities, or insufficient understanding of how to apply the knowledge effectively.

The engagement of hearts and minds, or what we call the affective dimension of practice and systems change, is not well explored in the literature but is a fundamental underpinning to the capacity of practitioners, organizations and systems to implement trauma-transformative practice. In addressing the affective dimension of change, attention must be paid to building capacity within the context of supportive and enabling environments characterized by empathy; paying attention to feelings, beliefs, values and assumptions; building trust, curiosity and openness; leading with honesty and transparency; acknowledging and addressing power differentials; and holding humility and tolerance (Metz *et al.*, 2021).

With this in mind, we turn to the broader issue of the 'capacity' of a practitioner, organization or system to engage in trauma-transformative practice. Brinkerhoff and Morgan (2010) define capacity as, 'the evolving combination of attributes, capabilities, and relationships that enables a system to exist, adapt, and perform' (p.3).

The development of capacity is dependent on the following five core capabilities (Baser and Morgan, 2008):

1. *The capability to commit and engage:* Stakeholders are able to mobilize resources (human and organizational); create space and autonomy for independent action; motivate unwilling or unresponsive partners; and, plan, decide and engage collectively to exercise their other capabilities.

2. *The capability to carry out technical, service delivery and logistical tasks*: Stakeholders are able to produce acceptable levels of performance; generate substantive outputs and outcomes; and add value for their clients.

3. *The capability to relate and attract support:* Stakeholders are able to

establish and manage linkages, alliances, and partnerships with others to leverage resources and actions; build legitimacy in the eyes of key stakeholders; and deal effectively with competition, politics and power differentials.

4. *The capability to adapt and self-renew:* Stakeholders are able to adapt and modify plans and operations based on monitoring of progress and outcomes; proactively anticipate change and new challenges, learn by doing; and cope with changing contexts and develop resiliency.

5. *The capability to balance diversity and coherence:* Stakeholders are able to develop shared short- and long-term strategies and visions; balance control, flexibility and consistency; integrate and harmonize plans and actions in complex, multi-actor settings; and cope with cycles of stability and change.

Pointing to the significant challenge of implementing a paradigm shift and echoing our earlier claims about the need to hold complexity, Brinkerhoff and Morgan (2010) noted the, 'complexity and inter-connectedness of the elements associated with capacity, which means that reductionist efforts to focus on separate components of capacity are unlikely to provide a sound basis for CD [capacity development] strategies and interventions' (p.3).

They go on to point to the utility of systems theory as a useful frame for understanding the multi-dimensional approach required in building capacity, suggesting that:

> ...systems thinking emphasises the multiple factors involved in creating and sustaining capacity, the connections among those factors, and the boundaries that distinguish them ... the systems perspective shows that no single factor or constituent element – incentives, financial support, trained staff, knowledge, organizational structure – can by itself explain the development of capacity. Thus, narrow interventions, such as staff training, are not likely to make a significant difference in performance ... CD design and implementation need to recognise the fallacy of one-best-way approaches, to incorporate flexibility and learning, and to pay attention to the specificities of context. (pp.7–9)

It is on this basis that we suggest that the effective implementation of trauma-transformative practice as the new operational paradigm is reliant on the following interrelated conditions within organizations and systems. While the focus here is the organizational and systems context, they also hold relevance for individual practitioners who operate outside an organizational environment.

Organizational/system culture and leadership

In our experience, the need to align organizational/system culture and leadership to the endeavour of changing paradigms in business-as-usual approaches is poorly understood and enacted. The key focus of their task is to ensure that the philosophy, goals, knowledge and skills related to the new paradigm are consistently and thoughtfully expressed throughout all levels of the organization or systems such that they use a shared language, focus on the same goals, and support and complement one another (Fixsen and Blasé, 2008). It requires a sustained commitment to the translation of trauma-transformative practice values and principles into daily practices of the organization/system in a manner that is accountable, responsible and in the best interests of those served. Far from a 'passive process' that suggests the dissemination of information about the required change to those who must make the change in practice, 'active' and sustained effort is required (Fixsen *et al.*, 2009). This commitment should be demonstrated across all levels of the organization/system from members of the board/executive to the operational staff. It should be evident in how the strategic vision and plan for an organization/system is articulated. It should be present in government policy, reform and funding agendas across all relevant departments – health, education, justice, housing, financial support, First Nations affairs, women's affairs and child welfare. It should be present in commitments to adequately resource the ongoing work required to realize the change. There are no quick fixes – change of this magnitude takes years not months to implement and embed into new and sustainable operating models and practices (Fixsen *et al.*, 2009). Organizations need to create the conditions for all staff, at all levels, to respond effectively to needs and complexity, and ensure that organization and system cultures (policies, practices and procedures at all levels) are congruent with the intent of trauma-transformative practice.

Leadership capability is often overlooked in the implementation of paradigm shifts in practice and service design and delivery, wrongly viewing that knowledge about practice is the domain of practitioners, rather than leaders. This could not be further from the truth. A comprehensive understanding of the philosophy, core constructs and relevant theoretical frameworks for trauma-transformative practice is critical to meaningful processes of practice integration and improvement, quality assurance and governance, and an appreciation of the needs of and challenges facing staff in their work with victims and survivors. Leadership requires a reflective and reflexive capability in order to achieve these complex activities. Indeed, practice leadership, as will be explained further under workforce capacity, is a critical element of leadership capability.

Participation and co-design

The ambition of trauma-transformative practice is its integration into existing and new service and system design. To ensure its relevance and applicability to the range of contexts and operating environments into which trauma-transformative practice may be applied, there is a critical need to involve key stakeholders in the design process, empowering them to play an active role in shaping the outcome of current service re-design and future service design. Using human-centred design thinking (Ructtinger, 2015), we need to privilege the expertise of lived and living experience and practice wisdom. By including a diverse range of perspectives, participation and co-design strategies help to generate trauma-transformative solutions that are culturally and contextually relevant and inclusive and for which there is a shared sense of trust, confidence and accountability.

Knowledge integration and translation

Trauma-transformative practice cannot and should not exist in a vacuum of other knowledge sources relevant to the broad purpose of a practitioner, organization or system. Thus, multiple sources of evidence must be integrated and translated into multi-dimensional systemic practices that generate improved outcomes for victims and survivors. We find utility in a definition of knowledge that is defined broadly as encompassing research and theoretical knowledge, procedural knowledge, cultural knowledge, self-knowledge and practice wisdom (Thompson and West, 2013). Each of these sources of knowledge contributes to professional practice. Theoretical knowledge in relation to trauma-transformative practice is the substance of this book and includes trauma theory, neurobiology, attachment, strengths-based theories and complexity theory. Practice wisdom in the context of trauma-transformative practice derives from the co-creation of meaning making with service users, and critical reflection. Research knowledge includes the outcomes of systematic literature reviews identifying critical evidence. This knowledge is considered alongside emerging evidence from exploratory research and the richness of data available from studies where the in-depth narratives of those with lived and living experience have been privileged. Procedural knowledge promotes organizational and contextual awareness, locating the new direction for practice within the context of the strategic and policy direction. This involves a working knowledge of policy, guidance procedure and process requirements to enable practitioner 'buy-in' to undertake new ways of working. Cultural knowledge privileges a cultural worldview within which there is an appreciation of cultural practices, norms, obligations and responsibilities. This includes an appreciation of culturally specific approaches to healing.

The critical task, then, is the integration of trauma-transformative practice knowledge with other knowledge and practices that are specific to the focus of particular organizations/systems. Education systems must integrate theory about teaching and learning with trauma-transformative practice to best serve their students. Substance abuse services cannot ignore critical addiction theories. Disability services must understand trauma-transformative practice in the context of disability support and practice. This step is often poorly understood or addressed and, at times, knowledge about trauma becomes divorced from the practice it is trying to transform. For this reason, we have made it a specific condition of successful trauma-transformative practice. Practitioners, organizations and systems must be resourced with the capacity to undertake knowledge integration and translation. Knowledge integration and translation are processes that facilitate the effective communication and application of knowledge across different disciplines, contexts and stakeholders. Knowledge integration involves bringing together the different types of knowledge described above to create a more comprehensive understanding of how to frame and respond to the needs of service users. Translation, on the other hand, involves converting knowledge from one context or language into another, making it more accessible and applicable to different audiences. This is critical in the context of system-wide change. Together, these processes help to bridge the gap between knowledge and practice, ensuring that knowledge is used to inform decision making and improve outcomes.

Workforce capacity

Building 'workforce' capacity is a critical aspect of the implementation of trauma-transformative practice. In this context, we consider the 'workforce' to be inclusive of practitioners, volunteers, carers, operational and senior leadership and executive management, representative of the whole of organization/system endeavour. The provision of training and professional development is but one of a range of critical mechanisms through which workforce capacity is built. The task begins at the recruitment stage with clear articulation of the desired workforce competencies, values and beliefs. It extends to how trauma-transformative practice is integrated into on-boarding, orientation and induction processes. This is the first step in a 'fit for purpose' workforce. Reflecting the experience of many child protection systems across Australia and internationally, Rycus and Hughes (2000) suggested that many staff hired to work in child welfare agencies are ill-prepared for the role, are largely unaware of its scope and complexity, and lack even basic knowledge of child welfare values, practice principles and intervention strategies. We would argue this is true of many areas of human services.

Training and professional development is an important but overly relied on means of building capacity. Training must be accessible, based on contemporary adult learning methodologies, and must accommodate individual training needs that will vary in response to differences in job and programme roles, the unique needs and attributes of victims and survivors, the social, geographic, and cultural composition of the local community, and employees' previous education, training and work experience (Walker, 2010; Rycus and Hughes, 2000). Training must clearly communicate the connectedness and relevance of policy, philosophy, theory and practice. Where many falsely believe the job is done with the delivery of training, it is the next steps that are the most important.

Workforce capability is built within a culture of continuous learning and reflection (APHSA, 2011). Engaging in trauma-transformative practice incorporates an intellectual and affective dimension which requires the workforce to employ sharp analytical and reflective skills to unravel presenting complexity, uncertainty and risk. Training programmes alone cannot ensure a highly skilled, effective workforce capable of achieving high-quality outcomes for victims and survivors and the organization (APHSA, 2011; Collins *et al.*, 2007; Bromfield and Ryan, 2006; Broad, 2000; Wall Williams, 2000). A range of support systems are also required to ensure that the workforce has ongoing and ready access to information and advice at the time it is required so that they are performing to the level and in the manner required of them (Wall Williams, 2000).

An organization/system that views itself as a learning organization/ system:

- places high value on individual, organizational and system learning as a prime asset
- works towards full utilization of all individual and group potential for learning and adapts itself to meet (and eventually set and review) organizational and system objectives
- does this in a way that also satisfies the needs and aspirations of the people involved
- identifies inhibitors or blocks to learning and removes them, while strong enhancers and structural support for sustained continuous learning are put in place
- creates a climate of continuous learning and improvement (Kandola and Fullerton, 2004).

Performance support systems differ from performance aids in that they are more complex systems that can provide multiple types of information, tutoring and advice. This must include practice leadership through the provision of high-quality supervision, coaching and mentoring, opportunities for reflective practice and strategies for self-care. Practice leadership is a distinct category of leadership and a unique domain of learning that differs from generic management training. It is conceived as a set of skills that leaders use to engage workers to consciously critique their practice and explore the interface between personal value judgement and professional decision making; manage risk; facilitate quality child protection decision making; facilitate strengths-base practice; lead multiple stakeholders in a statutory context; and provide coaching and supervisory processes and use research to inform practice. Practice leaders are strong operational managers and senior practitioners who demonstrate competent, safe and ethical practice, creative and critical thinking, have the ability to motivate individuals and teams, and are independent lifelong learners. They are tasked with serving as thought leaders and knowledge managers in a certain area of agency expertise, including policy advice, leadership in networks, overseeing practice quality and supporting career development for staff in the relevant professional practice area. Practice leaders develop and nurture expertise via the provision of professional advice and consultation, proactively sharing expertise with others on the team and in the agency, actively leading or participating in communities of practice, and contributing to the development of new practice resources and frameworks. Practice leadership is also demonstrated through the support of induction to protocols and guidelines, attention to administrative requirements, as well as staff orientation and supervision.

Processes and procedures

Policies and procedures are the procedural knowledge of organizations and systems that should support effective practice, promoting accountability and transparency. They must be aligned to the core constructs, philosophy and intent of trauma-transformative practice and ensure that all staff are working towards a common set of goals and objectives. By establishing clear policies and procedures, organizations can reduce confusion and ensure consistency in how work is performed. They also play an important role in risk management, helping to identify potential hazards or issues and outlining appropriate steps to address them.

Systems congruence and collaboration

Congruence and collaboration are key principles in the design and delivery of trauma-transformative practice. Trauma-transformative practice is, by definition, a multi-system undertaking and as such the conditions within the system are critical to the achievement of enhancing outcomes for victims and survivors, who most often engage with multiple services. Systems congruence speaks to the philosophical and conceptual alignment of how needs are understood and responded to and the generation of shared language and shared meaning making between organizations, practitioners and funding bodies that make up the system. Collaboration through the building of relationships, alliances and partnerships between organizations, practitioners, victims and survivors themselves and funding bodies is critical in the achievement of congruence and the development of creative solutions to the complex needs of victims and survivors.

Congruence and collaboration require strong leadership, effective communication and a commitment to shared goals. There is a need for systems to have their own reflective governance processes and ongoing mechanisms for practice improvement. These are required to maintain consistent practice and congruence between organizations, practitioners and other interfacing agencies such as funding bodies.

We suggest a range of strategies that promotes system congruence and collaboration, including:

- The development of interagency training, reflective practice and forums.
- Networking forums that bring together multidisciplinary agencies from a range of sectors in a geographical area to share information about services and intelligence about local needs, to collectivize action about creative solutions to address local need, and to consider the implications of broader political or sociocultural contexts for the work.
- Communities of practice as described by Atkinson and colleagues earlier in this book.
- Formalized processes for collaborative practice such as care teams described by Mitchell and Macnamara earlier in the book.

Conclusion

As Saleem approached the end of his story encompassing the experience of many of midnight's children, he reflected on all 30 pickle jars he had collected over the course of his life and observed that he had left one jar empty – for what was yet to come. At this point, he writes:

> ...the process of revision should be constant and endless; don't think I'm satisfied with what I've done... (Rushdie, 2010, p.643)

We have tried our best to offer a reconsideration of the trauma-informed paradigm because we believe in the endeavour. We hope that this book makes a valuable contribution in some way.

Children, young people, adults, families and communities with lived and living experiences of trauma need us to keep learning from them and other important sources of information and data so that we actively refresh what we think we know as practitioners, organizations and systems working to support them. This is a commitment to the ever-evolving understanding of how interpersonal violence profoundly scars the lives of victims and survivors and what it takes for sustained healing to occur. Trauma-transformative practice integrates the opportunity to embrace new knowledge as it emerges and keep itself open to change. It is a framework in which compassion, love and hope are deeply woven into its very fibre. It is these qualities that give it the best chance to succeed in changing practice, organizations and systems in their efforts to serve the needs and interests of all, and in particular those of victims and survivors of historical and ongoing forms of oppression and violation.

References

APHSA (2011). *A Guidebook for Building Organizational Effectiveness Capacity: A Training System Example*. Washington, DC: American Public Human Service Association.

Baser, H. and Morgan, P. (2008). *Capacity, Change and Performance. Study Report. Discussion Paper No.59B*. Maastricht, The Netherlands: European Centre for Development Policy Management.

Becker-Blease, K.A. (2017). As the world becomes trauma-informed, work to do. *Journal of Trauma and Dissociation*, 18(2), 131–138.

Birrell, P.J. and Freyd, J.J. (2006). Betrayal trauma: Relational models of harm and healing. *Journal of Trauma Practice*, 5(1), 49–63.

Bloom, S. (2016). Advancing a national cradle-to-grave-to cradle public health agenda. *Journal of Trauma and Dissociation*, 17(4), 383–396.

Brinkerhoff, D. and Morgan, P. (2010). Capacity and capacity development: Coping with complexity. *Public Administration and Development*, 30, 2–10.

Broad, M. (2000). Ensuring Transfer of Learning to the Job. In G. Piskurich, P. Beckschi and B. Hall (eds), *The ASTD Handbook of Training: A Comprehensive Guide to Creating and Delivering Training Programs – Instructor-led, Computer-based, or Self-directed* (pp.430–452). New York, NY: McGraw-Hill.

Bromfield, L. and Ryan, R. (2006). A National Comparison of Statutory Child Protection Training in Australian Communities. *Children and Families Australia*, 2, 59–72.

Collins, M., Amodeo, M. and Clay, C. (2007). Training as a factor in policy implementation: Lessons learned from a national evaluation of child welfare training. *Child and Youth Services Review*, 29, 1487–1502.

Dana, D. (2021). *Anchored: How to Befriend Your Nervous System Using Polyvagal Theory*. Sydney: Pan MacMillan.

Fixsen, D., Blasé, K., Naoom, S. and Wallace, F. (2009). Core implementation components. *Research on Social Work Practice*, 19(5), 531–540.

Fixsen, D.L. and Blasé, K.A. (2008). *Drivers Framework*. Chapel Hill, NC: The National Implementation Research Network, Frank Porter Graham Child Development Institute, University of North Carolina.

Foynes, M.M., Freyd, J.J. and DePrince, A.P. (2009). Child abuse: Betrayal and disclosure. *Child Abuse and Neglect*, 33(4), 209–217.

Freyd, J.J. (1996). *Betrayal Trauma: The Logic of Forgetting Childhood Abuse*. Boston, MA: Harvard University Press.

Harris, M. and Fallot, R.D. (2001). Envisioning a Trauma Informed Service System: A Vital Paradigm Shift. In M. Harris, and R.D. Fallot (eds), *Using Trauma Theory to Design Service Systems* (pp.3–22). San Francisco, CA: Jossey-Bass/Wiley.

Kaehler, L.A., Babcock, R., DePrince, A.P. and Freyd, J.J. (2013). Betrayal Trauma. In J.D. Ford and C.A. Courtois (eds), *Treating Complex Traumatic Stress Disorders in Children and Adolescents: Scientific Foundations and Therapeutic Models* (pp.62–78). New York, NY: Guilford Press.

Kandola, R. and Fullerton, J. (2004). *Diversity in Action: Managing the Mosaic*. London: Chartered Institute of Personnel and Development.

Metz, A., Albers, B., Burke, K., Bartley, L., Louison, K., Ward, C. and Farley, A. (2021). Implementation practice in human service systems: Understanding the principles and competencies of professionals who support implementation. *Human Service Organizations: Management, Leadership and Governance*. doi: 10.1080/23303131.2021.1895401.

Metz, A. and Bartley, L. (2012). Active implementation frameworks for program success: How to use implementation science to improve outcomes for children. *Zero to Three*, 34(4), 11–18.

Office for Health Improvement and Disparities (2022). *Working Definition of Trauma Informed Practice*. London: United Kingdom Government.

Pynoos, R.S., Fairbank, J.A., Steinberg, A.M., Amaya-Jackson, L. *et al.* (2008). The National Child Traumatic Stress Network: Collaborating to improve the standard of care. *Professional Psychology: Research and Practice*, 39(4), 389.

Ructtinger, L. (2015). *The Potential of Human-Centred Design (Thinking) for Education*. Fremantle: NSW Department of Education, AARE.

Rushdie, S. (2010). *Midnight's Children: A Novel*. Toronto: Vintage Canada.

Rycus, J. and Hughes, R. (2000). *What is Competency-Based Inservice Training?* www.ohsts. org/uploads/1/5/3/5/15354340/whatiscompetencybasedtraining.pdf.

Thompson, L.J. and West, D. (2013). Professional development in the contemporary educational context: Encouraging practice wisdom. *Social Work Education*, 32(1), 118–133.

Walker, S. (2010). Back to the future of social work: Child and adolescent mental health and the post qualifying curriculum in England and Wales. *Social Work Education*, 29, 616–632.

Wall Williams, S. (2000). Performance Support Systems and Job Aids. In G. Piskurich, P. Beckschi and B. Hall (eds), *The ASTD Handbook of Training: A Comprehensive Guide to Creating and Delivering Training Programs – Instructor-led, Computer-based, or Self-directed* (pp.415–429). New York, NY: McGraw-Hill.

Welsh Government (2022). *Trauma Informed Wales: A Societal Approach to Understanding, Preventing and Supporting the Impacts of Trauma and Adversity*. Cardiff: Traumatic Stress Wales.

Subject Index

Author Index